Handbook of Clinical Anesthesia

Handbook of Clinical Anesthesia

Editor: Norman Tucker

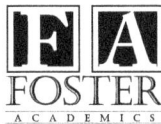

FA
FOSTER
ACADEMICS

www.fosteracademics.com

www.fosteracademics.com

FA
FOSTER
A C A D E M I C S

Cataloging-in-Publication Data

Handbook of clinical anesthesia / edited by Norman Tucker.
    p. cm.
Includes bibliographical references and index.
ISBN 978-1-63242-579-9
1. Anesthesiology. 2. Anesthesia. I. Tucker, Norman.

RD81 .H36 2019
61796--dc23

Foster Academics,
118-35 Queens Blvd., Suite 400,
Forest Hills, NY 11375, USA

ISBN 978-1-63242-579-9 (Hardback)

Contents

Permissions

List of Contributors

Index

Preface

This book has been a concerted effort by a group of academicians, researchers and scientists, who have contributed their research works for the realization of the book. This book has materialized in the wake of emerging advancements and innovations in this field. Therefore, the need of the hour was to compile all the required researches and disseminate the knowledge to a broad spectrum of people comprising of students, researchers and specialists of the field.

Anesthesia is a state of temporarily induced loss of awareness or sensation to achieve three primary goals of hypnosis, analgesia and muscle relaxation. There are varied drugs used for anesthesia such as general anesthetics, analgesics, neuromuscular-blocking drugs, etc. These drugs affect interconnected parts of the nervous system. An important stage of anesthesia is risk assessment, which is crucial for reducing anesthetic risks. It is a pre-operative procedure that covers the medical history, physical examination and lab tests, and obtains information about any medical conditions or genetic disorders that might afflict the patient. The various advancements in this field are glanced at in this book and their applications as well as ramifications are looked at in detail. It includes contributions of experts and scientists, which will provide innovative insights into the study of anesthesia. Researchers and students in this field will be assisted by this book.

At the end of the preface, I would like to thank the authors for their brilliant chapters and the publisher for guiding us all-through the making of the book till its final stage. Also, I would like to thank my family for providing the support and encouragement throughout my academic career and research projects.

Editor

Effect of Lidocaine Instillation into Endotracheal Tube on Intraocular Pressure during Extubation

Ahmed Hassanein[1*], Josef Zekrly[1] and Hosam Moharram[2]

[1]Department of Anesthesiology, Al-Minia University, Egypt
[2]Department of Ophthalmology, Al-Minia University, Egypt

*Corresponding author: Hassanein A, Department of Anesthesiology, Al-Minia University, Egypt, E-mail: ahmedhassanein10@yahoo.com

Abstract

Objectives: To study the effect of lidocaine instillation into endotracheal tube before extubation on intraocular pressure (IOP) and hemodynamics.

Patients and methods: 60 patients, (ASA) I-II, ages between 18 to 40 years were scheduled for elective unilateral ocular surgery (cataract, squint and ptosis). Patients were randomly classified into two groups of 30 patients each: lidocaine group; received 1 mg/kg lidocaine into the endotracheal tube before extubation, and control group; received saline into the endotracheal tube. IOP, systolic blood pressure (SBP), diastolic blood pressure (DBP) and heart rate (HR) were all measured before and after extubation.

Results: a significant increase of IOP in control group at 2, 5 and 10 minutes after extubation (P<0.01) when compared to baseline value (2 min. before extubation). The elevation in IOP in lidocaine group at 2 min was significantly less than that in control group (P<0.05), the readings of IOP at 5 and 10 min. was lower in lignocaine group compared to control group. Both groups showed significant increase in SBP and DBP after extubation compared to baseline (2 min. before extubation), and elevation in lignocaine group was significantly lower than that of control group (p=0.0001).

Conclusion: Instillation of lidocaine into endotracheal tube before extubation attenuates IOP after extubation

Keywords: Lidocaine; Endotracheal tube; Intraocular pressure; Extubation

Introduction

Increase in intraocular pressure (IOP) may have little adverse effects in patients with healthy eyes but has dangerous effects on a diseased or an injured eye. Efforts must be made to maintain intraocular tension at or below normal levels [1]. The stress response to tracheal intubation and extubation is associated with elevation in IOP mainly due to increased sympathetic stimulation [2,3]. Lower pharynx, epiglottis and larynx contain numerous sensory receptors which respond to chemical, thermal and mechanical stimuli. The mechanoreceptors are abundant especially in the lower pharyngeal wall, epiglottis and vocal cords. Stimulation of these mechanoreceptors during intubation or extubation can produce reflex motor responses like cough, hiccup and also reflex sympathetic stimulation and cardiovascular pressor response [4] and release of catecholamines from the adrenal medulla into the circulation [5]. The result of all these adrenergic outflow may cause vasoconstriction, tachycardia and an increase in central venous pressure which has a closer relationship to IOP than systemic pressure [6], this can produce an acute increase in IOP by increasing the resistance to the outflow of aqueous humor in the trabecular meshwork between the anterior chamber and the Schlemm's canal [7].

Although intubation has been regarded very much especially when there is a problem in airways, but extubation of patients has not been considered a lot. Anesthesia specialists know that the short time period after extubation is very harmful and causes several events such as laryngospasm, aspiration, lack of perfect opening of airways, lack of enough pulmonary rehabilitation, may result in marked increase IOP, and can develop myocardial ischemia especially in patients suffering from coronary artery disease [8]. Four urgent drugs including epinephrine, lidocaine, naloxan and atropine are injected into tracheal tube and are absorbed from endotracheal membrane because of its abundant vessels [9-12]. For avoidance of these complications, it is important to maintain IOP and cardiovascular condition at the end of general anesthesia, therefore, the aim of this study was to determine the effect of lidocaine instillstion into endotracheal tube before extubation on IOP and hemodynamics.

Patient and Methods

The study was conducted in Al-Minia university Hospital from April 2014 to February 2015. After approval by ethical committee and obtaining informed consents from patients, the study was carried out on sixty ASA grade I and II, patients of either sex , aged from 18 to 40 years, taken up for elective ophthalmic surgeries (unilateral cataract, squint, ptosis). Patients were divided into 2 equal groups (n=30 each group) by simple random sampling. Patients with history of glaucoma, suspected difficult airway, uncontrolled hypertension, diabetes mellitus and obesity were excluded. Monitoring included electrocardiography, heart rate (HR), pulse oximetry, end tidal carbon-dioxide measurement, and noninvasive blood pressure using the monitor (Spacelabs; model 90364, USA). An intravenous (IV) access was secured in operation room and all patients received fentanyl 1.0 μg/kg IV followed by induction of anesthesia with thiopentone sodium (5-7 mg/kg) to loss of eyelash reflex, atracurium bromide 0.5 mg/kg was given for neuromuscular (NM) blockade. Lungs were mask ventilated for 3 min with 100% oxygen with isoflurane, then endotracheal tube inserted with Macintosh laryngoscope and was fixed using adhesive tapes to the skin over maxilla and mandible, the patients were then connected to mechanical ventilation using positive intermittent mandatory ventilation (PIMV). Patients in whom more than one attempt was required for correct placement of the tube were excluded from the study. Anesthesia was maintained using isoflurane and atracurium top ups for NM blockade. Near the end of surgery, we asked the surgeon to till us when there is 10 min remaining before finishing the surgery to instill 1.0 mg/kg lidocaine (2%) inside the endotracheal tube in lidocaine group patients. At the end of the surgery, isoflurane was stopped and the residual NM blockade was antagonized with neostigmine and atropine in appropriate dosages. Lidocaine spray (10%, 10 mg/dose) was sprayed 2 sprayes (20 mg) inside the pharyngeal cavity one minute before extubation in patients of the 2 groups. Extubation was performed when the patient was able to open his healthy eye in reply to verbal orders. IOP was measured in the non-operated eye (previously prepared with lubricant eye drops) 2 min before extubation and subsequently three times at 2, 5, 10 minutes after extubation using Schiotz tonometer (The Diagnostic Company: Riester, Germany). Hemodynamic parameters which included heart rate, systolic and diastolic blood pressure were recorded simultaneously at the time of measuring IOP. These measurements were recorded by assistant anesthetist he was blinded to the study groups.

Statistical Analysis

Based on our pilot study of 5 patients in each group, a sample size of 30 patients per group was required to achieve a power of 80% with an alpha error of 5%, to detect a change in intraocular pressure of 35% from baseline value after extubation in control group versus 6% in lidocaine group.

For statistical analysis, Statistical Package for the Social Sciences (SPSS), version 16.0 (SPSS Inc., Chicago III) software was used. Continuous quantitative data were expressed as mean, standard deviation, median and range were calculated. Qualitative data were presented as number and proportion, and analyzed using Chi-square test or Fischer's exact test as appropriate. Normality test was used to identify a distribution as not normal when the distribution is skewed. Non-parameteric data were compared with Mann-Whitney test to compare independent groups and Wilcoxon test to compare related groups. $P<0.05$ was considered to be significant and $P<0.01$ was considered highly significant.

Results

In our study, 60 young adult patients, ASA class I and II were divided into 2 equal groups (30 patients each), selected to study the effects of lignocaine instillation into the endotracheal tube before extubation on IOP and hemodynamics. The two study groups were comparable with respect to weight, age, sex and surgical procedures (Table 1). Regarding hemodynamic changes (Table 2) both groups showed significant increase in SBP at 2 and 5 minutes after extubation when compared to baseline (2 min. before extubation), and the elevation in lidocaine group at 2 min was significantly lower than that of control group (p=0.0001). Both groups showed significant increase in DBP at 2 minutes after extubation when compared to base line (2 min. before extubation), and the elevation in lidocaine group at 2 and 5 min. was significantly lower than that of control group (p=0.002) and (p=0.003) respectively. HR showed non-significant differences neither within each group nor between the two groups.

Regarding IOP changes (Table 3), there was a significant increase in readings of IOP in control group at 2, 5 and 10 minutes after extubation (P<0.01) when compared to baseline value (2 min. before extubation). IOP showed a significant increase in lidocaine group at 2 min after extubation (P<0.05). The elevation in IOP in lidocaine group at 2 min was significantly less than that in control group (P<0.05), the readings of IOP at 5 and 10 min. was lower in lidocaine group compared to control group.

Discussion

We must avoid the increase in ocular congestion or increase of IOP during intraocular surgery because of undesirable and possibly dangerous effects, as expulsion of vitreous humor from the open eye. So, ideal anesthetic technique for intraocular surgery should produce a moderate reduction in IOP at near normal values and avoid marked fluctuations during surgery.

Variables	Control (n=30)	Lidocaine (n=30)	P-value
Age (years)	30.3 ± 6.2	31 ± 5.7	0.65
Sex (M/F)	19/11	16/14	0.43
Weight (kg)	69.6 ± 8.9	70 ± 12.3	0.88
ASA (I/II)	22/8	20/10	0.57
Operative time (min)	47.7 ± 14.6	51.5 ± 13.9	0.30
Operative type (Cataract/Ptosis/Squint)	16/8/6	18/7/5	0.87
Data are expressed as mean ± standard deviation for quantitative data or number for qualitative data. T-student test was used to compare quantitative data and Chi-square test was used to compare qualitative data.			

Table 1: Demographic data in the studied groups.

Parameters	Control (n=30)	Lidocaine (n=30)	P-value
SBP 2 min before extubation	113 ± 7.67 114 (95-126)	111 ± 6.73 110 (101-130)	0.14
SBP 2 min after extubation	130 ± 4.87° 130 (119-139)	120.96 ± 1.56° 121 (117-124)	0.0001*
SBP 5 min after extubation	114.96 ± 5.22 116 (103-125)	113.96 ± 6.59 113 (100-127)	0.50
SBP 10 min after extubation	112 ± 6.54 112 (102-126)	112.03 ± 3.25 112 (103-118)	0.85
DBP 2 min before extubation	69.03 ± 5.11 69 (61-80)	66.93 ± 4.07 67 (56-75)	0.16
DBP 2 min after extubation	75.10 ± 5.19° 74 (68-86)	71 ± 3.18° 71 (65-76)	0.002*
DBP 5 min after extubation	70.03 ± 4.29 70.5 (60-81)	67.83 ± 1.01 68 (66-70)	0.003*
DBP 10 min after extubation	67.96 ± 5.24 67.5 (54-81)	66.03 ± 2.55 66 (61-72)	0.09
HR 2 min before extubation	80.03 ± 10.78 80.5 (62-104)	78.03 ± 14.29 79 (45-107)	0.56
HR 2 min after extubation	85.96 ± 12.74 86 (62-104)	82.06 ± 12.10 79.5 (64-115)	0.15
HR 5 min after extubation	81.10 ± 9.88 79.5 (53-102)	78.96 ± 2.04 79 (74-83)	0.49
HR 10 min after extubation	81.93 ± 10.20 82 (62-108)	78 ± 3.22 77 (73-84)	0.12

Data are expressed as mean ± standard deviation and median (range); °Significant difference with baseline (within group); *Significant difference between groups; Mann-Whitney test was used for intergroups comparisons and Wilcoxon test was for within group comparison. SBP: Systolic Blood Pressure; DBP: Diastolic Blood Pressure; HR: Heart Rate.

Table 2: Comparison of hemodynamic changes before and after tracheal extubation in the studied groups.

Parameters	Lidocaine (n=30)	Control (n=30)	P-value
IOP 2 min before extubation	11.10 ± 1.76 11 (8-15)	11.56 ± 1.40 12 (9-14)	0.24
IOP 2 min after extubation	13.53 ± 1.07° 14 (11-15)	16.76 ± 1.10° 17(14-20)	0.0001*
IOP 5 min after extubation	11.53 ± 0.57 11.5 (11-13)	14.23 ± 0.56° 14 (13-15)	0.0001*
IOP 10 min after extubation	10.50 ± 0.50 11 (9-11)	12.40 ± 0.67° 12 (11-14)	0.0001*

Data are expressed as mean ± standard deviation and median (range); °Significant difference with baseline (inside group); *Significant difference between groups; Mann-Whitney test was used for intergroups comparisons and Wilcoxon test was for within group comparison; IOP: Intraocular Pressure.

Table 3: Comparison of intraocular pressure changes before and after tracheal extubation in the studied groups

In our study we selected the young adult age (18-40 years) as airway reflexes are attenuated by age and these reflexes are prominent in these middle ages than more old ages [13], intratracheal injection of lidocaine markedly attenuated the rise in IOP during the short period after extubation, and all IOP measurments (2, 5 and 10 min) after extubation were significantly lower in ledocaine than placebo. The hemodynamic responses in these times showed attenuation in lidocaine group when compared to placebo, SBP was significantly lower at (2 min), and DBP was significantly lower at (2 and 5 min) after extubation. HR readings were lower in lidocaine than placebo group.

In the study of Ebrahim N; the IOP readings were elevated after intubation and extubation, the highest level of IOP was at first minute after intubation and extubation. The increase of IOP was more after extubation than after intubation. The time passed after extubation till return the IOP to near base line was 10 minutes [14]. Also, similar observation by Pandya; who compared the effect of endotracheal tube versus laryngeal mask on IOP, they showed that IOP increased after extubation [15]. The previous studies coincide with our finding that extubation stress elevates IOP. We tried to avoid or attenuate this rise in IOP after extubation by instilling lidocaine inside the endotracheal tube before extubation; we found reduction and attenuation in this rise in lidocaine group.

Bidway and Stanly examined effects of lidocaine on blood pressure and HR in response to extubation. They injected 1.5 cc of lidocaine into tracheal tube 3 to 5 minutes before extubation and then they instilled 1cc (4%) lidocaine just before extubation. They showed no increase in blood pressure and HR during 1 to 5 minutes after extubation [16]. Tavakkol and his colleagues [17] studded the effect of lidocaine injection into endotracheal tube on incidence of cough and laryngospasm. In test group 100 mg (5 ml) of lidocaine 2% and in control group the same volume of placebo (normal saline) was injected into endotracheal tube. Using anesthesia drugs stopped 5 to 10minutes before end of the surgery and after ending the operation extubation took place. The number of coughs and laryngospasm assessed, recorded and compared. Numbers of coughs were higher in control group and the difference between 2 groups was significant. We decide to test this abolishing effect of lidocaine on IOP as it increased during intubation and extubation pharyngeal use of lidocaine to suppress the supraglottic origin of stress reflexes, but endotracheal lidocaine instillation attenuates manly infraglottic reflexes during extubation

We can conclude that lidocaine instillation into endotracheal tube before extubation can attenuate and prevent marked rise in IOP. It can be beneficial especially in open eye surgery.

References

1. Shah RJ, Kamdar V, Lala MN (1975) Effect of different anesthetic agents on intraocular pressur. Indian J Anaesth 64: 97-101.

2. Watcha MF, White PF, Tychsen L, Stevens JL (1992) Comparative effects of laryngeal mask airway and endotracheal tube insertion on intraocular pressure in children. Anesth Analg 75: 355-360.

3. Ghai B, Sharma A, Akhtar S (2001) Comparative evaluation of intraocular pressure changes subsequent to insertion of laryngeal mask airway and endotracheal tube. J Postgrad Med 47: 181-184.

4. Hagberg CA (2007) Benumof's Airway Management; Principles and Practice (2ndedn.) Mosby Elsevier.

5. Arthur C, Guyton (2000) Textbook of Medical Physiology (11thedn.) Elsevier Saunders Company, pp. 572-598.

6. Murphy DF (1985) Anesthesia and intraocular pressure. Anesth Analg 64: 520-530.

7. Langham ME, Kitazawa Y, Hart RW (1971) Adrenergic responses in the human eye. J Pharmacol Exp Ther 179: 47-55.

8. Miller KA, Harkin CP, Bailey PL (1995) Postoperative tracheal extubation. Anesth Analg 80: 149-172.

9. Sasaki CT, Isaacson G (1988) Dynamic anatomy of the larynx in physiology and consequences of intubation. In: Bishop MJ (ed.) Problems in anesthesia. JB Lippincot, Philadelphia 2:103.

10. Erskine RJ, Murphy PJ, Langton JA, Smith G (1993) Effect of age on the sensitivity of upper airway reflexes. Br J Anaesth 70: 574-575.

11. Kern MJ, Gudipati C, Tatineni S, Aguirre F, Serota H, et al. (1990) Effect of abruptly increased intrathoracic pressure on coronary blood flow velocity in patients. Am Heart J 119: 863-870.

12. Miller DR (2001) Local anesthesia. In: Latzung B (ed.) Basic and clinical pharmacology (8thedn.) McGraw-Hill companies, San Francisco, p. 43.

13. Land W, Steven James M (1999) Laryngospasm. In: John LA (ed.) Comlication in Anesthesia (1stedn.) Sanders Co., Philadelphia, pp. 623-625.

14. Ebrahim N, Seved J (2007) Comparative evaluation of intraocular pressure and hemodynamic changes during tracheal intubation and extubation. Res J Biol Sci 2: 344-347.

15. Pandya Malti J, Agarwal Geeta (2012) Comparative study of intraocular pressure changes with laryngeal mask airway and Endotracheal tube. National Journal of Community Medicine.

16. Bidwai AV, Stanley TH, Bidwai VA (1978) Blood pressure and pulse rate responses to extubation with and without prior topical tracheal anaesthesia. Can Anaesth Soc J 25: 416-418.

17. Tavakkol K, Ghaffarian Shirazi H (2009) Effect of lidocaine injection into endotracheal tube on incidence of cough and laryngospasm. Iranian Journal of Critical Care Nursing Spring 1: 23-26.

Inhaled Desflurane *vs.* Propofol for Postoperative Sedation Guided with Patient State Index of SEDLine in Mechanically Ventilated Liver Transplant Recipient

Khaled Ahmed Yassen[1*], Eman Kamal EL-Deen Awaad[2], Emad Kamel Refaat[3], Neveen Mostafa Soliman[4] and Magda Fouad Yehia[5]

Anaesthesia and Intensive Care Unit Department, National Liver Institute-Menoufiya University, Egypt

*Corresponding author: Khaled Ahmed Yassen, Anaesthesia and Intensive Care Unit Department, National Liver Institute-Menoufiya University, Egypt, E-mail: kyassen61@hotmail.com

Abstract

Background: Monitoring sedation depth with appropriate sedative choice can reduce over sedation and associated side effects.

Objectives: To compare Desflurane (Des) *vs.* Propofol (P) sedation with regards to, haemodynamics, recovery profiles, side effects and costs.

Design: A prospective randomized hospital based comparative study.

Setting: In a single centre between May 2012 and December 2014.

Patients: Sixty mechanically ventilated liver recipients were assigned randomly to receive postoperative sedation either with inhalational Des in air/oxygen 1 litre min-1 or intravenous P 4 mg/kg/hr.

Interventions: Recovery time and response to eye opening was recorded. Memorization of five words, Trieger dot test, and digit symbol substitution tests were applied. The Patient State Index (PSI) by SEDLine Sedation Monitor (Masimo, Irvin, CA) was used to target adequate depth of sedation (50-75) in both groups. Ramsay sedation score (RSS) was monitored. Fentanyl was used to assist sedation guided with PSI. The Transesophageal Doppler (TED) was recorded hourly; corrected flow time (FTc) of TED was used for fluid optimization.

Main outcome measures: Recovery profile was the primary end point. Secondary outcomes were haemodynamic events, side effects and cost.

Results: Recovery was faster with Desflurane than Propofol (2.0+1.1 *vs.* 13.1+4.4 min, $P<0.01$, respectively) regarding eye opening (PSI>75), five words recall, trieger dot test and digit symbol substitution test. Required duration of sedation was lower with Desflurane (6.83 ± 2.00 *vs.* 8.26 ± 1.68 hour, $P=0.004$). Systemic vascular resistance (SVR) and mean arterial blood pressure (MABP) were better maintained with Desflurane. Under comparable PSI readings between both groups at all measuring points (SVR, MABP and PSI after 2hrs sedation 908.93 ± 139.5 *vs.* 617.6 ± 104.5 dyn.sec.cm^{-5}, $P<0.01$ and 77.0 ± 3.8 *vs.* 63.4 ± 6.3 mmHg, $P<0.01$, 63.30 ± 6.374 *vs.* 62.2 ± 5.8, $P=0.517$ respectively), in contrast the mean RSS was consistently higher with Des compared to P, $P<0.01$ at all times. Less norepinephrine was required with Des (n=10) (33.3%) compared to P (n=23) (76.7%), ($P=0.001$). Ventilation duration shortened with Des vs, P (6.83 ± 2.00 *vs.* 8.26 ± 1.68 hour, $P=0.004$) with comparable arterial blood gases at start ($P>0.01$). Fentanyl was frequently combined with P to reduce its effect on SVR and MBP. (483.3+168.3 *vs.* 100 ± 0.00 μg, $P<0.05$). Total consumption of Des and P were (53.13 ± 10.30 ml *vs.* 1010.33 ± 205.06 mg). Cost was lower with Desflurane (0.9+0.3 *vs.* 1.6+0.4) Sterling £/hour, ($P=0.000$).

Conclusion: Postoperative Desflurane sedation guided with PSI enhanced recovery at a lower cost when compared to Propofol as well as preserving better the haemodynamics at a lower cost.

Keywords: Sedation; Liver transplantation; Propofol; Desflurane

Introduction

In the immediate postoperative period liver transplant recipients can require mechanical ventilation. An adequate level of sedation without over sedation is of significant importance for recipients with newly transplanted liver grafts and with anticipated haemodynamic and metabolic changes as a consequence of the procedure itself and of the graft performance. Careful drug choice with adequate sedative depth monitoring and analgesia can help reduce the unwanted side effects, and improve related morbidity and mortality with an enhancement in recovery [1].

In the immediate immediate post-liver transplant procedure management focuses on haemodynamic stability, protection of the newly transplanted graft from haemodynamic changes, as well as enhancing the weaning from mechanical support as early as possible. Propofol is commonly used for the sedation of patients in need for mechanical ventilation. Although, Propofol has been established as a safe and effective drug for the sedation of patients in the intensive care units, it's administration for liver transplant recipients has to be carefully monitored as most of these recipients suffer from a reduced systemic vascular resistance as a consequence of their long standing end stage liver disease [2].

Desflurane is one of the third generation inhaled anaesthetics. It is the halogenated inhaled anaesthetic with the lowest blood and tissue solubility's, which promotes its rapid equilibration and its rapid elimination following cessation of administration. Its benefits include rapid and predictable emergence and early recovery. In addition, the use of Desflurane promotes early and predictable extubation, which has a positive impact on patient turnover [3].

The aim of this study is to compare patient state index guided sedation with Propofol vs. Desflurane in mechanically ventilated adult living donor liver transplant recipients during their immediate postoperative period regarding their haemodynamics, sedation and recovery as well as cost.

Patients and Methods

Ethics

In this prospective hospital based randomized control study, a written informed consent and Institutional Research and Ethics Committee approval from National Liver Institute, Menoufiya University, Egypt (0070/2013, Chairperson Prof. Mohamed El Guindi) were obtained. The study was registered at the Cochrane research data base of South Africa (PACTR 201402000758402), (www.pactr.org).

Patients, groups and randomization

Sixty living donor liver recipients were categorized randomly using a simple random technique (closed envelopes) into two equal groups, for postoperative sedation either by Desflurane inhalation (group D) or Propofol infusion (group P). Inclusion criteria: written and informed consent , age 18–60 year, Model for End-Stage Liver Disease (MELD) score between 12-20, and living donor liver transplant recipients planned for weaning of ventilation normoxia, normothermia with no major intraoperative events. Exclusion criteria: severe haemodynamic instability at the end of the operation, patients in need for re-operation and unwilling to participate in the study.

Anaesthetic technique

After standard monitoring was in place, general anaesthesia was induced with intravenous (IV) Propofol 2 mg/kg with anaesthesia depth monitoring in place, Fentanyl 1 ug/kg and rocronium 0.6-0.9 mg/kg followed by endotracheal intubation.

Anaesthesia was maintained with (Desflurane) in O_2/Air mixture (FiO$_2$=0.4) rocuronium and fentanyl to keep Patient State Index (PSI) between 25-50 (SEDLine, Masimo, Irvine, CA, USA) to monitor and achieve surgical anaesthesia. Transesophageal Doppler probe (CardioQ Deltex Medical, Chichester, UK) was inserted via oral airway and used to monitor and measure haemodynamic variables.

Normothermia was achieved with a forced-air warming device. An arterial line was placed in the left radial artery, and central line was

inserted in the right internal jugular vein with triple lumen catheter and large-bore single lumen catheter 7.5F.

Fluid regimen consisted of Ringer acetate solutions at 6 ml/kg/h. Albumin 5% was given only to treat hypoalbuminaemia. Packed red blood cells were transfused to keep haematocrit above 25%. Other blood products were administered under guidance of Rotational Thromboelastometry (ROTEM). Hypervolemia was treated with bolus of colloid 5 ml/kg (130/0.4 Hydroxy ethyl statch (Voulven), Fresenius, Kabi). Boluses of colloid (maximum dose, 30 ml/kg) were administered, guided by an algorithm depending on the Doppler estimations of stroke volume and corrected flow time (FTc). This algorithm was similar to that used by Sinclair et al. [4].

Study protocol

At the end of surgery, patients were allocated randomly for sedation with either Desflurane (Group D) (Baxter,Erlangen, Germany) or Propofol (Group P). (Diprivan, Astra-Zeneca, Wedel, Germany).The study observation period started from arrival at the ICU to 2 hrs. post tracheal extubation.

Monitoring level of sedation was achieved by patient state index of the SEDLine Brain Function Monitor (Masimo, Irvine, CA, USA). Patients were monitored to assess the sedation status according to the Ramsay scale and keep the patient state index (PSI) between 50-75 hourly. All patients were ventilated with an anaesthesia ventilator (Cicero, Drager Medical, Lubeck, Germany). Ventilator offers synchronized intermittent mandatory ventilation. Fresh Soda Lime (Crane House, Molly Millars Lane, Wokingham, UK) was used for each patient and PEEP was set to 5 cm H_2O.

Desflurane was delivered (in group D) by a modified TEC-6 vaporisor (Dräger Medical). End-tidal concentration of 3 vol. % was used initially, and this could be changed in steps of up to 0.5 vol. %.

Ventilation was adjusted to maintain the $PaCO_2$ between 35-40 mmHg and the PaO_2 between 100 and 150 mmHg. End-tidal Desflurane and carbon dioxide concentrations were monitored by side-stream infrared spectroscopy.

In group P, Propofol infusions (range 0.5-6 mg/kg/h) were titrated to response guided by patient state index. Bolus doses of Propofol 40 mg were allowed.

In both groups, if there was a need for additive analgesia, Fentanyl was given and the requirements were recorded. The study drugs were adjusted to achieve target patient state index (PSI) of 50-75.

Before extubation study drugs were hold, and patients were addressed by their names, asked to open their eyes and to squeeze their hands.

Measurements

Preoperative data: Includes baseline score of five-word memory test, trigger's dot test and digit symbol substitution test.

Operative data include: Start time, end time and duration of operation (h), Volatile anesthetic (Desflurane) consumption (ml), Dosage of used opioids as Fentanyl (μg), Final core temperature (°C) and red blood cell transfusion requirements (units).

Postoperative data: Were monitored continuously from arrival at the intensive therapy unit until 2 h after tracheal extubation.

This includes; (1) Haemodynamic data; heart rate (HR), mean arterial blood pressure and transesophageal doppler parameters (cardiac output (COP), systemic vascular resistance (SVR) and corrected flow time (FTc). (2) An assessment of the sedation status according to both Ramsay Sedation scale and Patient State Index. (3) The Sedation profile; duration of sedation (hrs.), dosage and of additive analgesic drugs, as Fentanyl ((μg), dosage of study drugs; Desflurane (ml) and Propofol (mg/kg), the consumption of vasoactive drugs in both groups and the time from cessation of sedation to extubation was recorded in minutes. (4) The recovery profile; Time to early emergence (defined as verbal command responses [eye opening, hand squeezing], tracheal extubation, and orientation (defined as providing correct date of birth) and Psychometric tests; five-word memory test, Trigger's dot test and Digit symbol substitution test. (5) Side effects as nausea, vomiting, and agitation. (6) Total cost in both groups was calculated according to the British National Formula announced prices (www.bnf.org).

Statistical analysis

Design: Non-blind randomized prospective hospital based comparative study. In the present study α was set to 0.05, and maximum b accepted=20% with a minimum power of the study of 80% [5]. Primary outcome of this RCT is SVR with S.D. of 100 to 120, the effect size in SVR was set to 200, which resulted in a recommended sample size of 30 per group. Calculation of sample size was done using (IBM SPSS Sample power) software and was also confirmed using length Java Applets for Power and Sample Size (Computer software). Multiple samples will be normally-distributed, even if the source population is not normally-distributed, provided that the sample size is large enough (30 or more), so all variable included in the study considered to be normally distribution and parametric statistics were carried out.

- Exploration of the data: This yielded complete descriptive statistics including the minimum and maximum, range, mean, median and inter-quartile range for each variable.
- Data were described using minimum, maximum, mean and standard deviation.
- Comparisons were carried out between the two studied groups using independent t test (t test).
- Box and Whiskers graphs were carried out.
- Chi-square test and fisher exact test will be used to measure association between qualitative variables.

Correction of *P* value for multiple testing was set *P* to 0.01 to detect significant correlation (Bonforroni correction of multiple comparisons). So in the present study an alpha level was designed to 1% with a significance level of 99%, and a beta error accepted up to 20% with a power of study of 80%.

Results

A total of 63 patients were included, 2 patients were excluded due to haemodynamic instability during the immediate postoperative period and one due to relatives refusal. 60 recipients were randomized. 30 patients had been allocated to group Des and 30 to group P.

In Table 1 patients' characteristics of both groups, model of end stage liver disease (MELD), sex distribution, duration of operation, amount of blood loss, packed red blood cells transfusion requirements and total consumption of Fentanyl were comparable (P value>0.01).

	Propofol group (n=30)	Desflurane Group(n=30)	(*P*-value)
Age (yrs.)	43.70 ± 6.94	42.60 ± 8.18	0.577
Weight (kg.)	78.73 ± 8.58	78.13 ± 8.36	0.785
Height (cm.)	172.70 ± 6.22	170.16 ± 4.80	0.083
BMI	26.89 ± 2.73	26.63 ± 1.92	0.672
MELD Score	14.20 ± 1.90	14.36 ± 1.35	0.697
Males [n (%)]	26 (66.7%)	24 (80.0%)	0.488
Females [n (%)]	4 (13.3%)	6 (20.0%)	
Duration of surgery (hr.)	14.35 ± 1.86	14.78 ± 2.29	0.425
Blood loss (cc.)	1816.66 ± 1075.45	1883.33 ± 801.32	0.786
Dosage of Fentanyl (μg.)	1263.33 ± 403.84	1190.00 ± 325.20	0.442
Final core temperature (°C)	36.53 ± 0.39	36.57 ± 0.48	0.705
Packed RBCS transfused	6.43 ± 4.93	5.93 ± 4.19	0.674
Data are shown as mean ± standard deviation (mean ± SD)			

Table 1: Patient characteristics.

Postoperatively, the mean duration of sedation was significantly shorter in Desflurane group (6.83 ± 2.00 hrs.) compared to Propofol group (8.26 ± 1.68 hrs.) (P value<0.01).

Regarding the mean blood pressure, there were no statistically significant differences between both groups at T_0, P value>0.01 but a statistically highly significant differences at T_1-T_{11}, P value<0.01 was observed as presented in Figure 1.

As well as after extubation at $T_{1A.E}$ (82.46 ± 7.015) and $T_{2A.E}$ (83.20 ± 6.920) in Desflurane group *vs.* $T_{1A.E}$ (73.46 ± 4.297) and $T_{2A.E}$ (73.96 ± 3.011) in Propofol group, P value<0.01.

Regarding Transesophageal Doppler measured systemic vascular resistance, there were no statistically significant differences between both groups at T_0, P value>0.01 but statistically highly significant differences was present at T_1-T_{11}, (P value<0.01) Figure 2.

Both TED measured cardiac output and corrected flow time was comparable between both groups P>0.01.

The number of patients in need for catecholamine support (norepinephrine) were lower in Desflurane group (n=10) (33.3%) compared to Propofol group (n=23) (76.7%), P<0.01 Table 2.

No statistically significant differences between both groups regarding the patient state index as presented in Figure 3.

Mean values of Ramsay sedation scores were significantly lower in Propofol group compared to Desflurane group, P<0.01, starting from T_1 and afterwards Table 3.

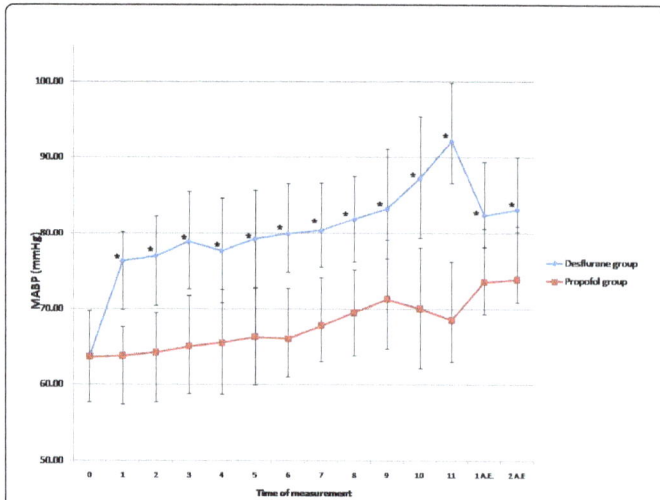

Figure 1: Changes overtime in mean arterial blood pressure (MBP) in both groups.T0, MBP before drug administration; T_1-T_{11}, MBP every hour till extubation; $T_{1A.E}$, $T_{2A.E}$, MBP one& two hours after extubation; *, significant ($P<0.01$).

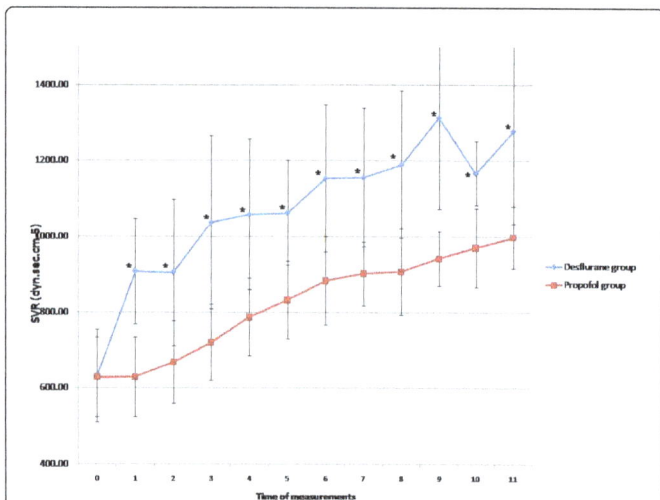

Figure 2: Changes overtime in systemic vascular resistance (SVR) in both groups.T0, SVR before drug administration; T_1-T_{11}, SVR every hour till extubation; *, significant (P<0.01).

Psychometric tests; Five wards memory test showed statistically significant difference between both groups at T_1 (one minute after extubation) $P<0.01$.

Both Triegar's dot test and Digit symbol substitution test also showed statistically highly significant difference at T60, (60 minute after extubation), (P value<0.01).

Nausea, vomiting, agitation and drowsiness were higher in number with in the Propofol group compared to the Desflurane group, $P<0.01$, while hypertension was reported once in the Desflurane group (n=1) (3.3%) compared to Propofol group (n=0) (0.0%).

Regarding mean sedation cost/hr. (£) in Sterling pounds was (0.985+0.332) with in the Desflurane group *vs.* (1.618+0.456) in Propofol group, P value<0.01.

Time from cessation of the study drug to eye opening (min), to hand squeezing (min), to verbal command(min) and to extubation were significantly shorter in Desflurane group than Propofol group, $P<0.01$ Table 4.

Discussion

The results of this current study demonstrated that recipients sedated with Desflurane preserved better their mean arterial blood pressure and systemic vascular resistance at all points of measurements during the period of mechanical ventilation and for two hours after extubation compared to the Propofol sedated group without causing any significant difference in cardiac output or heart rate between the two groups.

Groups	Norepinephrine	Frequency	Percent	X^2 test	P- value
P	Yes	23	76.7%		
	No	7	23.3 %		
	Total	30	100%	11.380	0.001*
D	Yes	10	33.3%		
	No	20	66.7		
	Total	30	100		

Table 2: Catecholamine (norepinephrine) support need differences between Propofol group (P) and Desflurane group (D).

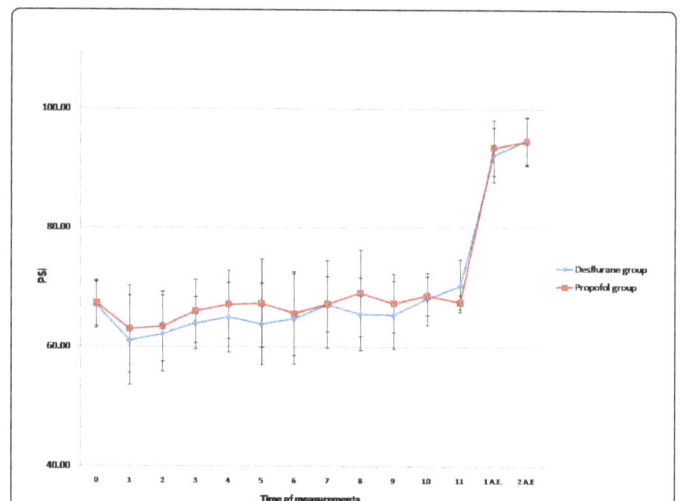

Figure 3: Changes overtime in Patient State Index in both groups.T_0, PSI before drug administration; T_1-T_{11}, PSI every hour till extubation; $T_{1A.E}$, $T_{2A.E}$, PSI one& two hours after extubation significant ($P<0.01$).

	T_0	T_2	T_4	T_6	T_8	T_{10}	T_{11}	$T_{1A.E}$	$T_{2A.E}$
Patient State Index (PSI)									
Group P	68.90 ± 7.674	63.30 ± 6.374	67.00 ± 5.842	65.64 ± 7.568	69.08 ± 6.067	68.63 ± 4.388	67.55 ± 4.390	93.40 ± 4.568	94.50 ± 3.892
Group D	69.90 ± 7.544	63.30 ± 6.374	65.03 ± 5.726	64.76 ± 6.998	65.60 ± 7.209	68.16 ± 3.188	70.40 ± 1.140	92.33 ± 4.603	94.73 ± 4.067
P value	0.349	0.517	0.193	0.662	0.117	0.821	0.187	0.371	0.821
Ramsay Sedation Score (RSS)									
Group P	4.46 ± 0.507	4.53 ± 0.507	4.63 ± 0.490	4.42 ± 0.572	4.47 ± 0.510	4.63 ± 0.504	4.33 ± 0.500		
Group D	4.46 ± 0.507	5.63 ± 0.490	5.53 ± 0.507	5.61 ± 0.571	5.66 ± 0.487	5.50 ± 0.547	5.60 ± 0.547		
P value	0.117	0.000*	0.000*	0.000*	0.000*	0.005*	0.001*		

Data were presented as mean ± SD, tested by student t-test, *P*-value<0.01 statistically significant. T_0: PSIand RSS before drug administration. T_2-T_{11}: PSIand RSS every hour till extubation. $T_{1A.E}$, $T_{2A.E}$: PSI one& two hours after extubation. SD: standard deviation

Table 3: Patient State Index (PSI) and Ramsay Sedation Score (RSS).

Measuring time	Groups	Min-max	Mean ± SD	t- test	*P*-value
To eye opening (min)	P	8.00-20.00	13.16 ± 4.472	13.175	0.000*
	D	0.25-5.00	2.07 ± 1.125		
To hand squeezing (min)	P	13.00-25.00	17.56 ± 4.903	15.442	0.000*
	D	0.50-6.00	2.98 ± 1.642		
Till verbal command (min)	P	15.00-45.00	22.60 ± 7.327	8.039	0.000*
	D	0.50-6.00	3.45 ± 1.656		
To extubation (min)	P	18.00-90.00	36.03 ± 18.214	13.213	0.000*
	D	3.00-15.00	8.93 ± 3.027		

Table 4: Time from cessation of drug to different parameters in the two study groups.

Several studies have explained these findings as the Propofol may lead to a reduction in the systemic vascular resistance, this Propofol induced hypotension is thought to be mediated by inhibiting the sympathetic nervous system and impairing the baroreflex regulatory mechanism, in addition Propofol is considered to have a direct relaxing effect on venous smooth muscles with an increase in venous capacitance which may contribute to the hypotension [6,7].

Similar results to our study were reported by Zahoor A and his colleagues [5]. They observed no change or decrease in the heart rate of their patients after a bolus or infusion of Propofol, in contrast, others have observed an initial tachycardia after Propofol administration [8].

Meiser et al. [9] showed that volatile anaesthetics act primarily on the more rostral brain structures like the cerebral cortex, and even at low concentrations may completely depress consciousness (MACawake) while leaving many autonomic functions (such as temperature control, blood pressure regulation or respiration) undisturbed.

The requirements for norepinephrine reported in this study were significantly lower in recipients sedated with Desflurane than with Propofol. Propofol/Fentanyl infusion resulted in a sustained decrease

in SVR due to its peripheral vasodilating effect, which was aggravated in cirrhotic patients already prone to peripheral vasodilation [10].

In this current study it was also noticed that the duration of required mechanical ventilation for liver transplant recipients was significantly longer for those receiving Propofol compared to patients receiving Desflurane. This can be partially explained by the rapid reversal of the sedating effect of Desflurane due to its pharmacokinetic properties. Minimal effects of Desflurane on circulation and cardiac performance lead to reduced demand for catecholamine support which preferable to be reduced prior to weaning from ventilator support, this helped in fulfilling the criteria for earlier extubation.

Kollef et al. [11] concluded in their study that the strategies targeted at reducing the use of continuous intravenous sedation could shorten the duration of mechanical ventilation for some patients.

It was also noticed that the mean dosage of additive sedative drug (Fentanyl) was lower in the Desflurane group than in the Propofol group. The haemodynamic changes after liver transplantation and the vasodilation effect of Propofol necessity the use Fentanyl to reduce the required Propofol dosage to achieve the targeted sedative effect while reducing the Propofol expected effect on MABP and SVR. Desflurane was not in need for any supplementations in this context due to it minimal haemodynamic effects in comparison to Propofol.

The need for analgesics in the current study is the Desflurane group was minimal in general. Several studies explained why liver transplant recipients are less in need for analgesics than other non-hepatic patients undergoing surgery. The changes in the level of endogenous neuropeptides, such as, beta-endorphins, meta-enkephalins, and substance P, are thought to be playing a part in reducing their requirements for intravenous opioids and even general anaesthetics, their levels are directly proportionate with the severity of liver disease and are reported to be higher in end stage liver disease patients [12,13]. Fentanyl was used more frequently in this study with Propofol to reduce its haemodynamic side effects.

All measured emergence times (defined as verbal command responses [eye opening, hand squeezing] tracheal extubation, and orientation (defined as providing correct date of birth) were more prolonged in Propofol group than in Desflurane group, this may be due to the peculiar nature of Desflurane which enjoys a low blood/gas solubility coefficient and low metabolic rate which can reach to 0.02% (the lowest in vivo metabolism of any available inhaled halogenated anaesthetics). Lendvay et al. [14] reported faster recovery with Desflurane anesthesia when compared with other intravenous anesthesia.

Similarly, Wachtel et al. [15] published a meta-analysis of average times and variability in times of extubation and following commands after Desflurane or Propofol anaesthesia. Their analysis showed distinct differences in favour of Desflurane.

In addition, the quick emergence times are indicators of greater control of sedation. If the level of sedation needs to be increased to perform unpleasant or painful procedures in the ICU, this can be achieved quickly by Desflurane. After the end of the procedure, the previous level of sedation may be restored immediately [16].

One of the limitations of our study was not using the Remifentanil instead of Fentanyl. Remifentanil seems to be the ideal partner for intravenous and inhalational sedation because of its better pharmacokinetics. Like the volatile anaesthetics, remifentanil will not accumulate even in patients with hepatic or renal insufficiency. Its use for ICU sedation has been described and it has been licensed for ICU sedation for up to 3 days, but unfortunately it is not yet available in the Egyptian market [17].

Interestingly, no patient in our study receiving Desflurane complained of nausea, a finding that contrasts with common experience from the post anaesthesia care unit where up to 30 or even 50% of patients after inhalational anaesthesia will complain of nausea or vomiting [16].

Meiser A et al. [16] compared Desflurane and Propofol for postoperative sedation in intensive care found similar results in their study.

Better cognitive functions were found after sedation with Desflurane. Patients in Desflurane group correctly stated their birth date earlier and were able to recall significantly more words at this time than patients in Propofol group with a better trieger dot test (TT) and digit symbol substitution test (DSST).

In contrast, Meiser A et al. [16] found that the TT and DSST did not detect differences in psychometric performance as many patients, in spite of being mentally competent, were not able to execute the tests

because of weakness, tremor, swollen hands, impaired vision (oedema of the conjunctiva or upper eye lids) and inability to sit up.

A frequently discussed adverse reaction to Desflurane is sympathetic hyperactivity [3]. Interestingly, in our study there wasn't any episode of tachycardia or hypertension attributable to an increase in Desflurane concentration probably because we never used more than 4 vol % Desflurane.

Ebert et al. [18] explained our finding that sympathetic activation only occurs when abruptly increasing the Desflurane concentration from 1 MAC (minimum alveolar concentration) (7.25 vol %) to 1.5 MAC (11 vol %), but not from 0.5 to 1 MAC.

In contrast, Ramsay scores were higher (more deeply sedated) in Desflurane group than in Propofol group. As an explanation, it is assumed that volatile anaesthetics may act like an on-off switch for consciousness, whereas with Propofol it may be easier to achieve intermediate levels of sedation as reported by Meiser et al. [16].

Schneider et al. [19], in a study among surgical intensive care patients receiving Propofol and Sufentanil, found the PSI to be highly predictive of the depth of sedation in mechanically ventilated patients. The PSI values showed significant differences between different levels of sedation as measured by the Ramsay sedation score (RSS).

A prospective blinded study of mixed ICU patients by Ramsay et al. [20] also found a strong correlation between the PSI and the RSS. Similarly in another study by Sessler et al. [21] investigating the relationship between PSI and the sedation/agitation level measured by Richmond Agitation-Sedation Scale score found significant associations between PSI and Richmond Agitation-Sedation Scale to support the validity of the PSI as a tool to monitor the level of sedation in the Intensive care Unit.

Higher costs for the Propofol group compared to the Desflurane group, this could be due to the low flow circuit used during Desflurane administration and the high dose of Propofol and Fentanyl consumed.

Similarly, Meiser et al. [16] showed that inhaled anaesthesia was associated with a lower cost when compared with the Propofol-based sedation.

No technical difficulties or problems in the use of the anaesthesia ventilator or the Desflurane vaporizer were reported in the Intensive Care. Anaesthesia Machines were equipped with a scavenging system using charcoal adsorption.

Sackey et al. [22] demonstrate that the occupational load from the volatile anaesthetic, in the presence of anaesthetic gas scavenging system at the bedside, is minimal and within the international standard (mean of 0.1 ppm), using isoflurane.

In conclusion Des sedation guided with PSI preserved better the haemodynamic parameters, enhanced recovery at a lower cost compared to Propofol. Patient state index (PSI) was able to provide a consistent and comparable depth of sedation with two different sedative drugs as Des and P in contrast to Ramsay sedation score (RSS). Further multicenter studies on a larger scale are recommended.

Acknowledgement

Number for the registry: PACTR201402000758402

Name of registry: South African Cochrane Centre

References

1. Brush DR, Kress JP (2009) Sedation and analgesia for the mechanically ventilated patient.Clin Chest Med 30: 131-141.

2. Ypsilantis P, Mikroulis D, Politou M, Tsoukali H, Pitiakoudis M, et al. (2006) Tolerance to Propofol's sedative effect in mechanically ventilated Rabbits.Anesth Analg 103: 359-365, table of contents.

3. Jakobsson J (2012) Desflurane: a clinical update of a third-generation inhaled anaesthetic.Acta Anaesthesiol Scand 56: 420-432.

4. Sinclair S, James S, Singer M (1997) Intraoperative intravascular volume optimisation and length of hospital stay after repair of proximal femoral fracture: Randomised controlled trial. BMJ 315: 909–912.

5. Field A (2006) Sample Size Calculation: In: Discovering Statistics Using SPSS (2nd edn.) London, California, New Delhi: SAGE Publications Ltd 143-217.

6. Zahoor A, Ahmed N (2010) The effects of duration of Propofol injection on hemodynamics. Middle East J Anaesthesiol 20: 845-850.

7. Barker P, Langton JA, Murphy P, Rowbotham DJ (1991) Effect of prior administration of cold saline on pain during propofol injection. A comparison with cold propofol and propofol with lignocaine. Anaesthesia 46:1069-1070.

8. Tham CS, Khoo ST (1995) Modulating effects of lignocaine on propofol. Anaesth Intensive Care 23: 154-157.

9. Meiser A, Laubenthal H (2005) Inhalational anaesthetics in the ICU: theory and practice of inhalational sedation in the ICU, economics, risk-benefit.Best Pract Res Clin Anaesthesiol 19: 523-538.

10. Wahr JA, Plunkett JJ, Ramsay JG, Reeves J, Jain U, et al. (1996) Cardiovascular responses during sedation after coronary revascularization. Incidence of myocardial ischemia and hemodynamic episodes with Propofol vs. midazolam. Institutions of the McSPI Research Group. Anesthesiology 84: 1350-1360.

11. Kollef MH, Levy NT, Ahrens TS, Schaiff R, Prentice D, et al. (1998) The use of continuous i.v. sedation is associated with prolongation of mechanical ventilation. Chest 114: 541-548.

12. Donovan KL, Janicki PK, Striepe VI, Stoica C, Franks WT, et al. (1997) Decreased patient analgesic requirements after liver transplantation and associated neuropeptide levels. Transplantation 63: 1423-1429.

13. Hasanin AS, Mahmoud FM, Yassen KA (2013) Entropy-guided end-tidal Desflurane concentration during living donor liver transplantation. Saudi J Anaesth 7: 399-403.

14. Lendvay V, Draegni T, Rostrup M, Arvid K (2010) Propofol/Remifentanil vs. Desflurane/Fentanyl in Open Hemicolectomy Surgery. J Anesthe Clinic Res 1: 102-107.

15. Wachtel RE, Dexter F, Epstein RH, Ledolter J (2011) Meta-analysis of Desflurane and propofol average times and variability in times to extubation and following commands. Can J Anaesth 58: 714-724.

16. Meiser A, Sirtl C, Bellgardt M, Lohmann S, Garthoff A, et al. (2003) Desflurane compared with propofol for postoperative sedation in the intensive care unit. Br J Anaesth 90: 273-280.

17. Dahaba AA, Grabner T, Rehak PH, List WF, Metzler H (2004) Remifentanil vs. morphine analgesia and sedation for mechanically ventilated critically ill patients: a randomized double blind study. Anesthesiology 101: 640-646.

18. Ebert TJ, Perez F, Uhrich TD, Deshur MA (1998) Desflurane-mediated sympathetic activation occurs in humans despite preventing hypotension and baroreceptor unloading. Anesthesiology 88: 1227-1232.

19. Schneider G, Heglmeier S, Schneider J, Tempel G, Kochs EF (2004) Patient State Index (PSI) measures depth of sedation in intensive care patients. Intensive Care Med 30: 213-216.

20. Ramsay MA, Huddleston P, Hamman P, Tai S, Greg M (2004) The Patient State Index Correlates Well with the Ramsay Sedation Score in ICU Patients. Anesthesiology 101: A338.

21. Sessler CN, Kollef M, Hamilton A, Grap MJ, Jefferson D (2005) Comparison of depth of sedation measured by PSA 4000 and richmond agitation-sedation scale (RASS). CHEST Journal 128: 151S-152S.

22. Sackey PV, Martling CR, Nise G, Radell PJ (2005) Ambient isoflurane pollution and isoflurane consumption during intensive care unit sedation with the Anesthetic Conserving Device. Crit Care Med 33: 585-590.

3

Intraoperative Transthoracic Echocardiography is a Feasible Technique Used in Morbidly Obese Patients for Non-Invasive Cardiovascular Monitoring

María Carolina Cabrera Schulmeyer[*], **Jaime De la Maza**, **Ignacio Fernández**, **Cristián Ovalle and Carlos Farias**

Anesthesiology Department, Universidad de Valparaíso, Hospital Clínico FACH, CINTO Santiago de Chile, Chile

[*]**Corresponding author:** Maria Carolina Cabrera Schulmeyer, Anesthesiology Department, Universidad de Valparaíso, Hospital Clinico FACH, CINTO Santiago de Chile, Chile, E-mail: carol218@vtr.net

Abstract

Background and objectives: To evaluate the feasibility of an abbreviated focus-assessed transthoracic echocardiography protocol in morbidly obese patients. The purpose of this study was to evaluate whether good images could be obtained from this particularly difficult group of patients for whom acoustic imaging is often poor. Heart imaging could be helpful for cardiopulmonary screening and real-time monitoring.

Materials and methods: The study included 106 morbidly obese patients, who were undergoing laparoscopic bariatric surgery. The mean patient age was 32 years (range 21- 52), and there were 35 males. The parasternal long and short axes, apical 4 and 5 chambers were evaluated.

Results: In 95% of the patients, at least one view was obtained. In 78% two views were obtained and in 31% of the patients, all views and measurements could be performed.

Discussion: In obese patients, the major advantage of having a non-invasive cardiac monitoring device is the ability to perform anesthesia delivery.

Conclusion: Focused echocardiogaphy examination performed by anesthesiologists in the intraoperative period of morbid obese patients is feasible for almost all patients. Echocardiography offers non-invasiveness and speed for assessing the hemodynamic state and heart function of an obese patient. The image quality of the heart is sufficient to undergo interpretation and, therefore can contribute to intraoperative clinical decision-making

Keywords: Anesthesia; Obese patient; Transthoracic echocardiography

Introduction

Obese patients are always challenging for anesthesiologists [1-3]. The effect of obesity and its associated comorbidities, such as hypertension, diabetes, dyslipidemia and obstructive apnea syndrome, induce a different spectrum of pathologies [4,5]. In particular obesity produces the obesity cardiomyopathy, which alters diastolic and systolic functions. In addition, obesity is associated with 30 % increase in ischemic heart disease and sudden death [6]. Laparoscopic bariatric surgery is considered an effective and economical treatment for promoting and maintaining weight lost, thereby decreasing comorbidities, such as heart disease. The preoperative cardiovascular evaluation of the morbid obese patients is challenging, because these patients have exercise intolerance, and there are weight limitations for imaging tests [7]. Therefore, many obese patients arrive in the operating room with limited cardiovascular evaluations and there are known hemodynamic changes that will occur during general anesthesia [8,9]. Physiologic changes occur also because of the pneumoperitoneum and the patient position [10]. Echocardiography is the only technique that provides dynamic and real-time bedside imaging of the heart [11,12].

Small portable ultrasound machines with transthoracic echocardiographic (TTE) probes are now readily available in the operating room. The use of focused transthoracic echocardiography by anesthesiologists has shown that they are able to obtain rapid diagnostic quality images and good assessments of the ventricular load and valvular function [13,14]. The aim of focused intraoperative TTE is to noninvasively enhance the clinical cardiac assessment and immediately evaluate the hemodynamic condition, which is not easily detectable by traditional intraoperative non-invasive monitors.

The aim of the study was to evaluate and assess the feasibility of intraoperative image quality and limitations in morbidly obese patients during laparoscopic bariatric surgery using a focused TTE protocol performed by anesthesiologists.

We hypothesized that current TTE imaging equipment was adequate for identifying the cardiac chambers, valves, and volume status of these patients despite their obesity.

Materials and Methods

The study was conducted with approval from the Human Ethics Committee of the Hospital (FACh A, 131-009), and written informed consent was obtained from all patients.

Prospectively, patients with body mass index (BMI) over 40 undergoing laparoscopic bariatric surgery, between November 2010 and December 2012 were included in the study.

All of the studies were performed or supervised by an anesthesiologist with extensive TTE experience using the Turbo (Sonosite, Fujifilm, Bothell, WA, USA). A 1.5-3.6 MHz phased array transducer was used.

Echocardiography and measurements were obtained with the patient placed in a supine position, anesthetized and intubated. An electrocardiogram, an automated non-invasive blood pressure monitor and a pulse oximeter were continuously used.

The focused echocardiography protocol was divided following the same order:

Parasternal long axis view

The transducer was placed on the third or fourth intercostal space, adjacent to the left lateral margin of the sternum. Here the left atrial size, left and right ventricular contraction and dimension of the left ventricular outflow tract (LVOT) diameter were measured (Figure 1).

Parasternal short axis view

By rotating the transducer 90° from the parasternal long axis view, the short axis view was displayed to evaluate the left ventricular (LV) contractility (Figure 2).

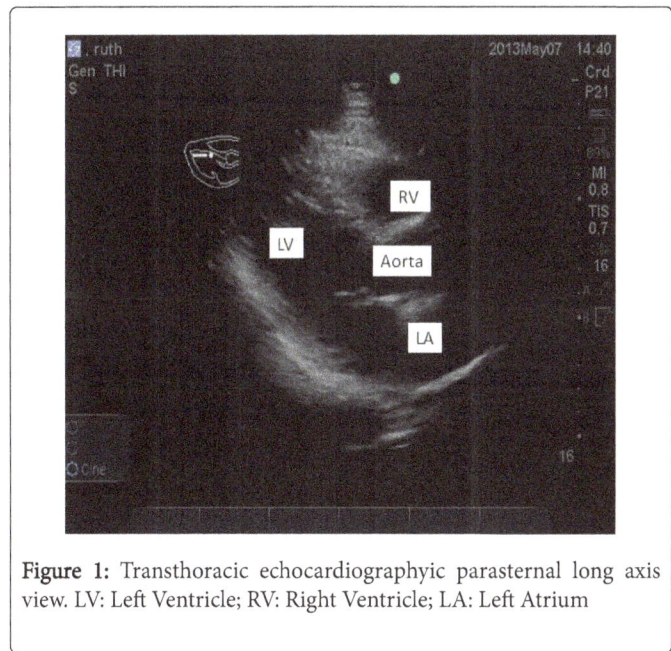

Figure 2: Transthoracic short axis view. LV: Left Ventricle; RV: Right Ventricle.

At the level of the mitral valve, the diastolic function was assessed measuring the LV inflow (Figure 3). Rotating the probe counter clockwise, a 3-chamber view was obtained for measuring the velocity of the outflow tract

Subcostal views were omitted because of the interference with the surgical field.

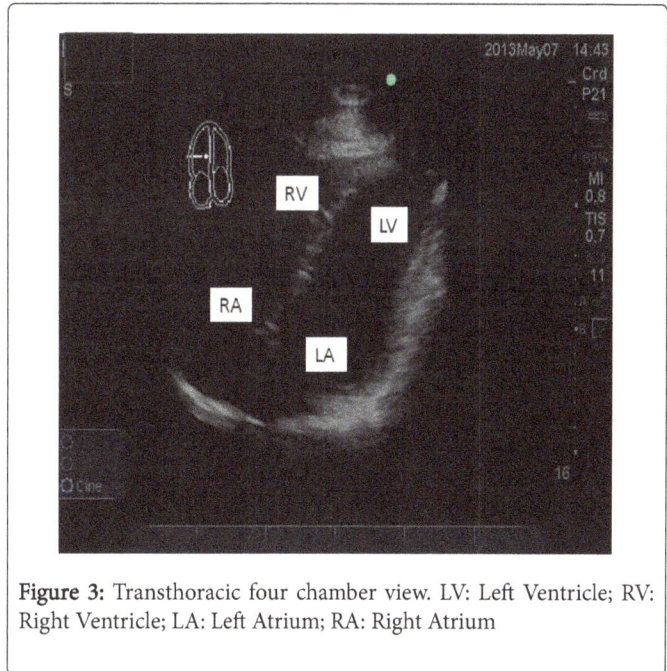

Figure 1: Transthoracic echocardiographyic parasternal long axis view. LV: Left Ventricle; RV: Right Ventricle; LA: Left Atrium

Apical 4-chamber view

The transducer was placed over the apex of the heart, and the ultrasound beam was directed parallel to the long axis. Here, it was important to observe the atrial and ventricular cavities.

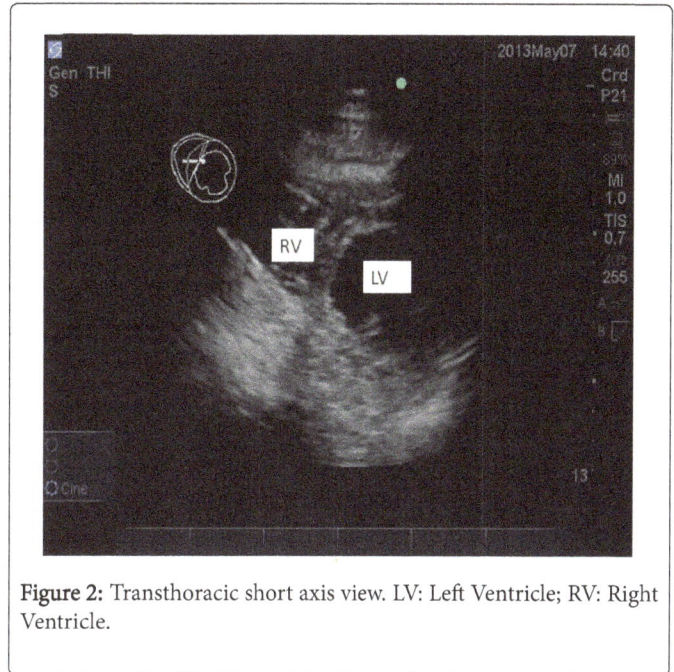

Figure 3: Transthoracic four chamber view. LV: Left Ventricle; RV: Right Ventricle; LA: Left Atrium; RA: Right Atrium

Statistical analysis

Continuous data were expressed as a mean value ± SD or as a percentage. Descriptive data were analyzed using STATA 10.0 (StataCorp LP4905 Lakeway DriveCollege Station, Texas, USA).

Results

Hundred-six obese patients with BMI of 43 ± 12 were included in the study. There were 35 males and 21 females. The average patient age was 32 ± 10 years.

In 95% of patients, it was possible to obtain at least one usable window of the proposed views to assess the heart.

In 78% of patients it was possible to obtain 2 of the proposed views. Subsequently, in 56% of patients, 3 views were found, and in 31% all proposed views and measurements were found. In only 3 patients (5%) no images could be taken.

The parasternal long axis view with the patient lying supine provided the best cardiac window in most patients, with an 81% success rate.

The presence of pneumoperitoneum did not significantly influence the achievability of a successful examination.

With a 34 % success rate the 5-chamber apical view was the most difficult view to obtain.

Discussion

This study was designed to assess the feasibility of a focused TTE in morbidly obese patients. In this study, we found that the 2D TTE images were useful for obtaining at least one acceptable quality view that could be used to directly assess the hearts of morbidly obese patients. Despite all of the limitations of this study population and the prejudgment that it would not be possible to obtain any views, because of the poor window quality in morbidly obese patients, the success rate was considerable (>one-third), and all cardiac windows were obtained. As illustrated by our patients, the parasternal transducer positions provided the highest yields, despite the supine position of the patient. With this view, substantial information about dimensions and contractility was obtained. According to the literature, this result was positive [15,16].

Previous data in perioperative populations undergoing non-cardiac surgery have supported the concept of a limited TTE and its ability to provide additional information that is not obtainable with standard clinical examination [17,18]. This process can be performed in approximately 10 minutes.

Having TTE monitoring during a laparoscopic bariatric surgery can lead to different scenarios. The heart can be completely normal during the entire procedure. TTE had the effect of reassuring the anesthesiologist, which led to a reduced requirement for further investigation and, reduced invasive monitoring and postoperative level of care. The goal is to avoid the insertion of more invasive monitoring tools, such as an arterial line or a central venous catheter, with the known risks and difficulties associated with both procedures, particularly in obese patients.

Another completely different scenario might occur if a clinically important hemodynamic or valvular abnormality is diagnosed in an obese patient with intraoperative TTE; this images can alert the anesthesiologist to an increased cardiac risk, leading to an increase in the level of intraoperative hemodynamic monitoring and treatment or postoperative care. The unique nature of anesthesia practice with sudden changes in patient physiology in the operating room means that having anesthesiologists with some TTE capability is invaluable.

It must be clearly stated that focused echocardiographic examinations are not a substitute for formal accredited TTE assessments. Instead they are designed for situations where limited examinations formats also assess intraoperative volume status, LV contractility and function and to exclude significant pathology. There have been several models for limited cardiac assessment such as the FATE (focused assessment with transthoracic echocardiography) examination in intensive care [19]. The HEART (hemodynamic echocardiographic assessment in real time) scan [20] is an assessment of ventricular filling, function and pressures: it is repeatable, as required, to allow for dynamic changes (e.g. intraoperatively).

As yet, there are no formal training guidelines for physicians wishing to incorporate TTE into their anesthesia practice. Recent data in the ICU literature suggest that non-cardiologists may acquire basic skills in focused critical care echocardiography with approximately 10 hours of didactic and practical teaching [21]. One of the problems with performing a limited or goal directed TTE is the failure to recognize significant pathology that might be observed during a formal TTE. Focused TTE, however, accurately identifies major cardiac abnormalities compared to non- invasive monitoring. Royse et al. [22] found that a novice operator could reach agreement with an expert operator in as few as 20 studies for basic hemodynamic state measurements and in 40 studies for all of the measurements performed.

This study has several limitations. The correct acquisition, processing and interpretation data require a thorough understanding of the possible pitfalls, along with an understanding of the limitations related to the patients, equipment and examiner. Another major limitation of an abbreviated goal directed TTE protocol is the subjective and qualitative nature of the assessment. With experience and training, however, the ability to extract increasingly large amounts of data has improved. Another important limitation of the study included the observational nature of the design, which was aimed at establishing proof of the concept of focused TTE examination in obese patients, rather than the effect on patient outcomes, which will be the subject of future investigations for our study group.

Conclusion

In conclusion the focused performed echocardiogaphic examination of morbidly obese patients performed by anesthesiologists in the intraoperative period is feasible for nearly all patients. One or more acoustic windows were obtained in 80% of the patients. Echocardiography is non-invasive and can quickly assess the hemodynamic state and function of the hearts of obese patients. The image quality of the heart is sufficient for interpretation and, therefore, can contribute to intraoperative clinical decision-making in morbidly obese patients. Further studies will be needed to study the impact and changes in patient management based on the echo images.

Competing Interests

The authors have reported no external funding or conflicts of interest.

References

1.   Donohoe CL, Feeney C, Carey MF, Reynolds JV (2011) Perioperative evaluation of the obese patient. J Clin Anesth 23: 575-586.

2.   Cheah MH, Kam PC (2005) Obesity: basic science and medical aspects relevant to anaesthetists. Anaesthesia 60: 1009-1021.

3. Bergland A, Gislason H, Raeder J (2008) Fast-track surgery for bariatric laparoscopic gastric bypass with focus on anaesthesia and peri-operative care. Experience with 500 cases. Acta Anaesthesiol Scand 52: 1394-1399.

4. Tung A (2010) Anaesthetic considerations with the metabolic syndrome. Br J Anaesth 105 Suppl 1: i24-33.

5. Bagry HS, Raghavendran S, Carli F (2008) Metabolic syndrome and insulin resistance: perioperative considerations. Anesthesiology 108: 506-523.

6. Tchernof A, Despres JP (2013) Pathophysiology of human visceral obesity: an update. Physiol Rev 93: 359-404.

7. Poirier P, Alpert MA, Fleisher LA, Thompson PD, Sugerman HJ, et al. (2009) Cardiovascular evaluation and management of severely obese patients undergoing surgery: a science advisory from the American Heart Association. Circulation 120: 86-95.

8. Reinius H, Jonsson L, Gustafsson S, Sundbom M, Duvernoy O, et al. (2009) Prevention of atelectasis in morbidly obese patients during general anesthesia and paralysis: a computerized tomography study. Anesthesiology 111: 979-987.

9. Pelosi P, Gregoretti C (2010) Perioperative management of obese patients. Best Pract Res Clin Anaesthesiol 24: 211-225.

10. Sprung J, Whalley D, Tommaso F, Warner D, Hubmayr R, et al. (2002) The impact of morbid obesity, pneumoperitoneum, and posture on respiratory system mechanics and oxygenation during laparoscopy. Anesth Analg 94:1345-1350.

11. Joseph MX, Disney PJ, Da Costa R, Hutchison SJ (2004) Transthoracic echocardiography to identify or exclude cardiac cause of shock. Chest 126: 1592-1597.

12. Cowie B (2009) Focused cardiovascular ultrasound performed by anesthesiologists in the perioperative period: Feasible and alters patient management. J Cardiovasc Thorac Anesthesia 23: 450-456.

13. Manasia A, Nagraj H, Kodali R, Croft LB, Oropello JM, et al. (2005) Feasibility and potential clinical utility of goal- directed transthoracic echocardiography performed by noncardiologist intensivists using asmall handcarried device in crtically ill patients. J Cardiovasc Vasc Anesth 19:155-159.

14. Cowie BS (2010) Focused transthoracic echocardiography in the perioperative period. Anaesth Intensive Care 38: 823-836.

15. Canty DJ, Royse CF, Kilpatrick D, Williams DL, Royse AG (2012) The impact of pre-operative focused transthoracic echocardiography in emergency non-cardiac surgery patients with known or risk of cardiac disease. Anaesthesia 67: 714-720.

16. Manecke GR Jr, Vezina DP (2009) Perioperative transthoracic echocardiography: "universal acid"? J Cardiothorac Vasc Anesth 23: 447-449.

17. Beaulieu Y (2007) Specific skill set and goals of focused echocardiography for critical care clinicians. Crit Care Med 35: S144-149.

18. Royse C (2009) Ultrasound-guided haemodynamic state assessment. Best Practice & Research Clinical Anesthesiology 23:273-283.

19. Jensen MB, Sloth E, Larsen KM, Schmidt MB (2004) Transthoracic echocardiography for cardiopulmonary monitoring in intensive care. Eur J Anaesthesiol 21: 700-707.

20. Canty DJ, Royse CF (2009) Audit of anaesthetist-performed echocardiography on perioperative management decisions for non-cardiac surgery. Br J Anaesth 103: 352-358.

21. Lemola K, Yamada E, Jagasia D, Kerber R (2003) A hand-carried personal ultrasound device for rapid evaluation of left ventricular function: use after limited echo training. Echocardiography 20: 309-312.

22. Royse C, Seah J, Donelan L, Royse G (2006) Point of care ultrasound for basic haemodynamic assessment: novice compared with an expert operator. Anaesthesia 61: 849-855.

4

Intravenous Acetaminophen Administration in Patients Undergoing Craniotomy - A Retrospective Institutional Study

Hoefnagel AL, Lopez M *, Mitchell K, Smith DI, Feng C and Nadler JW

University of Rochester Medical Center, Rochester, NY, USA

*Corresponding author: Mathew J Lopez, MD, University of Rochester Medical Center, 601 Elmwood Avenue, Rochester, NY 14642, USA, E-mail: mathew_lopez@urmc.rochester.edu

Abstract

Introduction: Patients undergoing craniotomy for tumor resection often experience moderate to severe postoperative pain. Intravenous acetaminophen has been proposed as an analgesic adjunct to potentially decrease opioid requirements and incidence of nausea in these patients allowing for prompt postoperative neurological evaluations. At this time, however, there is no evidence to show that acetaminophen reduces patient pain or opioid consumption after craniotomy.

Methods: A retrospective analysis of 81 patients undergoing craniotomy was done to evaluate the effect of IV acetaminophen (APAP) administration on reported pain scores, opioid usage, time in the post-anesthesia care unit (PACU), and incidence of nausea within the first 24 hours.

Results: No significant differences in patient reported pain scores, opioid consumption within the first 24 hours, anti-emetic use, or time in PACU were found in patients who received intravenous acetaminophen compared to those who received opioids alone.

Discussion: Our investigation represents the first evidence looking for an effect of acetaminophen on post-craniotomy pain and nausea. There are randomized and blinded trials currently in progress that will add to our knowledge on this topic. Acetaminophen is a relatively safe intervention. However, until those randomized trials are completed and reported, we cannot uniformly recommend the intraoperative administration of intravenous acetaminophen to patients undergoing craniotomy.

Keywords: Acetaminophen; Intravenous; Craniotomy; Pain; Opioid; Nausea

Introduction

Patients undergoing elective craniotomy often experience moderate to severe post-operative pain; the management of which is believed suboptimal and continually evolving [1-5]. Historically, post-craniotomy pain has been undertreated for fear of opioid interference with prompt postoperative neurologic examinations [6,7]. Opioids have several well-established, dose-dependent side effects: sedation, hypoventilation, hypercarbia, and impaired cognition [8,9]. These adverse effects can result in increased cerebral blood flow and concomitant rise in intracranial pressure, possibly leading to additional poor outcomes [9,10]. Opioids may also exacerbate post-operative nausea and vomiting (PONV), a common complication of intracranial surgery [11-13], and treatment with anti-emetics can further depress mental status and perpetuate a negative cycle [14]. Opioid selection during craniotomy (and the subsequent effects on postoperative recovery) has been reviewed in detail [15]. Still, it is essential to maintain adequate analgesia in neurosurgical patients. Insufficient treatment of pain can result in decreased patient satisfaction [16]. More alarmingly, uncontrolled pain may lead to increased agitation, shivering, hypertension, and vomiting, which may increase intracranial pressure and risk of bleeding [17].

The ideal anesthetic in craniotomies remains one that provides a fast offset to aid in post-operative neurological examinations as well as providing adequate analgesia. This had led physicians to pursue other modalities to reduce opioid requirements in the perioperative period. Scalp infiltrations with local anesthetics have demonstrated mixed results with little effect on intraoperative opioid administration [18-20]. Recent work has shown that dexmedetomidine can reduce pain after craniotomy [21], but dexmedetomidine also has sedative and hemodynamic effects that may not be desirable. More promisingly, non-steroidal anti-inflammatory drugs (NSAIDs) can also be used as adjuncts in the multi-modal approach to pain management [22,23]. NSAIDs are shown to reduce post-operative analgesic requirements and limit narcotic-related side effects, particularly PONV, but may negatively impact surgical hemostasis, and thus cannot be used universally [22]. Acetaminophen has a well-established safety profile, relatively few side effects or contraindications, and intravenous administration can provide fast and predictable analgesia along with a significant opioid sparing effect [24,25]. Acetaminophen alone is not likely to provide adequate pain relief after supratentorial craniotomy: oral acetaminophen has been shown to provide adequate relief postoperatively in only 27% of patients [26], and another study that included a paracetamol arm stopped enrollment in that arm due to inadequate pain control [27]. But while it also compares unfavorably with opioids when administered post-operatively for craniotomy pain [28], it may make for a suitable adjunct.

Intravenous acetaminophen (Ofrimev*) has been available for use in the United States for quite a while. However, its increased cost in recent months prompts further investigation into its utility. Here we aim to investigate whether a single dose of Ofrimev*, given at the time of dural closure, impacts patient reported pain score, overall usage of opioid medications within 24 hours, post-operative nausea and vomiting, or anti-emetic usage. It is our hypothesis that patients who received intraoperative intravenous acetaminophen will have less post-operative pain and nausea than those patients who did not.

Materials and Methods

After obtaining IRB approval, records of 225 patients, aged 18 and older, undergoing craniotomy at a single tertiary care hospital, during an 8-month period in 2014 were reviewed. Patients were excluded from analysis if they were on chronic opioids or anti-emetics defined as daily medication intake for a period of greater than 2 weeks prior to date of surgery. Patients were also excluded from analysis if they could not participate in an assessment of their pain scores, which involved a comparative number scale. Forty-two patients received IV APAP intra-operatively in addition to traditional anesthetic management during this time period. Thirty-nine age-matched controls were selected from this same time period.

All patients received 10 mg of dexamethasone and 4 mg of ondansetron intravenously for PONV prophylaxis. Patients with a history of PONV and those undergoing posterior fossa surgery also had a scopolamine patch placed prior to being transferred to the operating room.

General anesthesia with an endotracheal tube in place was used in 79 patients; while an asleep-awake-asleep [19] technique was used for 3 patients (2 in the APAP group, 1 in the standard group). Anesthetic management was accomplished with infusions of propofol, dexmedetomidine, and/or remifentanil as needed to facilitate neurophysiologic monitoring [22]. Location of tumor and surgical approach also determine pain severity, which is why patients were matched for procedure location [14] (Table 1).

		APAP	Standard	p value
Gender	Male	19	17	0.88
	Female	23	22	
Mean		53.4 ± 16.5	52.9 ± 17.9	0.91
BMI		29 ± 6.9	29.5 ± 7.2	0.76
ASA Status	2	27	7	0.06
	3	23	25	
	3E	1	1	
	4	1	5	
	4E	1	1	
Craniotomy Type	S	30	30	0.09
	O	6	4	

Table 1: Patient characteristic; SD: Standard Deviation; in craniotomy type S: Supratentorial; O: Suboccipital; P: Posterior fossa; APAP: Acetaminophen.

Following extubation, patients were transferred to the PACU for recovery from general anesthesia and monitoring of hemodynamic and neurologic status. Patient pain scores using a verbal 10-point scale or visual analog scale (VAS) were recorded every 15 minutes by the PACU nurse. Uncontrolled pain (>5/10) or discomfort visualized by the PACU RN were treated with intravenous opioids. Presence of nausea requiring anti-emetic medications was also documented during PACU stay. Total amounts of medications administered in PACU were noted. Following transfer from PACU to the neurosurgical inpatient unit, pain scores were recorded by floor RNs every 2 hours. Total amounts of opioid and anti-emetic medications received on the floor were reviewed in the electronic medical record and 24-hour totals were obtained.

Results

A total of 81 patients were included in the data analysis. Primary outcomes were highest pain score in PACU and in the first 24 hours, length of stay in PACU, opioid use in PACU and within the first 24 hours, and use of anti-emetics in PACU and within 24 hours. The mean and standard deviation of pain score in each treatment group was calculated and the two-sample t-test used to compare the mean pain scores between two groups. Linear regression analysis was utilized to compare treatment effect controlling for patient factors (age, gender, ASA physical status), and the surgical procedure.

The mean high pain score in PACU was 3.8 in the acetaminophen group, and 4.6 in the opioid only group (p=0.29). The mean 24-hour pain score was 3.4 vs. 3.9 (p=0.21) in the respective groups, and 24-hour administration of opioids in morphine equivalents was not significantly different in the patients who had received APAP intra-operatively (23.1 mg/18.9 mg, p=0.47). No difference in the amount of time in PACU was observed between the groups (p=0.21). Similarly there was no difference in anti-emetic use in the PACU or in the first 24 hours post-operatively between the two groups (p=0.19, 0.17) (Table 2).

	APAP	Standard	p value
PACU high pain score	3.7 ± 3.4	4.6 ± 3.8	0.29
Opioid PACU (mg)	7.9 ± 6	7.2 ± 5	0.67
24hr pain mean	3.4 ± 1.9	3.9 ± 2.4	0.21
Opioids 24hr (mg)	20.1 ± 18.6	22.9 ± 15.6	0.57
Mean time in PACU (min)	167 ± 117	138 ± 87	0.21
Antiemetic PACU %	38	55	0.19
24hr antiemetic %	42	56	0.17

Table 2: Primary outcomes; Opioid dose are reported in milligrams (mg) of morphine equivalents. APAP: Acetaminophen; PACU: Post-Anesthesia Care Unit.

Dexmedetomidine has been shown to provide analgesic effect [28-32]. This was identified as a potential confounding variable. There was significantly more dexmedetomidine use in the group that also received IV APAP (p=0.002).

Discussion

Decreasing post-operative pain and nausea are goals in the management of any anesthetic, but it is especially important for patients undergoing craniotomy. This report suggests that administration of a single dose of intravenous acetaminophen during anesthesia does not reduce pain or nausea following craniotomy.

Given the cost of intravenous acetaminophen, it is important to demonstrate that a reduction in pain score is not just statistically significant, but also clinically relevant. This study had a 0.8 power of detecting a 30% decrease in our primary outcome of peak PACU pain scores. It is possible that acetaminophen did alleviate pain to a smaller degree than our study was powered to detect. For the most common measure of pain intensity; the 11-point pain intensity numerical rating scale (as used in this study); a reduction of approximately 30% represents a clinically important difference [33]. A larger study would have been more likely to return a significantly different result, but that result may not have been clinically relevant.

This study has several limitations. First, we cannot rule out the possibility that there may have been a sizable percentage of individual patients or subgroups that experienced a clinically important pain reduction despite the lack of a mean difference between our groups at the population level. For example, infratentorial procedures are associated with more pain than supratentorial craniotomies [34], and so perhaps that subgroup would benefit more from the addition of adjunctive pain medications. Likewise, age, gender and the presence of preoperative opioid requirements affect post-craniotomy pain [4,7,34], and these groups might have difference responses to the addition of acetaminophen. Second, our investigation only examined the effect of a single dose of intravenous acetaminophen administered intra-operatively. Third, some patients received a combination of oral medications that included acetaminophen with an opioid within the first 24 hours post-operatively. This may have lowered the pain scores, opioid requirements, and anti-emetic usage in both groups, making any difference more difficult to detect. Fourth, there are limitations inherent in any retrospective study, including selection bias on the part of practitioners who may have based their administration of acetaminophen on patient or surgical factors not captured by our review or recall bias that may exist in the capture of data from medical record [35].

In 2014 the cost of a dose of intravenous acetaminophen increased by 140% [36]. This has prompted a much closer look into value-added and case-by-case results for intravenous acetaminophen versus alternative therapies. Our investigation represents the first evidence looking for an effect of acetaminophen on post-craniotomy pain and nausea. We had hypothesized that patients who received intraoperative intravenous acetaminophen would have had less pain and nausea than those who did not, but this was not the case. Using our chosen metrics, there was no difference between the group that received intraoperative acetaminophen and the group that did not.

There are randomized and blinded trials currently in progress that will add to our knowledge on this topic. Acetaminophen is a relatively safe intervention; however, until those randomized trials are completed and reported, we cannot uniformly recommend the intraoperative administration of intravenous acetaminophen to patients undergoing craniotomy.

References

1. Gottschalk A (2009) Craniotomy pain: trying to do better. Anesth Analg 109: 1379-1381.

2. Roberts GC (2005) Post-craniotomy analgesia: current practices in British neurosurgical centres--a survey of post-craniotomy analgesic practices. Eur J Anaesthesiol 22: 328-332.

3. Hansen MS, Brennum J, Moltke FB, Dahl JB (2013) Suboptimal pain treatment after craniotomy. Dan Med J 60: A4569.

4. De Benedittis G, Lorenzetti A, Migliore M, Spagnoli D, Tiberio F, et al. (1996) Postoperative pain in neurosurgery: a pilot study in brain surgery. Neurosurgery 38: 466-469.

5. Hansen MS, Brennum J, Moltke FB, Dahl JB (2011) Pain treatment after craniotomy: where is the (procedure-specific) evidence. A qualitative systematic review. Eur J Anaesthesiol 28: 821-9.

6. Stoneham MD, Walters FJ (1995) Post-operative analgesia for craniotomy patients: current attitudes among neuroanaesthetists. Eur J Anaesthesiol 12: 571-575.

7. Mordhorst C, Latz B, Kerz T, Wisser G, Schmidt A, et al. (2010) Prospective assessment of postoperative pain after craniotomy. J Neurosurg Anesthesiol 22: 202-206.

8. Berde C, Nurko S (2008) Opioid side effects--mechanism-based therapy. N Engl J Med 358: 2400-2402.

9. Cold GE, Felding M (1993) Even small doses of morphine might provoke "luxury perfusion" in the postoperative period after craniotomy. Neurosurgery 32: 327.

10. Weinstabl C, Spiss CK (1993) Fentanyl and sufentanil increase intracranial pressure in head trauma patients. Anesthesiology 78: 622-623.

11. Watcha MF, White PF (1992) Postoperative nausea and vomiting. Its etiology, treatment, and prevention. Anesthesiology 77: 162-184.

12. Fabling JM, Gan TJ, Guy J, Borel CO, el-Moalem HE, et al. (1997) Postoperative nausea and vomiting. A retrospective analysis in patients undergoing elective craniotomy. J Neurosurg Anesthesiol 9: 308-312.

13. Maxwell LG, Buckley GM, Kudchadkar SR, Ely E, Stebbins EL, et al. (2014) Pain management following major intracranial surgery in pediatric patients: a prospective cohort study in three academic children's hospitals. Paediatric Anaesth. 24: 1132-40.

14. Braude D, Crandall C (2008) Ondansetron versus promethazine to treat acute undifferentiated nausea in the emergency department: a randomized, double-blind, noninferiority trial. Acad Emerg Med 15: 209-215.

15. Ayrian E, Kaye AD, Varner CL, Guerra C, Vadivelu N, et al. (2015) Effects of anesthetic management on early postoperative recovery, hemodynamics and pain after supratentorial craniotomy. J Clin Med Res 7: 731-41.

16. Leslie K, Troedel S, Irwin K, Pearce F, Ugoni A, et al. (2003) Quality of recovery from anesthesia in neurosurgical patients. Anesthesiology 99: 1158-1165.

17. Kim YD, Park JH, Yang, Kim IS, Hong JT, et al. (2013) Pain assessment in brain tumor patients after elective craniotomy. Brain Tumor Res Treat 1: 24-27.

18. Bloomfield EL, Schubert A, Secic M, Barnett G, Shutway F, et al. (1998) The influence of scalp infiltration with bupivacaine on hemodynamics and postoperative pain in adult patients undergoing craniotomy. Anesth Analg 87: 579-582.

19. Batoz H, Verdonck O, Pellerin C, Roux G, Maurette P (2009) The analgesic properties of scalp infiltrations with ropivacaine after intracranial tumoral resection. Anesth Analg 109: 240-244.

20. Williams DL, Pemberton E, Leslie K (2011) Effect of intravenous parecoxib on post-craniotomy pain. Br J Anaesth 107: 398-403.

21. Peng K, Hiao JH, Si LL, Fu JH (2015) Effect of intraoperative dexmedetomidine on post-operative craniotomy pain. Clin Therap 37: 1114-21.e1.

22. Marret E, Kurdi O, Zufferey P, Bonnet F (2005) Effects of nonsteroidal antiinflammatory drugs on patient-controlled analgesia morphine side effects: meta-analysis of randomized controlled trials. Anesthesiology 102: 1249-60.

23. Kehlet H, Dahl JB (1993) The value of "multimodal" or "balanced analgesia" in postoperative pain treatment. Anesth Analg 77: 1048-1056.

24. Delbos A, Boccard E (1995) The morphine-sparing effect of propacetamol in orthopedic postoperative pain. J Pain Symptom Manage 10: 279-286.

25. Macario A, Royal MA (2011) A literature review of randomized clinical trials of intravenous acetaminophen (paracetamol) for acute postoperative pain. Pain Pract 11: 290-296.

26. Nair S, Rajshekhar V (2011) Evaluation of pain following supratentorial craniotomy. Br J Neurosurg 25: 100-103.

27. Verchère E, Grenier B, Mesli A, Siao D, Sesay M, et al. (2002) Postoperative pain management after supratentorial craniotomy. J Neurosurg Anesthesiol 14: 96-101.

28. Hassani E, Mahoori A, Sane S, Tolumehr A (2015) Comparison the effects of paracetamol with sufentanil infusion on postoperative pain control after craniotomy in patients with brain tumor. Adv Biomed Res 4: 64.

29. Burnand C, Sebastian J (2014) Anesthesia for awake craniotomy. Contin Educ Anaesth Crit Care Pain 14: 6-11.

30. Sloan TB, Heyer EJ (2002) Anesthesia for intraoperative neurophysiologic monitoring of the spinal cord. J Clin Neurophysiol 19: 430-443.

31. Bekker A, Sturaitis MK (2005) Dexmedetomidine for neurological surgery. Neurosurgery 57: 1-10.

32. Fairbanks CA, Stone LS, Kitto KF, Nguyen HO, Posthumus IJ, et al. (2002) alpha(2C)-Adrenergic receptors mediate spinal analgesia and adrenergic-opioid synergy. J Pharmacol Exp Ther 300: 282-290.

33. Farrar JT, Young JP Jr, LaMoreaux L, Werth JL, Poole RM (2001) Clinical importance of changes in chronic pain intensity measured on an 11-point numerical pain rating scale. Pain 94: 149-158.

34. Flexman AM, Ng JL, Gelb AW (2010) Acute and chronic pain following craniotomy. Curr Opin Anaesthesiol 23: 551-557.

35. Lambert J (2011) Statistics in brief: how to assess bias in clinical studies? Clin Orthop Relat Res 469: 1794-1796.

36. Prince JS, Dungy D (2015) When IV acetaminophen cost skyrocketed, the heathy system did some new math. Drug Topics.

5

Is Epidural Analgesia a Predictor of Low Newborn Apgar? A Hospital-Based Observational Study

Alexandra Saraiva[1], Sónia Duarte[1], Filipa Lagarto[1], Helena Figueira[1], Catarina S Nunes[2], Paulo Lemos[1] and Humberto S Machado[1]*

[1]*Departamento de Anestesiologia, Emergência e Cuidados Intensivos, Centro Hospitalar do Porto, Porto, Portugal*

[2]*Universidade Aberta, Departamento de Ciências e Tecnologia, Delegação do Porto, Porto, Portugal*

*Corresponding author: Humberto S Machado, Anesthesiology Department, Centro Hospitalar do Porto, Largo Abel Salazar, 4099-001 Porto, Portugal, E-mail: hjs.machado@gmail.com

Abstract

A painful labor induces adverse maternal effects and increases fetal stress, yet evidence of lack of adverse effect of epidural anesthesia to the newborn Apgar score has been inconsistent.

The aim of this study was to investigate maternal, newborn and anesthetic factors associated with a low Apgar score, in particular the effect of modality and timing of epidural analgesia, since this may allow for an appropriate neonatal care planning.

We retrospectively analyzed the labor process of 1850 out of 2006 parturients/participants/deliveries at Centro Hospitalar do Porto in 2014.

Our primary outcome was newborn Apgar score at fifth minute post-partum. Statistical significance was set as a p value inferior to 0.05.

Seventy-one newborns (3.8%) had Apgar score below 7 and 1779 (96.2%) above or equal to 7 at fifth minute. None of the variables identified as maternal age, BMI, previous labor, gestational age, cervix dilation and newborn weight have proved to be different between groups of Apgar below and above 7 (t-test). There was also no significant difference between newborns with Apgar above or below 7 in what concerned initiation of labor, mode of epidural analgesia, previous cesarean, type of delivery and newborn sex (Chi-squared). Median hour of birth and median labor length since beginning of epidural analgesia were not different between the two groups of outcome (Kruskall Wallis). The multivariable model showed that the risk for low Apgar was not independently associated with any of the variables analyzed (Chi-squared Omnibus).

In our study, modality and timing of epidural analgesia was not a predictor of low neonate Apgar score at fifth minute postpartum. Nonetheless, we demonstrated that epidural analgesia of low concentration local anesthetics with opioids was non-inferior to the opioid-free variety.

Keywords: Low APGAR predictive factors; Epidural anesthesia and APGAR

Introduction

The Apgar score is a quick and standardized assessment tool for clinical evaluation of the newborn at birth. Developed in the 1950s by the anesthesiologist Dr. Virginia Apgar, it remains useful until present days as a survival prediction score at 28 days of life [1-3].

The score is calculated by assigning a value of zero to two points for each of the five indices of well-being: heart rate, respiratory effort, reflex irritability, muscle tone and color [3]. In practice, Apgar score should be assessed at 1st and 5th minute. A score more than or equal to 7 is considered normal, while if less than 4 is considered severely low, at the 5th minute [4]. Fifth minute Apgar seems a better predictor compared with 1st minute Apgar, as it already signifies newborn answer to resuscitation maneuvers. Fifth minute Apgar score has been shown to be a better predictor of neonatal outcome than umbilical-artery blood pH [2]. The predictive strength of the Apgar score seems to stand beyond the neonatal period as a low value at fifth minute has been associated with cognitive impairment measured by academic achievement in adolescence [5,6].

Previous studies reported several predictors of low apgar score including maternal age [7,8], parity [9,10] smoking [11-15], obesity [16-19] and delivery by C-section [20]. Newborn factors included gestational age [10,21-23], low birth weight [10,22] and breech presentation [20].

The influence of anesthetic factors on neonatal well-being has also been questioned. Epidural analgesia is nowadays considered the standard for labor analgesia, unless contraindicated. It should be offered to all pregnant women, and despite conflicting results on its impact on instrumental delivery incidence, a 2011 Cochrane review concluded it has no significant impact on the rates of cesarean section neither on the newborn outcome assessed by the Apgar score [24,25].

The moment of initiation of epidural analgesia has also been questioned as a potential factor to modify labor progression and clinical maternal and neonatal outcomes. However, recent studies and a 2014 Cochrane review advocate that epidural analgesia should be initiated as soon as requested by the mother, without impact on Apgar score or cord pH [26-29].

Although Apgar score has been used worldwide for many years to evaluate early neonatal condition, it has been questioned if it is still relevant with all the advances in health-care service provision, neonatal resuscitation and infant care. Few data support its use as isolated criteria to predict mortality and morbidity, especially in preterm neonates [30].

Furthermore, Apgar score presents several limitations. The variables included depend on the newborn physiologic maturity, and no consistent data proved its applicability in preterm infants, so a false low Apgar score could be erroneously attributed to a healthy preterm infant; it could be affected by external factors as drugs, infections, trauma, and other non-controlled factors; and finally the evaluation of some of its components could be significantly subjective [30].

Moreover, neonatal resuscitation guidelines applied today are beyond the scope of the Apgar score and its prediction power. During neonatal resuscitation maneuvers, Apgar score should not be applied, as it was assigned for infants breathing spontaneously and not for neonates under resuscitation. In these newborns, score should be mentioned as "assisted", however no predictive power has been tested for this new concept [30,31].

Despite all this recent discussion around Apgar score, understanding its multiple limitations, it continues to present to date as a worldwide easy, standardized and immediate tool for neonatal assessment [30].

The aim of this study was to investigate if mode and timing of epidural labor analgesia is associated with a low Apgar score, since this may allow for an appropriate neonatal care planning.

Methods

Study design and sample

We performed a retrospective analysis of all labors occurred in our Obstetric Department in Centro Hospitalar do Porto, between 1st January and 31st December 2014. Centro Hospitalar do Porto is a grade-1 public hospital, offering all medical and surgical specialties, with the exception of cardiothoracic surgery.

Elective cesarean sections were excluded. To avoid possible bias, twins were excluded from the analysis. All labors that were converted into urgent cesareans due to fetal stress or other maternal related factors, as well as breech deliveries were included in the analysis. Women submitted to intravenous analgesia for labor were also excluded, as this regimen is only an option in parturient with specific pathologies that prevent the use of regional analgesia techniques. Maternal associated pathology and obstetric conditions (e.g. placenta previa, placental abruption, premature membrane rupture, cord prolapse) were not registered in the analyzed charts and these variables were not taken into account in this analysis. Importantly, all women with previous cesareans that were included in the analysis had only one previous cesarean, as the trial of scar is not performed in out maternity in women who had had 2 or more cesarean deliveries.

Data were collected in charts designed to register all steps of labor analgesia in our Department, fulfilled by an anesthesiologist attending or resident. All data were posteriorly transcripted and analyzed in Excel - Microsoft Windows*.

Variables

The following variables were registered: maternal age (years), maternal body mass index (BMI) (kg/m^2), parity(n), previous labor (n), gestational age (weeks), previous cesarean (yes or no), birth weight (g), beginning of labor (spontaneous or induced), cervix dilatation at beginning of analgesia (inferior or equal to 4 cm and superior to 4 cm), mode of epidural analgesia (Ropi+S: patient-controlled epidural analgesia (PCEA) with ropivacaine 0.1% and sufentanil 0.25 ug/mL (10 ml/h), with 5 mL bolus (lockout time: 30 min) Or the same mixture but in continuous infusion; Ropi 0.2%: continuous epidural infusion with high local anesthetic concentration, ropivacaine 0.2% (6-8 ml/h) and bolus given by the anesthesiologist as needed; others: including other choices of combination of local anesthetics and opioid or mixed options with more than one mode of analgesia), type of delivery (eutocic, dystocic, cesarean) delivery hour (hh:mm:ss) and labor length since beginning of analgesia (hh:mm:ss).

Outcome

Our primary outcome was to analyze predictive factors of newborn Apgar score below 7 at fifth minute post-partum.

Statistical analysis

Statistical analysis was performed using IBM SPSS statistics version 22.

Categorical variables are presented as frequency and percentage and continuous variables are presented as mean ± standard deviation (SD). For comparison between groups, the t-student's test was used for continuous variables; chi-squared test was used for categorical variables. Levene's test was used to check the homogeneity of variances. Non parametric Kruskal-Wallis test was used to compare the delivery time of day, and duration of delivery. Logistic Regression was used to identify independent risk factors for low Apgar score (below 7). A p-value<0.05 was considered to be statistically significant.

Results

Two thousand and six labors were performed in our Department in 2014 (excluding elective cesareans). Twins, newborns from mothers who received intravenous analgesia and registers with missing outcome data were excluded (n=156).

One thousand eight hundred and fifty newborns were included in the analysis. Among those, 3.8% (n=71) had Apgar score below 7 and 1779 (96.2%) above or equal to 7 at fifth minute. 906 (48.4%) were female. Demographic data of study population is presented in Table 1.

Initiation of labor was spontaneous in 1282 (79.8%) patients and medically induced in 325 (20.2%).

Epidural analgesia was initiated early in labor with cervix dilation inferior to 4 cm in 239 (13.3%) women. Ropi+S were the analgesic option in 953 (49.1%) women, Ropi 0.2 in 587 (30.3%). Four hundred (20.6%) parturients received other treatments.

Delivery was eutocic in 1080 (58.4%) cases, dystocic in 568 (30.7%) from which 294 (26,7%) were vaginal instrumented and 274 (14.8%)

ended in cesarean section. Among the parturients, 152 (8.6%) had a previous cesarean.

	Media	APGAR<7	APGAR>7	P
Maternal age	30.06 ± 6.333	29.63 ± 7.539	30.06 ± 6.293	>0.05
BMI	29.2180 ± 4.44777	28.8294±4.301883	29.2058±4.42733	>0.05
Para	0.65 ± 1.265	0.57 ± 1.258	0.65 ± 1.260	>0.05
Idade gestacional	38.371 ± 2.4893	38.460 ± 2.1984	38.369 ± 2.4923	>0.05
Cervix dilation	4.63 ± 1.245	4.63 ± 1.112	4.63 ± 1.248	>0.05
Newborn weight	3166.67 ± 487.203	3111.96 ± 552.966	3173.31 ± 473.600	>0.05
APGAR - 5° minute	9.326 ± 1.4534			

Table 1: Demographic data.

The median hour of birth was 13h46m00s and the median labor length since beginning of epidural analgesia was 3h09m00s.

None of the variables identified as maternal age, BMI, previous labor, gestational age, cervix dilation and newborn weight have proved to be different between groups of Apgar below and above 7 (t-test p>0.05).

There was also no significant difference between newborns with Apgar above or below 7 in what concerned initiation of labor, mode of epidural analgesia, previous cesarean, type of delivery and newborn sex (Chi-squared p>0.05).

Median hour of birth and median labor length since beginning of epidural analgesia were not different between the two groups of outcome (Kruskall wallis p>0.05).

The multivariable model showed that the risk for low Apgar was not independently associated with any of the variables analyzed (Chi-squared Omnibus p>0.05) (Table 2).

Discussion

Identifying independent and modifiable predictors of low Apgar is warranted to improve medical care. With this observational study, we were not able to identify any factor independently associated with newborn Apgar score below 7.

In a recent study, low Apgar score at fifth minute has been shown to be strongly associated with the risk of neonatal and infant death [32], remaining an important indicator of neonatal well-being.

In our study the global prevalence of Apgar score below 7 at fifth minute postpartum of 3.8% was substantially higher than described in other European developed countries [29]. For this high value may have contributed the high heterogeneity of our sample. We did not exclude high-risk pregnancies, such as babies from diabetic mother, advanced maternal age and previous cesarean delivery, nor have we excluded premature neonates or with severe malformations, or babies born from emergent cesarean sections. Most studies do exclude these

confounding variables and some only included nulliparous mother to achieve a more homogenous low-risk sample.

Variables		Co-efficient (β-values)	Standard Error (SE)	P-value	Odds Ratio (OR)	95% CI of odds ratios	
						Lower limit	Upper limit
IMC		0.008	0.042	0.850	1,008	0.928	1.095
Parity		-0.108	0.178	0.544	0.897	0.633	1.272
Gestational Age		0.009	0.073	0.905	1.009	0.874	1.165
Baby's weight		0.000	0.000	0.578	1.000	0.999	1.001
Baby's Gender	Female	0.092	0.351	0.792	1.097	0.551	2.183
	Male (RC)						
Beginning of Labor	Spontaneous	-0.817	0.548	0.136	0.442	0.151	1.294
	Induced (RC)						
Cervix dilation		0.231	0.557	0.679	1.260	0.422	3.756
Type of Labor	Eutocic	0.455	0.464	0.327	1.576	0.635	3.914
	Cesarean	-0.020	0.422	0.963	0.980	0.429	2.242
	Dystocic (RC)						
Type of epidural analgesia	PCEA	0.364	0.522	0.485	1.439	0.517	4.005
	Ropi 0.2	0.164	0.564	0.771	1.179	0.390	3.563
	Others (RC)						
Time of Labor		0.000	0.000	0.319	1.000	1.000	1.000
Duration of Anesthesia		0.000	0.000	0.521	1.000	1.000	1.000

Table 2: Results of logistic regression of risk factors for APGAR<7. *P<0.05; RC: Reference Category.

Advanced maternal age has been associated with poor neonatal outcomes [33], including low Apgar score. However, this has not been confirmed in other studies [5]. In our study, no relation was evident between maternal age and low Apgar score. This opposite result may have turned from the fact that the impact of this variable is significantly influenced by socioeconomic factors, namely level of education. It has been shown that a high level of education for women over 41 years-old mitigates the higher risk that these mother would present when compared to younger individuals, showing that the risk increment is probably multifactorial [33].

Obesity is one of the most concerning public health issues, and maternal overweight has been associated with adverse perinatal events and, neonatal death. In our study, we did not find a significant association between maternal obesity and low Apgar score. Nonetheless, most studies document an increased risk of low Apgar score in babies born from these parturients [34,35]. The precise mechanisms by which obesity negatively influences newborn outcome are not completely understood. As we have a high percentage of overweighed mothers in our sample, we would expect a significant result as described in literature. This showed that probably other important non-controlled factors might have dissuaded the impact of maternal obesity in outcome.

The association of multiparty and poor neonatal outcome has not been consistent for decades. In some studies, the odds of a low Apgar score were higher for women with no previous live births compared to those without previous live births [2,28], but others did not share similar results. According to the literature, having more than 6 childbirths is associated with an increased prevalence of maternal and neonatal complications such as malpresentation, meconium-stained liquor, placenta previa and a low Apgar score, comparing with other multiparous women [36]. In our sample 1066 (58.5%) of women are nulliparous. We were not able to show any effect of parity on Apgar score and further studies seem necessary to better clarify this subject.

Nowadays, it is consensual that women who have had a previous cesarean section can safely go through a vaginal labor, as it is assumed that the risk for the mother and newborn are low [37]. Furthermore, there is no difference in neonatal outcome among those delivered by trial of scar (VBACS) compared to those who underwent emergency CS due to failed trial of scar. Despite this agreement, the risks are still higher than those associated with repeated elective cesareans [38]. In fact, babies born from women with one previous cesarean seem to be at increased risk of low Apgar score and perinatal death, when compared with neonates from mothers with history of one previous vaginal delivery [39]. In our study, history of previous cesarean was not an independent risk factor for low Apgar score. Further studies are needed for professionals to provide their patients with better counseling regarding the choice of the most appropriate route of delivery.

As it was previously stated, the Apgar score suffers the influence of many factors, one of the most important being the gestational age [30]. In our study, this variable was not a predictor of Apgar score inferior to 7 at fifth minute. This might reflect the high efficacy of the current neonatal resuscitation maneuvers immediately instituted after birth, and the generalized availability of invasive mechanical support in our hospital.

The Apgar score has been traditionally inversely related to neonate birth weight [40]. Nowadays, with the increase of maternal metabolic risk factors and neonatal overweight, it has been shown that the heaviest infants are also at risk for low apgar score, that can be six-fold higher than for infants with normal birth weight. Furthermore, this has been proved even after exclusion of mothers with pre-existing and gestational diabetes mellitus [28]. Also, newborn sex has been investigated as a risk factor for low Apgar score. In one study, girls had a reduced risk for low 5-minute Apgar score than boys, and the difference remained significant even after stratification for birth weight [28]. The predisposition for preterm delivery in male gestations has been implied it the low Apgar score that neonatal boys present. However, this phenomenon has been shown even when preterm boys are compared with preterm girls [41]. In our study neither birth weight nor newborn gender was associated with low Apgar score. In what concerns the sex issue in particular, the relevance of this matter may be more of the statistical and academic field than of the clinical setting interest.

Controversy has been following the indication for elective induction of labor before 41 weeks of gestation. It was previously stated that elective induction of labor at 37 weeks of pregnancy, without medical indication was associated with increased cesarean rates [42]. In fact, a recent systematic review concludes that only induction of labor at 41 weeks of gestation and beyond is associated with low risk of cesareans. In that review, thirteen studies contributed to show no difference if Apgar score at fifth minute between elective induction of labor and expectant management [43]. However, in another study, induction of labor at 37 to 40 weeks of gestation was associated with low incidence of cesarean section. The authors further demonstrated that this practice was not related with increased perinatal mortality or neonatal admission to intensive care unit, when compared with expectant management [44]. In our center, induction of labor is currently performed after 41 weeks of gestation, being anticipated only if there is a valid medical indication. In the present study, we found no difference in Apgar scores between inducted and spontaneous labors.

In this study we also investigated whether the hour of birth was associated with differences in Apgar scores. It has been reported an increased risk of being born with a low Apgar score during "non-office hours" and during the periods of general holiday [28]. Also, a Welsh study found that infant death was higher for babies delivered at night and during July and August [45]. Although we have not found any difference in neonatal Apgar score at any hour of the day, these results should alert the medical community to the importance and significance of maintaining an elevated and irreprehensible high standard of care, especially in such a sensitive field of clinical practice.

Impact of labor analgesia techniques on neonatal apgar score

A painful labor induces adverse maternal effects and increases fetal stress. For the mother, there will be an increase of circulating catecholamines, hyperventilation during contractions and hypoventilation during rest. Those mechanisms can induce deterioration in pH and base excess both in babies and mother, which can easily be attenuated by adequate analgesia [29].

Neuraxial analgesia is the actual gold standard for maternal pain relief during labor. However, controversy still follows the exact moment in labor when it should be performed, and its influence of maternal and neonatal outcomes.

Meta-analysis of the literature determined that the timing of neuraxial analgesia does not affect Apgar scores at first and fifth minutes [26]. Nonetheless, the definition of early epidural varies among studies, being typically defined as initiation of epidural analgesia when cervix dilation is inferior to 4 to 5 cm. According to the American Society of Anesthesiologists' guidelines for obstetric anesthesia; the insertion of a spinal or epidural catheter may precede the onset of labor or a patient's request for labor analgesia [46]. In our study, we considered an early epidural as that performed with cervix dilation inferior to 4 cm. As according to the literature, we found no influence on Apgar scores at fifth minute.

In the past few years, many studies have searched for evidence of the best epidural analgesic regimens for labor. Meta-analysis of the literature concluded that low concentrations of local anesthetics with opioids presents as one of the best options for labor analgesia, improving its quality and duration. It also allows for sparing of higher local anesthetics concentration, reducing adverse effects, such as motor block. Furthermore, the use of opioids in neuraxial infusions until the moment of birth does not increase fetal or neonatal side effects [46]. In our study, no difference was found between epidural infusion of high concentration of local anesthetics and lower concentrations with opioids.

Limitations

As a retrospective study there are inherent limitations in data collection that cannot be controlled. The ideal study design to better investigate predictive factors of low Apgar score in what concerns the impact of epidural analgesia would be a randomized controlled trial. However, these are very difficult, if not unethical, to perform, as epidural is a gold standard for labor analgesia nowadays. For most of the factors that can possibly affect neonatal Apgar score, such as maternal and biological factors, no randomization is ever possible.

We chose to work on a more comprehensive and heterogeneous sample, so we did not exclude from out study preterm infants, high-risk pregnancies or multiparous mothers. With this approach, we intended to have more generalizable results; however we cannot avoid a bias effect induced by this miscellaneous sample.

Also, the size or our sample, although high in absolute and reflecting only one year of clinical practice in our institution, may not be sufficient to adequately investigate such a rare event, as an Apgar score inferior to 7 at fifth minute. We chose not to include data from previous years, as obstetric and anesthetic practice has been changing, and misleading conclusion could arise from such analysis.

The impact of the socioeconomic factors may be of great importance on this issue and the study was not controlled for these variables.

Furthermore, maternal satisfaction is an important endpoint of quality and it is assessed in our institution in a subjective way. As we do not routinely use international validated instruments for this assessment, we did not use these data in our study. In a near future, we intend to establish an objective method of evaluation of this important outcome.

Conclusions

In our study we did not find any maternal, newborn, obstetric and anesthetic-related predictive factors for low neonate Apgar score at fifth minute postpartum. In particular, modality and timing of epidural analgesia was not a predictor of worse neonatal outcome.

Importantly, we were able to demonstrate the non-inferiority on neonatal Apgar score of epidural analgesia with infusion of low concentration local anesthetics with opioids until the moment of delivery, when compared to an opioid-free approach.

Controversy still surrounds which factors may be implicated in a worse fetal outcome, as assessed by Apgar score, as important methodological barriers hinder flawless investigations. Baring this challenges in mind, future studies are required to achieve conclusions to support changes in clinical practice towards improved neonatal well-being.

References

1. APGAR V (1953) A proposal for a new method of evaluation of the newborn infant. Curr Res Anesth Analg 32: 260-267.

2. Casey BM, McIntire DD, Leveno KJ (2001) The continuing value of the Apgar score for the assessment of newborn infants. N Engl J Med 344: 467-471.

3. Rubarth L (2012) The apgar score: simple yet complex. Neonatal Netw 31: 169-177.

4. Odd DE, Doyle P, Gunnell D, Lewis G, Whitelaw A, et al. (2008) Risk of low Apgar score and socioeconomic position: a study of Swedish male births. Acta Paediatr 97: 1275-1280.

5. Salustiano EM, Campos JA, Ibidi SM, Ruano R, Zugaib M (2012) Low Apgar scores at 5 minutes in a low risk population: maternal and obstetrical factors and postnatal outcome. Rev Assoc Med Bras 58: 587-593.

6. Stuart A, Otterblad Olausson P, Källen K (2011) Apgar scores at 5 minutes after birth in relation to school performance at 16 years of age. Obstet Gynecol 118: 201-208.

7. Haines CJ, Rogers MS, Leung DH (1991) Neonatal outcome and its relationship with maternal age. Aust N Z J Obstet Gynaecol 31: 209-212.

8. Kilsztajn S, de Souza Lopes E, Nunes do Carmo MS, de Andrade Reyes AM (2007) [Apgar score associated with mode of delivery in São Paulo State, Brazil]. Cad Saude Publica 23: 1886-1892.

9. Mongelli M, Rogers MS, Brieger GM (1997) Obstetric determinants of low Apgar scores in a Chinese population. Int J Gynaecol Obstet 57: 67-68.

10. Andrejevic A, Cvetkovic S, Vitosevic Z, Andrejevic L, Relic G (2011) Multiparity, perinatal morbidity and mortality. Clin Exp Obstet Gynecol 38: 71-75.

11. Hingson R, Gould JB, Morelock S, Kayne H, Heeren T, et al. (1982) Maternal cigarette smoking, psychoactive substance use, and infant Apgar scores. Am J Obstet Gynecol 144: 959-966.

12. Garn SM, Johnston M, Ridella SA, Petzold AS (1981) Effect of maternal cigarette smoking on Apgar scores. Am J Dis Child 135: 503-506.

13. Hübner F, Schonlau H, Stumpf C (1988) [Effect of risk factors on premature labor and neonatal condition following delivery]. Z Geburtshilfe Perinatol 192: 91-95.

14. Aviram A, Raban O, Melamed N, Hadar E, Wiznitzer A, et al. (2013) The association between young maternal age and pregnancy outcome. J Matern Fetal Neonatal Med 26: 1554-1558.

15. Lamminpää R, Vehviläinen-Julkunen K, Gissler M, Heinonen S (2012) Preeclampsia complicated by advanced maternal age: a registry-based study on primiparous women in Finland 1997-2008. BMC Pregnancy Childbirth 12: 47.

16. Minsart AF, Buekens P, De Spiegelaere M, Englert Y (2013) Neonatal outcomes in obese mothers: a population-based analysis. BMC Pregnancy Childbirth 13: 36.

17. Sekhavat L, Fallah R (2013) Could maternal pre-pregnancy body mass index affect Apgar score? Arch Gynecol Obstet 287: 15-18.

18. Gilead R, Yaniv Salem S, Sergienko R, Sheiner E (2012) Maternal "isolated" obesity and obstetric complications. J Matern Fetal Neonatal Med 25: 2579-2582.

19. Chen M, McNiff C, Madan J, Goodman E, Davis JM, et al. (2010) Maternal obesity and neonatal Apgar scores. J Matern Fetal Neonatal Med 23: 89-95.

20. De Zorzi Pde M, Madi JM, Rombaldi RL, de Araújo BF, Zatti H, et al. (2012) [Perinatal factors associated with pH<7.1 in umbilical artery and Apgar 5 min <7.0 in term newborn]. Rev Bras Ginecol Obstet 34: 381-385.

21. Catlin EA, Carpenter MW, Brann BS 4th, Mayfield SR, Shaul PW, et al. (1986) The Apgar score revisited: influence of gestational age. J Pediatr 109: 865-868.

22. Rogers JF, Graves WL (1993) Risk factors associated with low Apgar scores in a low-income population. Paediatr Perinat Epidemiol 7: 205-216.

23. Erdemoglu E, Mungan T, Tapisiz OL, Ustunyurt E, Caglar E (2003) Effect of inter-twin delivery time on Apgar scores of the second twin. Aust N Z J Obstet Gynaecol 43: 203-206.

24. Scherer R, Holzgreve W (1995) Influence of epidural analgesia on fetal and neonatal well-being. Eur J Obstet Gynecol Reprod Biol 59 Suppl: S17-29.

Is Epidural Analgesia a Predictor of Low Newborn Apgar? A Hospital-Based Observational Study

25

25. Anim-Somuah M, Smyth RM, Jones L (2011) Epidural versus non-epidural or no analgesia in labour. Cochrane Database Syst Rev 12: CD000331.

26. Sng BL, Leong WL, Zeng Y, Siddiqui FJ, Assam PN, et al. (2014) Early versus late initiation of epidural analgesia for labour. Cochrane Database Syst Rev 10: CD007238.

27. Ohel G, Gonen R, Vaida S, Barak S, Gaitini L (2006) Early versus late initiation of epidural analgesia in labor: does it increase the risk of cesarean section? A randomized trial. Am J Obstet Gynecol 194: 600-605.

28. Thorngren-Jerneck K, Herbst A (2001) Low 5-minute Apgar score: a population-based register study of 1 million term births. Obstet Gynecol 98: 65-70.

29. Törnell S, Ekéus C, Hultin M, Håkansson S, Thunberg J, et al. (2015) Low Apgar score, neonatal encephalopathy and epidural analgesia during labour: a Swedish registry-based study. Acta Anaesthesiol Scand 59: 486-495.

30. American Academy of Pediatrics, Committee on Fetus and Newborn; American College of Obstetricians and Gynecologists and Committee on Obstetric Practice (2006) The Apgar score. Pediatrics 117: 1444-1447.

31. Bharti B, Bharti S (2005) A review of the Apgar score indicated that contextualization was required within the contemporary perinatal and neonatal care framework in different settings. J Clin Epidemiol 58: 121-129.

32. Iliodromiti S, Mackay DF, Smith GC, Pell JP, Nelson SM (2014) Apgar score and the risk of cause-specific infant mortality: a population-based cohort study. Lancet 384: 1749-1755.

33. Almeida NK, Almeida RM, Pedreira CE (2015) Adverse perinatal outcomes for advanced maternal age: a cross-sectional study of Brazilian births. J Pediatr (Rio J) pii: S0021-7557(15)00067-4.

34. Papile LA (2001) The Apgar score in the 21st century. N Engl J Med 344: 519-520.

35. Suka M, Sugimori H, Nakamura M, Haginiwa K, Yoshida K (2002) Risk factors of low APGAR score in Japanese full-term deliveries: a case-control study. J Epidemiol 12: 320-323.

36. Mgaya AH, Massawe SN, Kidanto HL, Mgaya HN (2013) Grand multiparity: is it still a risk in pregnancy? BMC Pregnancy Childbirth 13: 241.

37. García-Benítez CQ, López-Rioja Mde J, Monzalbo-Núñez DE (2015) [Vaginal birth after cesarean. A safe option?]. Ginecol Obstet Mex 83: 69-87.

38. Sentilhes L, Vayssière C, Beucher G, Deneux-Tharaux C, Deruelle P, et al. (2013) Delivery for women with a previous cesarean: guidelines for clinical practice from the French College of Gynecologists and Obstetricians (CNGOF). Eur J Obstet Gynecol Reprod Biol 170: 25-32.

39. Carlsson Wallin M, Ekström P, Marsál K, Källén K (2010) Apgar score and perinatal death after one previous caesarean delivery. BJOG 117: 1088-1097.

40. Hegyi T, Carbone T, Anwar M, Ostfeld B, Hiatt M, et al. (1998) The apgar score and its components in the preterm infant. Pediatrics 101: 77-81.

41. Nagy E, Orvos H, Bakki J, Pal A (2009) Sex-differences in Apgar scores for full-term neonates. Acta Paediatr 98: 898-900.

42. Stock SJ, Ferguson E, Duffy A, Ford I, Chalmers J, et al. (2012) Outcomes of elective induction of labour compared with expectant management: population based study. BMJ 344: e2838.

43. Caughey AB, Sundaram V, Kaimal AJ, Gienger A, Cheng YW, et al. (2009) Systematic review: elective induction of labor versus expectant management of pregnancy. Ann Intern Med 151: 252-263, W53-63.

44. Darney BG, Snowden JM, Cheng YW, Jacob L, Nicholson JM, et al. (2013) Elective induction of labor at term compared with expectant management: maternal and neonatal outcomes. Obstet Gynecol 122: 761-769.

45. Stewart JH, Andrews J, Cartlidge PH (1998) Numbers of deaths related to intrapartum asphyxia and timing of birth in all Wales perinatal survey, 1993-5. BMJ 316: 657-660.

46. American Society of Anesthesiologists Task Force on Obstetric Anesthesia (2007) Practice guidelines for obstetric anesthesia: an updated report by the American Society of Anesthesiologists Task Force on Obstetric Anesthesia. Anesthesiology 106: 843-863.

6

O₂ and N₂O: Between the Rock and the Hard Place

Humberto S Machado*

Serviço de Anestesiologia, Centro Hospitalar do Porto, Portugal

***Corresponding author:** Humberto S Machado, Serviço de Anestesiologia, Centro Hospitalar do Porto, Portugal, E-mail: hjs.machado@gmail.com

Abstract

The use of oxygen and nitrous oxide is part of anesthetic practice since ever. These gases follow anesthetic practice in almost all types of clinical settings, procedures and patients. Their indications and limitations of use are well known.

In recent years a great debate either in literature or in scientific meetings has been addressed, concerning the potential poor outcomes related to the use of certain amounts of oxygen and the use of nitrous oxide.

The objective of this review is to gather information related to these two topics, based on the recent most relevant publications (2000-2016).

Results show that both drugs have its advantages and drawbacks, and it is the clinical objective, the procedure, and the type of patient that will contribute the most for the anesthesiologist final decision.

As a conclusion it was found that, 1) oxygen is a lifesaving drug on one side, but its use should be judicious since its high inspired fraction may have direct implications on that lung wellbeing, and 2) nitrous oxide has its known contraindications that should be taken into consideration and preclude its use when not clinically appropriate, however no evidence exists that indicates a formal discontinuation of its use, and in certain clinical scenarios it can be of relevant utility.

Keywords: Oxygen toxicity; Nitrous oxide indications; Contraindications

Introduction

The practice of anaesthesia has been evolving astonishingly fast in the last decades. From the great monitoring progresses to the new ultra short-acting drugs currently available, most have happened in recent years. In addition, the global awareness on what anaesthesia is and could provide to patients makes our specialty particularly exposed and vulnerable to the public opinion. It is not uncommon that our patients and their families, nowadays specially informed, continually evaluate anesthetic practice.

Evidence is being gathered by publications worldwide, in that anaesthesia is no longer innocuous. This idea is growing in several areas, namely about the indication and safety to anesthetize pediatric patients [1], the use of intravenous infusions of opioids that might be related to the development of hyperalgesia [2], the advantages and drawbacks of the amount of oxygen to use [3] or even the current indication for the use of nitrous oxide [4].

Patient satisfaction with overall healthcare provision in a certain clinical scenario relies very often on non-clinical issues, like nontangible factors of the medical profession and the maintenance of almost like-home routine and comfort. These current needs and expectations are some of the great challenges of the modern medical practice.

Anesthesia as a specialty that is focused on patient safety and satisfaction has improved in several areas that meet these needs, namely the control of postoperative acute pain (POAP), the perioperative management of the occurrence of postoperative nausea and vomiting (PONV), the prevention of intraoperative awareness and many others.

The adoption of certain work methodologies and the avoidance of some special practices that directly or indirectly may compromise a good result, have been growing among anaesthesiologists. The choice of the correct inspired fraction of oxygen during anesthesia, or the use of nitrous oxide as part of the anesthetic technic have been subject of huge debates either in the published literature and the scientific meetings worldwide. This editorial commentary will address a summary of the main arguments on these two topics.

Oxygen

The use of oxygen during anesthesia is ubiquitous; everyone uses it with various inspired fractions (FiO_2). Its use starts before anesthesia, as to pre-oxygenate the patient in order to have some reserve for the apnea period of laryngoscopy and intubation [3]. The first choice starts at this moment, what FiO_2 should one use? One hundred percent is a very attractive choice since, a very good reserve will allow some time for laryngoscopy and intubation, and we all know this is a quite thrilled moment [5], nevertheless there is a price for this relief. Atelectasis are prone to develop with the choice of pre-oxygenation with 100% FiO_2 [3], and this is a major issue, that needs a special intervention, namely the use of positive end expiratory pressure

(PEEP) to maintain the lungs open [3], since even recent investigation have shown that if this is not instituted to the patient, the lung will certainly be poorly aerated [6].

During anesthesia, another conflict decision arises. Should a high FiO_2 be used and promote a decreased probability of surgical site infection [7]. Or, in case of a documented high pulmonary vascular resistance, should a high FiO_2 be used to try and mitigate this situation [8]. These problems may be overcome by high-inspired fractions of oxygen, but this again has a price. Animal studies have shown that oxygen itself, as a supplement in spontaneous ventilation, induced higher lung inflammatory infiltrates when compared to room air ventilation [9]. Furthermore, the connection between high-inspired fractions of oxygen and the development of oxidative stress and the occurrence of an inflammatory lung lesion, formerly designated as acute lung injury, has been extensively documented [10,11].

At the end of procedure, before emergence from anesthesia, another critical period is imminent. On this regard, anesthesiologists frequently use high-inspired fractions of oxygen again to assure some reserve for the immediate post-extubation period. This decision is often critical, since this promotes again the occurrence of reabsorption atelectasis [3], which is a major cause of shunt that will accompany the patient to post-anesthetic care unit and the ward. Physiology principles teach us that the natural supporter of open alveoli is the atmospheric nitrogen, since at sea level it is not absorbed to blood stream; the removal of this supporter by high inspired fractions of oxygen will certainly induce alveolar collapse and the formation of atelectasis areas.

Perhaps, the most prudent and advisable practice, when oxygen is to be used, will be to think of it as a lifesaving drug with its undeniable advantages and uses, and at the same time a gas that has to be handle with special care. The thought that hypoxia may be managed by several means (PEEP, recruitment maneuvers) before the decision of a high-inspired fractions of oxygen should be always in our minds. Table 1 summarizes oxygen uses, side effects and complications.

Positive Actions	Reference	Negative actions	Reference
Pre-oxygenation to prevent hypoxia during laryngoscopy	[3]	Formation of atelectasis & shunt	[3]
Post-oxygenation to reduce emergence hypoxia	[3]	Alveolar collapse & shunt	[3]
May decrease surgical wound infection	[7]	Risk of Acute Lung Injury	[10]
Decrease pulmonary vascular resistance	[8]	Higher lung inflammation in spontaneous ventilation	[9]
Use oxygen judiciously, if possible find other means to improve oxygenation before increasing FiO2, remember the advantages of PEEP and recruiting maneuvers [3].			
FiO2-Oxygen inspired fraction; PEEP – Positive end-expiratory pressure			

Table 1: Oxygen actions.

Nitrous Oxide

Nitrous oxide (N_2O) accompanies anesthesiologists for several centuries now. It is a more soluble gas than nitrogen, in large concentrations is associated to a second gas effect, diffusion hypoxia and expansion of air-filled spaces in the body [12]. Its role has evolved greatly, since a sole anesthetic to a volatile anesthetic vehicle, and it has its place in common practice. A kind of smoothness has been linked to N_2O action when used with volatiles for mask induction; a unique technic used by anesthesiologists for patients with such a need, like children or especially needle scared adults. These characteristics make of N_2O a key tool, which goes in favour of the patient satisfaction.

Nitrous oxide has several pharmacodynamic effects that include: increases respiratory rate, reduces the ventilatory response to hypoxia and hypercapnia, reduces mucociliary function and neutrophil chemotaxis, impels some myocardial depression (despite increasing sympathetic out flow), increases pulmonary vascular resistance, increases cerebral blood flow, cerebral metabolism and intracranial pressure [12]. It has analgesic effect thought to be mediated by activation of opioid receptors in the periaqueductal grey matter of the midbrain, which leads to modulation of nociception pathways and activation of α2 adrenoreceptors in the dorsal horn of the spinal cord [12].

Recent years' evidence has questioned the use of N_2O on several potential or actual negative actions, namely: Inhibition of methionine synthetase (inactivation B12 vitamin) [13], increase closed spaces volume and pressure [14], reduce protein synthesis promoting surgical site infection [15,16], increase vascular risk in perioperative period [17], increase in PONV [16], and a contribution to degradation of ozone layer as a greenhouse effect gas [18].

Believing that the previous experiences with the use of N_2O were not so devastating, the scientific community was impelled to investigate and try and sort out the true impact of N_2O.

Several studies have been published centering the issue in a quite moderate approach; with a prudent stand, addressing that may be, it is still not the time for the N_2O retirement.

Some studies found that the surgical infection rate was somehow similar with and without N2O use [13,19]. Sanders et al found that the occurrence of cardiovascular events did not increase with N2O [20], results aligned with other authors' studies [17,19]. The PONV linked with N_2O were investigated and it was found that there may be a time relation (longer expositions lead to higher incidence of PONV) [21].

A critical global problem is the sustainability of the planet. It is known that N_2O is several times more dangerous for the ozone layer than for example carbon dioxide. Nevertheless, the contribution of N_2O medical use is almost negligible when compared to the major contributors (industry, agriculture and motor cars) that clearly should be regulated [22].

Concern has been raised if the use of N_2O might have any advantages over its non-use. Several studies have shown some usefulness on the prevention of a potential hyperalgesia related to perfusion of some opioids [2], and the decreased occurrence of postoperative chronic pain [23]. Moreover, the use of N_2O has been established has a good practice [24], namely for promoting faster recoveries in the ambulatory surgery scenario [24].

Apart from all these results, care has been taken on the utilization of N_2O and key opinion leaders from scientific societies have sorted out very prudent and reasonable guidelines for its use, which simple state that it has its place and indication. In addition, no evidence exists that recommends, without any doubt, its discontinuation and, most importantly, health professionals are not at risk when N_2O is used in modern, state of the art operating rooms with adequate scavenging systems [4,24]. Table 2 summarizes the uses of N_2O in clinical practice, its side effects and complications.

Positive actions	Reference	Reported Negative actions	References	Unproven Negative actions	Reference
Decreases hyperalgesia of opioids	[2,23]	Inhibition of methionine synthetase	[13]		
Decreases chronic postsurgical pain	[23]	Increase bowel volume and pressure in closed spaces	[14]		
Good vehicle of volatiles (less dose)	[24]	Reduce protein synthesis promoting surgical site infection	[15,16]	Similar infection rate	[13,19]
		Increased vascular risk in perioperative period	[17]	No increase in cardiovascular effects	[20,19]
		Increase PONV	[16]	Small increase (resolved with one anti-emetic) Depends on duration	[21]
		Greenhouse effect	[17]	Anesthetic use is not a problem compared to agriculture & industry	[22]
Not enough evidence to support Nitrous Oxide exclusion from clinical practice. No effect no health professionals [4,25]					
PONV-Post-operative nausea and vomiting					

Table 2: Nitrous oxide actions.

Conclusion

Regarding the use of oxygen, care should be taken on the decision about what level of inspired fraction should be used. From one side oxygen is needed in order to assure patient safety in key critical moments, but very high oxygen inspired fractions might induce some type of lung lesion.

N_2O has its known contraindications and should not be used in such clinical settings; nevertheless, evidence is lacking that supports its complete discontinuation since in selected patients and /or procedures it might be of great help.

References

1. Saraiva A, Duarte S, Machado HS (2015) Anesthetic Neurotoxicity to the Fragile Young Brain: Where Do We Stand? J Pregnancy Child Heal 2: 2-5.
2. Echevarria G, Elgueta F, Fierro C, Bugedo D, Faba G, et al. (2011) N2O reduces postoperative opioid-induced hyperalgesia after remifentanil-propofol anaesthesia in humans. Br J Anaesth 107: 959-965.
3. Hedenstierna G (2014) Effects of anaesthesia on ventilation/perfusion matching. Eur J Anaesthesiol 31: 447–449.
4. Buhre W, Cerny V, De Hert S, Disma N, Habre W, et al. (2015) The current place of nitrous oxide in clinical practice. Eur J Anaesthesiol 32: 1-4.
5. Doleman B, Blackwell J, Karangizi A, Butt W, Bhalla A, et al. (2016) Anaesthetists stress is induced by patient ASA grade and may impair non-technical skills during intubation. Acta Anaesthesiol Scand.
6. Borges JB, Porra L, Pellegrini M, Tannoia A, Derosa S, et al. (2016) Zero expiratory pressure and low oxygen concentration promote heterogeneity of regional ventilation and lung densities. Acta Anaesthesiol Scand.
7. Hovaguimian F, Lysakowski C, Elia N, Tramer MR (2013) Effect of intraoperative high inspired oxygen fraction on surgical site infection, postoperative nausea and vomiting, and pulmonary function: systematic review and meta-analysis of randomized controlled trials. Anesthesiology 119: 303–316.
8. Roberts D, Lepore JJ, Maroo A, Semigran M, Ginns L (2001) Oxygen therapy improves cardiac index and pulmonary vascular resistance in patients with pulmonary hypertension. Chest 120: 1547-1555.
9. Machado HS, Nunes CS, Sá P, Couceiro A, Da Silva ÁM, et al. (2014) Increased lung inflammation with oxygen supplementation in tracheotomized spontaneously breathing rabbits: an experimental prospective randomized study. BMC Anesthesiol 14: 86.
10. Guarracino F (2012) Anesthesia & Clinical Perioperative Acute Lung Injury: Reviewing the Role of Anesthetic Management. J Anesth Clin Res 4.
11. Licker M, Fauconnet P, Villiger Y, Tschopp JM (2009) Acute lung injury and outcomes after thoracic surgery. Curr Opin Anaesthesiol 22: 61-67.
12. Banks A, Hardman JG (2005) Nitrous oxide. Contin Educ Anaesthesia, Crit Care Pain 5:145-148.
13. Fleischmann E, Lenhardt R, Kurz A, Herbst F, Fülesdi B, et al. (2005) Nitrous oxide and risk of surgical wound infection: a randomised trial. Lancet 36: 1101-1107.
14. Akça O, Lenhardt R, Fleischmann E, Treschan T, Greif R, et al. (2004) Nitrous oxide increases the incidence of bowel distension in patients undergoing elective colon resection. Acta Anaesthesiol Scand 48: 894-898.
15. Chen Y, Liu X, Cheng CHK, Gin T, Leslie K, et al. (2013) Leukocyte DNA damage and wound infection after nitrous oxide administration: a randomized controlled trial. Anesthesiology 118: 1322–1331.
16. Myles PS, Leslie K, Chan MT, Forbes A, Paech MJ, et al. (2007) Avoidance of nitrous oxide for patients undergoing major surgery. Anesthesiology 107: 221–231.
17. Leslie K, Myles PS, Chan MT V, Forbes A, Paech MJ, et al. (2011) Nitrous oxide and long-term morbidity and mortality in the ENIGMA trial. Anesth Analg 112: 387-393.
18. Søvik A, Augustin J, Heikkinen K, Huttunen J, Necki J, et al. (2006) Emission of the greenhouse gases nitrous oxide and methane from constructed wetlands in europe. J Env Qual 35: 2360-2373.

19. Myles PS, Leslie K, Chan MT V, Forbes A, Peyton PJ, et al. (2014) The safety of addition of nitrous oxide to general anaesthesia in at-risk patients having major non-cardiac surgery (ENIGMA-II): a randomised, single-blind trial. Lancet 384: 1446–1454.

20. Sanders R, Graham C, Lewis S, Bodenham A, Gough M, et al. (2012) Nitrous oxide exposure does not seem to be associated with increased mortality, stroke, and myocardial infarction: a non-randomized subgroup analysis of the General Anaesthesia compared with Local Anaesthesia for carotid surgery (GALA) trial. Br J Anaesth 109: 361-367.

21. Peyton P, Wu C (2014) Nitrous oxide-related postoperative nausea and vomiting depends on duration of exposure. Anesthesiology 120: 1137-1145.

22. Inventory of US Greenhouse gas emissions (2013) N2O greenhouse effect.

23. Chan M, Wan A, Gin T, Leslie K, Myles P (2011) Chronic postsurgical pain after nitrous oxide anesthesia. Pain 152: 2514-2520.

24. Smith I (2006) Nitrous oxide in ambulatory anaesthesia: does it have a place in day surgical anaesthesia or is it just a threat for personnel and the global environment? Curr Opin Anaesthesiol 19: 592-596.

25. Turan A, Mascha EJ, You J, Kurz A, Shiba A, et al. (2013) The association between nitrous oxide and postoperative mortality and morbidity after noncardiac surgery. Anesth Analg 116: 1026-1033.

7

Obesity Surgery Mortality Risk Score: Can we Go Beyond Mortality Prediction?

Sílvia Pinho, Marta Carvalho, Maria Soares, Daniela Pinho, Carla Cavaleiro and Humberto S Machado*

Department of Anaesthesiology, Intensive Care and Emergency, Centro Hospitalar do Porto, Portugal

Corresponding author: Humberto S Machado, Department of Anesthesiology, Centro Hospitalar do Porto, 4099-001, Portugal, E-mail: hjs.machado@gmail.com

Abstract

Introduction: High morbidity and low mortality has been linked to bariatric surgery. The Obesity surgery mortality risk score (OS-MRS) is a validated scale for mortality risk assessment. The aim of this study was to evaluate if OS-MRS scale can also be used as a predictor of postoperative complications in obese patients submitted to primary laparoscopic gastric bypass.

Methods: Retrospective study including all patients submitted to primary laparoscopic gastric bypass between January and December 2014. The OS-MRS scale was applied preoperatively, and postoperative to access morbidity and mortality at 30 and 90 days. Complications were classified according to Clavien-Dindo's grades (I to V). The association between different OSMRS classes and the occurrence of adverse events was analyzed.

Results: 85 patients were included and classified as class A (n=33; 38.8%), class B (n=48; 56.5%) and class C (n=4; 4.7%). No mortality cases were registered. The morbidity rate at 30 days was 23.5% (n=20), and 25.9% at 90 days (n=22). The complications rate in each of OS-MRS subgroups, was 9.1% in class A (both at 30 and 90 days), 31.3% and 35.4% in class B (at 30 and 90 days respectively), and 50% in class C (both at 30 and 90 days). There was a statistically significant independent relationship between OS-MRS scale, ASA physical status and the risk of developing pulmonary embolism, both at 30 and 90 postoperative days. Patients from classes B and C showed a greater risk of complications when compared to class A (at 30 days, OR 4.9, 95% IC: 1.3-18.2; p=0.019 and at 90 days, OR 5.8, 95% IC: 1.5-21.4; p=0.009).

Conclusion: There is increasing evidence that OS-MRS scale is a useful tool to predict morbidity after gastric laparoscopic bypass in morbidly obese patients.

Keywords: Obesity; Morbidity; Bariatric surgery; Predictive factors; OS-MRS; Laparoscopic gastric bypass; Complications

Introduction

Obesity is a global health problem defined as a body mass index (BMI) greater than 30 kg/m². World Health Organization states that worldwide obesity more than doubled since 1980 and in 2014 it was estimated that about 13% of the adult population were obese. In Portugal, this prevalence reached 20.1% [1].

Bariatric Surgery experienced new developments in the last few decades, and with the advent of laparoscopy become progressively less invasive. Laparoscopic gastric bypass (LGB) is currently the most common procedure for the treatment of morbid obesity [2]. Bariatric surgery, even as an elective procedure, is associated with considerable morbidity, even though it presents low mortality (under 1.5%) [3]. Values reported for morbidity are quite discrepant varying from 3 to 20% [4].

Recently, many scoring systems have been used to predict the mortality risk of patients proposed to bariatric surgery. Obesity surgery mortality risk score (OS-MRS) is used for patient's risk stratification and mortality risk assessment at 90 days postoperatively, and is validated by multiple centers [5-8]. Simplicity is its main advantage, consisting in assigning 1 point for each of the following preoperative variables: male, age ≥ 45 years, BMI ≥ 50 kg/m², and

arterial hypertension (ATH), known risk factors for pulmonary thromboembolism (PTE). Patients with 0-1 points are classified as class A (low risk), with 2-3 points as class B (moderate risk) and with 4-5 points as class C (high risk).

Given the low mortality described for this type of surgery, stratifying patients according to their risk of postoperative complications, rather than mortality, seems a more logical and useful approach. However, only few authors have studied the possibility of using the OS-MRS with morbidity's prediction as an end point. Sarela et al. concluded that the patients included in OSMRS class C presented more adverse events, when compared to those from classes A+B, [9]. Lorente et al [10] found complications in patients from classes B+C to be more frequent then in those from class A. However, these studies had several limitations: patients were submitted to different bariatric surgical procedures, there were multiple interventions at the same operative time, and post-operative records were analyzed only in the first 30 days.

The aim of this study was to evaluate OS-MRS as a predictor of complications at 30 and 90-days postoperative in morbidly obese patients submitted to primary laparoscopic gastric bypass.

Methods

A retrospective study was performed including all consecutive patients who underwent primary laparoscopic gastric bypass between

January 1st and December 31st 2014, at Centro Hospitalar do Porto, Portugal.

The usual multidisciplinary preoperative evaluation (including Surgery, Endocrinology, Anesthesia, Psychiatry and Nutrition) took place in our institution, which is considered national reference for laparoscopic bariatric surgery. Patients with co-existing surgical procedures besides LGB were excluded. Most patients were admitted one day before surgery and were discharged on the 3rd postoperative day. Anesthesia technique included induction with propofol and maintenance with desflurane to a bispectral index (BIS®) target of 40-60. A perfusion of remifentanil was used during the procedure. Muscle relaxation was achieved with rocuronium and reversed with sugammadex, under train-of-four neuromuscular monitoring.

Clinical electronic records were accessed to evaluate age, gender, preoperative weight, height, BMI, American Society of Anaesthesiology physical status (ASA), ATH and increased risk of PTE, defined as if there was previous history of PTE, hypoventilation ($PaCO_2$>45mmHg), presence of inferior vena cava filter or a diagnosis of pulmonary hypertension.

Morbidity and mortality at 30 and 90 days following surgery were recorded. If there was not a medical appointment during this period, patients were contacted by telephone to clarify their clinical status.

Complications were classified according to Clavien-Dindo's grades [11-13]. This classification stratifies adverse events into one of 5 grades: grade I includes any deviation from normal postoperative course without the need for pharmacological or other treatment (allowing antiemetics, analgesics, diuretic, electrolytes and physiotherapy); grade II complications require blood transfusion, total parenteral nutrition or pharmacological treatment besides the one allowed on grade I; grade III requires surgical, endoscopic or radiological intervention; grade IV are life-threatening complications; and finally grade V refers to the death of a patient.

The OS-MRS was calculated, as previously described. Patients were then classified into three groups according to their score.

Microsoft Excel® (2010) was used for statistical analysis. Odds Ratio was used to analyze the influence of OS-MRS classes on the development of postoperative complications. The chi-square test or the Fisher's test was used to analyze the association between different individual risk factors and the development of postoperative complications.

Results

Eighty-five consecutive patients submitted to primary laparoscopic gastric bypass were included, of which 70 (82.4%) were female. The mean age was 44 years old (range 20-65) and the mean BMI was 44.3 ± SD 5.8 kg/m². Concerning the ASA physical status, 56 patients (65.9%) were classified as ASA II, and the remaining as ASA III. The prevalence of the risk factors included in OS-MRS and their co-existence, is presented in Tables 1 and 2.

On the OS-MRS scale, 33 patients were classified as class A (38.8%), 48 as class B (56.5%) and 4 as class C (4.7%).

No mortality cases were registered. Twenty patients (23.5%) presented at least one complication during the first 30 days. A total of 22 patients had some complication by the 90th postoperative day (25.9%) (Table 3). It should be noted that one patient presented one grade I complication at the first 30 days, and another of grade III during the 90 postoperative days.

	Total of patients	%
Age ≥ 45	44	51.8
Body mass index ≥ 50 kg/m2	15	17.6
Male	15	17.6
Arterial Hypertension	52	61.2
Risk of Pulmonary Thromboembolism	23	27.1
Totality of Patients included	85	100

Table 1: Prevalence of the risk factors used to calculate OS-MRS.

	Age ≥ 45	BMI ≥ 50	Male	AHT	Risk of PTE
Age ≥ 45	44	5	6	36	13
BMI ≥ 50		15	4	9	4
Male			15	13	4
AHT				52	15
Risk of PTE					23

BMI: Body Mass Index; AHT: Arterial Hypertension; PTE: Pulmonary Thromboembolism

Table 2: Relation and frequency of risk factors used to calculate OS-MRS in the 85 patients.

For statistical analysis purposes, at 90 days, this patient was considered only once, with the complication of higher grade. Of the registered complications, 5% (n=1) at 30 days, and 9% (n=2) at 90 days, were considered major, requiring surgical or endoscopic intervention.

Unimodal analysis showed statistical significance for OS-MRS scale, ASA physical status and the risk of developing PTE, regarding the occurrence of postoperative complications, both at 30 and 90 postoperative days (Table 4).

The rate of complications in each of OS-MRS subgroups at 30 and 90 days was: 9.1% in class A (both evaluations), 31.3% and 35.4% in class B (at 30 and 90 days, respectively) and 50% in class C (both evaluations).

Due to the small sample of high-risk patients, classes B (moderate risk) and C (high risk) were grouped together for analysis. When patients classified as class A were compared to those from classes B and C, we found that the risk of general complications was significantly greater in the last group, with an odds ratio of 5.8 at 90 days (95% IC: 1.5-21.4; p=0.009). Similar results were obtained at 30 days with an odds ratio of 4.9 (95% IC: 1.3-18.2; p=0.019).

However, when excluding minor adverse events (Clavien-Dindo grade I) the results did not show the same statistically significant difference between Class A and Classes B+C, with an OR=1.5 at 90 days (95% IC: 0.37-6.49; p=0.54) and an OR=2.4 at 30 days (95% IC: 0.47-12.39; p=0.29).

Type	Complication	At 30 days	Cumulative at 90 days
I	Accentuated nutritional deficit	0	1
	Persistent vomiting requiring postponing discharge, non-scheduled medical consultation or hospital readmission	11*	11*
II	Surgical wound infection	2	2
	Dysrhythmia	1	1
	Digestive haemorrhage with transfusion	1	1
	Respiratory insufficiency with noninvasive ventilation	2	2
	Respiratory infection	1	1
	Acute Kidney Injury with dehydration	1	1
III	Anastomosis dehiscence	1	1
	Anastomosis stenosis	0	1*
Total of Patients with Complications		20	22*

*Note that one patient presented episodes of vomit at 30-days and anastomosis stenosis at 90 days. For analysis purposes at 90 days it was considered only once, with the highest grade complication.

Table 3: Postoperative complications at 30 and 90 postoperative days, divided according to Clavien-Dindo's classification.

Discussion

In our series, there were no cases of mortality, which seems to be in line with the extremely low mortality rate described in other studies.

Although our complications' rate was higher when compared to the existing literature, only 2 major complications (2.4%) were registered, which is consistent with other studies [10,14]. In addition, even though most complications occurred in the first 30 days, we analyzed a longer time period (90 days).

Although there are some scores designed for predicting morbidity in bariatric surgery, such as the ones developed by Gupta et al. and Turner et al., some limitations have been reported [15,16]. Some are not exclusively designed for LGB, or are difficult to apply and their calculation is time-consuming, others are not validated in multiple centers or do not stratify patients in risk groups. OS-MRS, previously only a tool for estimating mortality, is a much simpler tool, as most of its variables are routinely gathered in a preoperative consultation. We found that OS-MRS is useful in predicting the risk of postoperative complications after laparoscopic gastric bypass, which is of great importance both for selection, patient information and decisions regarding the perioperative period and the follow-up. This seems to be in accordance with findings of both Sarela et al. and Lorente et al. [9,10].

In our study, when different risk factors were individually analyzed, only the risk of PTE, OS-MRS and ASA classification were related to the occurrence of complications. However, previous studies also found correlations with age, BMI, sex and ATH [16-19].

Regarding both periods analyzed (30 versus 90 days) the conclusion reached for each of them are similar; thus, although there is an advantage of predicting morbidity at 90 days, future studies for

validation of this score may draw conclusions from a shorter follow-up period such as 30 days.

The OS-MRS score was useful in predicting general morbidity; the same was not valid when excluding minor complications. This, however, does not minimize its importance in the preoperative setting as a tool to stratify patients. In fact, complications of grade I, even though not demanding specific or invasive therapeutics, require postponing discharges, patients' re-admissions or additional complementary laboratorial and imagiologic exams, bringing important social and economic implications for both the patient and the institution.

			At 30 days		At 90 days	
		Total	Complications	P	Complications	P
Age ≥ 45 years	Yes	44	13	0.279	15	0.123
	No	41	7		7	
	Total	85				
BMI ≥ 50 kg/m^2	Yes	15	3	1	4	1
	No	70	17		18	
	Total	85				
Male	Yes	15	5	0.3301	5	0.521
	No	70	15		17	
	Total	85				
Arterial Hypertension	Yes	52	15	0.1929	17	0.0818
	No	33	5		5	
	Total	85				
Risk of PTE	Yes	23	12	0.0005*	12	0.002*
	No	62	8		10	
	Total	85				
ASA physical status	II	56	9	0.0474*	9,0	0.0091*
	III	29	11		13,0	
	Total	85				
OS-MRS	A	33	3	0.0172*	3,0	0.0052*
	B+C	52	17		19,0	
	Total	85				

BMI: Body Mass Index; PTE: Pulmonary Thromboembolism; ASA: American Society of Anaesthesiology; OS-MRS: Obesity Surgery Mortality Risk Score; *p<0.05.

Table 4: Analysis of the association between each risk factor individually and the occurrence of postoperative complications.

The study presents some limitations: small sample size, patients from only one institution, retrospective design. Even though it clearly demonstrates the ability to identify the patients with higher risk of postoperative adverse events, a larger sample might be needed to address the possibility of predicting high-grade complications. However, the prevalence of higher-grade complications in our sample seems in accordance with the literature [10,14]. Lastly, although retrospective, the study variables included in OS-MRS are routinely assessed and registered in the clinical anesthesia pre-operative assessment of these patients.

In conclusion, there is increasing evidence that OS-MRS scale might be a useful tool to predict general morbidity after gastric laparoscopic bypass in morbidly obese patients.

This evidence allows physicians to better inform patients and decide on which strategies they could benefit for in the perioperative period.

References

1. WHO (2015) Obesity and overweight.

2. Gilbert EW, Wolfe BM (2012) Bariatric surgery for the management of obesity: state of the field. Plast Reconstr Surg 130: 948-954.

3. Thomas H, Agrawal S (2012) Systematic review of obesity surgery mortality risk score-preoperative risk stratification in bariatric surgery. Obes Surg 22: 1135-1140.

4. Martins-Filho ED, Katz L, Amorim M, Ferraz AA, Ferraz EM (2011) Prediction of severe complications and death in superobese patients undergoing open gastric bypass with the Recife Score. Arq Gastroenterol 48: 8-14.

5. Arterburn D, Johnson ES, Butler MG, Fisher D, Bayliss EA (2014) Predicting 90-day mortality after bariatric surgery: an independent, external validation of the OS-MRS prognostic risk score. Surg Obes Relat Dis 10: 774-779.

6. DeMaria EJ, Portenier D, Wolfe L (2007) Obesity surgery mortality risk score: proposal for a clinically useful score to predict mortality risk in patients undergoing gastric bypass. Surg Obes Relat Dis 3: 134-140.

7. DeMaria EJ, Murr M, Byrne TK, Blackstone R, Grant JP, et al. (2007) Validation of the Obesity Surgery Mortality Risk Score in a Multicenter Study Proves It Stratifies Mortality Risk in Patients Undergoing Gastric Bypass for Morbid Obesity. Ann Surg 246: 578-584.

8. Mansour S, Kaur V, Vasilikostas G, Reddy KM, Wan A (2010) Relevance of the Obesity Surgery Mortality Risk Score in Patients Undergoing Roux-en-Y Gastric Bypass. Internet J Surg 25: 2.

9. Sarela AI, Dexter SP, McMahon MJ (2011) Use of the obesity surgery mortality risk score to predict complications of laparoscopic bariatric surgery. Obes Surg 21: 1698-1703.

10. Lorente L, Ramón J, Vidal P, Goday A, Parri A, et al. (2014) Obesity Surgery Mortality Risk Score for the Prediction of Complications After Laparoscopic Bariatric Surgery. Cir Esp 92: 316-23.

11. Dindo D, Demartines N, Clavien PA (2004) Classification of surgical complications: a new proposal with evaluation in a cohort of 6336 patients and results of a survey. Ann Surg 240: 205-213.

12. Clavien PA, Sanabria JR, Strasberg SM (1992) Proposed classification of complications of surgery with examples of utility in cholecystectomy. Surgery 111: 518-526.

13. Clavien PA, Barkun J, de Oliveira ML, Vauthey JN, Dindo D, et al. (2009) The Clavien-Dindo classification of surgical complications: five-year experience. Ann Surg 250: 187-196.

14. Young MT, Gebhart A, Phelan MJ, Nguyen NT (2015) Use and Outcomes of Laparoscopic Sleeve Gastrectomy vs Laparoscopic Gastric Bypass: Analysis of the American College of Surgeons NSQIP. J Am Coll Surg 220: 880-885.

15. Turner PL, Saager L, Dalton J, Abd-Elsayed A, Roberman D, et al. (2011) A nomogram for predicting surgical complications in bariatric surgery patients. Obes Surg 21: 655-662.

16. Gupta PK, Franck C, Miller WJ, Gupta H, Forse RA (2011) Development and validation of a bariatric surgery morbidity risk calculator using the prospective, multicenter NSQIP dataset. J Am Coll Surg 212: 301-309.

17. Qin C, Luo B, Aggarwal A, De Oliveira G, Kim JY (2015) Advanced age as an independent predictor of perioperative risk after laparoscopic sleeve gastrectomy (LSG). Obes Surg 25: 406-412.

18. Livingston EH, Huerta S, Arthur D, Lee S, De Shields S, et al. (2002) Male gender is a predictor of morbidity and age a predictor of mortality for patients undergoing gastric bypass surgery. Ann Surg 236: 576-582.

19. O'Rourke RW, Andrus J, Diggs BS, Scholz M, McConnell DB, et al. (2006) Perioperative morbidity associated with bariatric surgery: an academic center experience. Arch Surg 141: 262-268.

8

Paravertebral Block *vs.* Caudal Block Using Dexmedetomidine Plus Local Anesthetics for Inguinal Hernia Repair in Pediatrics: A Randomized Prospective Trial

Naglaa Khalil and Hesham M Marouf*

Faculty of Medicine, Tanta University, Egypt

***Corresponding author:** Hesham M Marouf, Faculty of Medicine, Tanta University, Egypt, E-mail: heshammarouf@hotmail.com

Abstract

Aim: We aimed to compare the effects of caudal block (CB) and paravertebral block (PVB) using dexmedetomidine plus local anesthetics on postoperative pain and analgesia requirements in pediatrics after inguinal hernia surgery.

Methods: This randomized prospective study was carried out on 80 pediatric patients underwent inguinal hernia repair. Two groups (each 40 patients) were included in the study: group CB and group PVB. After a standardized general anaesthesia, caudal or lumbar paravertebral block was performed using bupivacaine (0.25%) and dexemetomidine 1 µg/kg . We recorded FLACC score, number of patients needed rescue analgesia, the total number of doses of rescue analgesia, the duration of postoperative analgesia, parents satisfaction and adverse events.

Results: FLACC score was higher in group (CB) compared with group (PVB) at 12 h and 16 h postoperative. The total number of patients need postoperative analgesia and the total number of doses of postoperative analgesia were higher in group (CB) compared with group (PVB). The duration of postoperative analgesia was significantly longer in group (PVB) than group (CB) (16.25 ± 1.66 *vs.* 10.69 ± 1.34). Parent satisfaction was higher in group (PVB) than group (CB). No major complications were detected in both groups.

Conclusion: paravertebral block (using dexmedetomidine+local anaesthetics) was associated with better postoperative analgesia and higher parents satisfaction compared to caudal block (using dexmedetomidine+local anaesthetics) for inguinal hernia repair in children.

Keywords: Paravertebral; Caudal; Dexmedetomidine; Hernia; Pediatric

Introduction

One of the most common surgical procedures in pediatrics is inguinal hernia repair. This surgery lead to different degree of pain postoperative [1].

Regional anesthetic procedures can reduce intra-operative anaesthetic requirement, allow rapid recovery, and decrease postoperative pain and opioids use [2].

Caudal block is the most popular regional anaesthesia technique used to relieve pain in children after surgery of the lumbosacral to midthoracic dermatomal level. Caudal block using single shot technique is associated with short duration of analgesia [3].

Paravertebral block (PVB) is a regional anaesthesia technique where local anesthetic is injected close to the site where the nerves come out from the intervertebral foramina. Paravertebral block affords a good analgesia after thoracotomy and abdomen surgery [4,5].

Both caudal and paravertebral blocks were used successfully in pediatrics to improve postoperative analgesia [6,7].

Dexmeditomidine is an Alpha (α)-2-adrenergic receptor agonist which has sedative, sympatholytic, and analgesic effects. Adding dexmedetomidine to local anesthetics during peripheral nerve blockade and regional anesthesia procedures is proved to be effective for the surgical patient [8].

The aim of the present study was to compare the effects of caudal block and paravertebral block using dexmedetomidine plus local anesthetics on postoperative pain and analgesia requirements in pediatric patients after unilateral inguinal hernia surgery

Pan African Clinical Trials Registry (PACTR) registration number : PACTR201611001695146.

Methods

After approval by local ethical committee, this randomized prospective study was performed in Tanta University Hospital for 6 months from 1/4/2016 to 1/10/2016 on 80 pediatric patients (ASA I-II) scheduled for elective unilateral inguinal hernia surgery. A written and informed consent was obtained from the parent of each patient.

Patients were randomly allocated into 2 equal groups (each 40 patients)

- Caudal group (group CB) (40 patients)

- Paravereberal group (group PVB) (40 patients)

Randomization was performed using computer generated block randomization to create a list of numbers, each number referred to one of the 2 groups. Then each number was sealed in opaque envelope. Each parent asked to choose one of the envelopes and was given it to the anesthesiologist who compared the number with computer generated list and accordingly assigned the patient to one of the 2 groups.

Inclusion criteria

Patients were involved in the study if they were aged 3-7 years, had ASA I-II, and scheduled for elective unilateral inguinal hernia surgery.

Exclusion criteria

Patients were omitted from the study if they had contraindication to regional anesthesia, such as congenital abnormalities of spine and meninges, coagulopathy or anticoagulation therapy, infection at the site of injection, mental retardation or history of developmental delay and allergy to local anaesthetics drugs.

Procedure

On arrival of the patients to the operative theatre, and after placement of the standard monitoring (including ECG, noninvasive blood pressure, and pulse oximetry, capnograph), general inhalational anesthesia was induced by face mask with sevoflurane (Kahira pharmaceuticals and chemical industries company, Egypt under license of Abbvie UK) (4-8%) in 100% oxygen, IV canula was secured then intravenous Propofol [9] (Astra Zeneca UK) 1-2 mg/kg was injected. No muscle relaxant or intraoperative opioids were given. All children were allowed to breathe spontaneously *via* a laryngeal mask airway. Anesthesia was maintained with isoflurane (Kahira pharmaceuticals and chemical industries company, Egypt under license of Abbvie UK (0.5-2%) in oxygen-air mixture. Paracetamol [10] (Pharco B international, Egypt) 15 mg/kg was given intravenously.

Caudal or lumbar paravertebral block was performed prior to surgery with patients in the lateral decubitus position.

In group (CB) patients were placed in a lateral position and povidone iodine solution was used to clean the skin over the sacrum, then under complete aseptic precautions 25 G needle was used to perform single dose caudal block. To confirm the correct position of the needle pop sensation should be noticed during penetration of the sacro-coccygeal ligament, which was followed by the whoosh test [11] using 0.5 ml of air. After needle insertion and negative aspiration of blood or cerebrospinal fluid, bupivacaine (Aldebeiky phrma Egypt) (0.25%) 1 ml/kg and dexemetomidine [10] (Pfizer, USA) 1 mic/kg were injected.

In group (PVB) PVB was performed as previously described by Hadzic and Vloka [12]. Graduated epidural needle was inserted perpendicularly to the skin (1 to 2 cm lateral to the spinal process at the level of second lumbar vertebra) and when the needle reached the transverse process it was withdrawn to the subcutaneous tissue and redirected to walk off the caudal edge of the transverse process. When the needle reached the paravertebral space (which was identified by loss of resistance to air) and after negative (aspiration to be sure it is not intravascular) a bolus of 0.5 ml/kg of bupivacaine (0.25%) [13] and dexmetomidine 1 mic/kg [14] were injected.

We used blind technique for both PVB and CB as the ultrasound machine was not working well during our study (due to maintenance problem). Fifteen min after performing PVB or CB, surgery was initiated. Cardioacceleration changes (increasing noninvasive mean arterial pressure and heart rate >15% in response to painful surgical stimulation) and/or patient movement of his limbs were interpreted as insufficient analgesia. In such instances, PVB or CB was considered failed, then 1-2 μg/kg IV fentanyl were administered, and the patient was excluded from the study.

Postoperatively the patients were given regular paracetamol (E.I.P.I.CO. Egypt) 15 mg/kg [10] every 6 h intravenous.

FLACC score and other data were collected by anesthesiologist who is blind to the group of the patients.

Postoperative pain was assessed in both groups by FLACC [15] score to evaluate the effectiveness of the block (face, legs, activity, cry and consolability) at 15 min, 1 h, 4, 8, 12, 16, 20, and 24 h postoperative.

If a FLACC score was more than 3, the child was managed nonpharmacologically (position changing, tactile stimulation, etc) if no effect after 5 min, intravenous fentanyl [16] (Sunny pharmaceutical, Egypt under license of Hameln pharmaceutical, Germany) as rescue analgesia was given in a dose 0.5 mic/kg if FLACC score still more than 3 after 10 min another 0.5 mic/kg of fentanyl was given.

Primary outcome

Primary outcome included number of patients needed rescue analgesia.

Secondary outcome

Secondary outcome included FLACC score, the total number of doses of rescue analgesia, the duration of postoperative analgesia (time from recovery to first dose of fentanyl) and parents satisfaction (Parents were asked to rate their degree of satisfaction on scale from 1 to 10 where 1=completely dissatisfied and 10=completely satisfied). Any postoperative adverse events were documented as bradycardia (heart rate less than 65 beat/min) hypotension (blood pressure less than 20% of base line reading), and respiratory depression (SpO_2 less than 95%).

The minimally required sample size to detect 30% difference in the number of children needed rescue analgesia between the PVB and CB groups was 34 patients in each study group assuming power of 80% and an alpha error of 0.05. We aimed to include 40 patients in each group.

Statistical analysis

Statistical analysis was done using SPSS programme version 20 (IBM, Armonk, NY, United States of America). Quantitative data were expressed as mean ± standard deviation (SD) and analyzed using Independent-samples t-test. Qualitative data were expressed as frequency and percentage and analyzed using Chi-square (X^2) test.

Results

Our result showed that one patient in PVB group had failure of paravertebral block because it was difficult to detect the paravertebral space, another patient in CB group had vascular puncture during the procedure. Both patients were excluded from the study and the study was done on 39 patients in each group. Table 1 shows that no significant differences were detected among the two groups in terms of demographic data including age, sex; body weight and duration of the surgery (p>0.05) (Table 1).

Variables	Group (CB)	Group (PVB)	P value
Age, years	4.69 ± 1.32	4.74 ± 1.37	0.86
Weight, kg	16.58 ± 2.77	17.48 ± 2.96	0.17
Sex M/F	23/16	24/15	0.82
Duration of surgery min	70.2 ± 6.7	71.4 ± 7.03	0.44
Data are presented as mean ± SD or ratio.			
(*) significant p value<0.05			

Table 1: Patients' characteristic.

Table 2 shows that there was insignificant difference regarding FLACC score between both groups at 15 min, 1 h, 4 h, 8 h, 20 h, and 24 h postoperative but there was a significant increase in FLACC scores in group (CB) compared with group (PVB) at 12 h postoperative (2.87 ± 0.97 *vs.*1.69 ± 0.69 respectively) and at 16 h postoperative (3.1 ± 0.91 *vs.* 2.10 ± 1.03 respectively).

FLACC scores	(CB) group	(PVB)	P value
At 15 min	1.41 ± 0.49 (1.24-1.57)	1.23 ± 0.42 (1.09-1.36)	0.09
At 1 h	1.07 ± 0.48(0.92-1.23)	1.2 ± 0.46 (1.05-1.35)	0.24
At 4 h	1.79 ± 0.65(1.58-2)	1.74 ± 0.67 (1.52-1.96)	0.73
At 8 h	1.89 ± 0.63(1.68-2.1)	1.74 ± 0.64 (1.53-1.95)	0.29
At 12 h	2.87 ± 0.97(2.57-3.17)	1.69 ± 0.69 (1.46-1.91)	0.00*
At 16 h	3.1 ± 0.91(2.8-3.39)	2.10 ± 1.03 (1.79-2.46)	0.00*
At 20 h	2.71 ± 0.75(2.43-2.89)	2.61 ± 0.98 (2.24-2.77)	0.61
At 24 h	1.79 ± 0.69(1.56-2.02)	1.41 ± 0.49 (1.24-1.57)	0.006
Data are presented as mean ± SD (95% confidence interval).			
(*) significant p value<0.05.			

Table 2: FLACC scores.

Table 3 showed that the total number of patients need analgesia were more in group (CB) compared with group (PVB) (21 *vs.* 7) (P=0.001). Fifteen patients in group (CB) needed single analgesic dose *vs.* six patients in group (PVB) (P=0.022). Patients needed two doses were significantly higher in group (CB) (6 patients) compared to group (PVB) (1 patient) (P=0.048) (Table 3). The duration of postoperative analgesia was significantly longer in group (PVB) than group (CB) (16.25 ± 1.66 *vs.* 10.69 ± 1.34). Parents satisfaction was higher in group (PVB) than group (CB) (7.23 ± 2.52 *vs.* 6.07 ± 1.43) (Table 3).

No major complications were detected in both groups. Two patients in paravertebral group complained from pain at the site of injection and in CB group three patients complained from shivering.

Variables	Group (CB)	Group (PVB)	P value
Total number of patients needed rescue analgesia	21/39 (53.8%)	7/39 (17.9%)	0.001*
Number of patients needed single dose of rescue analgesia	15/39 (38.5%)	6/39 (15.4%)	0.022*
Number of patients needed two doses of rescue analgesia	6/39 (15.4%)	1/39 (2.6%)	0.048*
Duration of postoperative analgesia (h)	10.69 ± 1.34 (10.12-11.25)	16.25 ± 1.66 (15.71-16.79)	0.001*
Parents satisfaction	6.07 ± 1.43	7.23 ± 2.52	0.001*
Data are presented as mean ± SD, mean ± SD (95% confidence interval) or number and percentage.			
(*) significant p value<0.05.			

Table 3: Postoperative data.

Discussion

Our study showed that group (PVB) (using dexmedetomidine+local anaesthetics) was associated with lower FLACC score (at 12 h and 16 h postoperative), fewer number of patients who needed rescue analgesia, longer duration of postoperative analgesia, less postoperative rescue analgesia requirements and higher parents satisfaction as compared to group (CB) (using dexmedetomidine+local anaesthetics). In the present study we gave paracetamol as base line analgesia and we measured number of patients who needed rescue analgesia (fentanyl) and duration postoperative analgesia which was defined as time from recovery to first dose of fentanyl.

The relative avascularity of the paravertebral space and hence the slow uptake of local anaesthetic explained the prolonged duration of analgesia in PVB than CB [17].

Our result was supported by the study done by Tug R et al. [18] who found that the number of patients who did not need postoperative analgesia was higher in (PVB) group compared to (CB) group, and the duration of analgesia was longer in (PVB) group than (CB) group. But regarding FLACC score Tug R et al. [18] reported that no difference was recorded between both groups while in our study FLACC score was lower in (PVB) group compared to (CB) group. Also our result was in line with the study done by Akçaboy et al. [19] who reported that PVB had effective and prolonged analgesia compared with spinal block in adult patients. Our results agreed with the study done by Lonnqvist and Olsson [6] who compared lumbar epidural blocks with somatic paravertebral block in children and reported that the number of patients who required no morphine was lower in paravertebral group than the epidural group.

Berta et al. [7] studied the effect of PVB on postoperative pain in children undergoing renal surgeries under general anaesthesia and reported that the median duration of postoperative analgesia was 600 min (range 180-720 min) and 10 patients (41.7%) did not need analgesia while 14 patients (58.3%) needed analgesia during the first 12 postoperative hours, but in our study the duration of postoperative analgesia was 16.25 ± 1.66 h (mean ± sd) and 7 patients (17.9%) needed analgesia during the first 24 postoperative hours. The differences between our results and Berta' s results may be due to different type of surgeries in both studies also in our study we used local anaesthetic drug pluse dexmetomidine which is known to potentiate the effect of local anaesthetics as reported by Esmaoglu A et al. [20].

In contrast to our results Davies et al. [21] reported (in their systemic review and meta–analysis) that analgesia was similar in epidural group and paravertebral group but paravertebral group was associated with less complications. The differences between our results and Davies' s results may be due to difference in the techniques (thoracic epidural and caudal block) or differences in type of surgery.

No major complications were recorded in both groups in the present study, similar results have been reported in other studies [18,22].

Our study showed that parent satisfaction was significantly higher in PVB group compared to CB group. This result was supported by the studies done by Tug R et al. [18] and Naja ZM at al. [23].

Conclusion

In conclusion, paravertebral block (using dexmedetomidine+local anaesthetics) in combination with general anaesthesia resulted in improved and prolonged postoperative analgesia, higher parents satisfaction compared to caudal block (using dexmedetomidine+local anaesthetics) for inguinal hernia repair in children.

Limitations

Limitations from our point of view there are 2 limitations to the study. The first is absence of control group. The second is that blindness to the group was impossible for the anaesthesiologist during surgery. But we think that these limitations did not affect the strength of the study.

References

1. Goyal V, Kubre J, Radhakrishnan K (2016) Dexmedetomidine as an adjuvant to bupivacaine in caudal analgesia in children. Anesth Essays Res 10: 227-232.

2. Johr M (2013) Practical pediatric regional anesthesia. Curr Opin Anaesth 26: 327-332.

3. Rapp HJ, Folger A, Grau T (2005) Ultrasound-guided epidural catheter insertion in children. Anesth Analg 101: 333-339.

4. Rorarius MG, Kujansuu E, Baer GA, Suominen P, Teisala K, et al. (2001) Laparoscopically assisted vaginal and abdominal hysterectomy: comparison of postoperative pain, fatigue and systemic response. A case-controlled study. Eur J Anaesthesiol 18: 530-539.

5. Thompson TK, Hutchison RW, Wegmann DJ, Shires GT 3rd, Beecherl E (2008) Pancreatic resection pain management is combining PCA therapy and a continuous local infusion of 0.5% ropivacaine beneficial? Pancreas 37: 103-104.

6. Lonnqvist PA, Olsson GL (1994) Paravertebral vs. epidural block in children. Effects on postoperative morphine requirement after renal surgery. Acta Anaesthesiol Scand 38: 346-349.

7. Berta E, Spanhel J, Smakal O, Smolka V, Gabrhelik T, et al. (2008) Single injection paravertebral block for renal surgery in children. Paediatr Anaesth 18: 593-597.

8. Khan ZP, Ferguson CN, Jones RM (1999) Alpha-2 and imidazoline receptor agonists. Their pharmacology and therapeutic role. Anesthesia 54: 146-165.

9. Splinter WM, Thomson ME (2010) Somatic paravertebral block decreases opioid requirements in children undergoing appendectomy. Can J Anaesth 57: 206-210.

10. Fares KM, Othman AH, Alieldin NH (2014) Efficacy and Safety of Dexmedetomidine Added to Caudal Bupivacaine in Pediatric Major Abdominal Cancer Surgery. Pain Physician 17: 393-400.

11. Lewis MP, Thomas P, Wilson LF, Mulholland RC (1992) The 'whoosh' test. A clinical test to confirm correct needle placement in caudal epidural injections. Anesthesia 47: 57-58.

12. Hadzic A, Vloka J (1997) Thoracolumbar Paravertebral Block. In: Hadzic A, Vloka J, eds. Periperal Nerve Blocks: Principles and Practice. New York, NY: McGraw Hill 2004. p. 208-217. in young children. Pediatr Nurs 23: 293-297.

13. Chalam KS, Patnaik SS, Sunil C, Bansal T (2015) Comparative study of ultrasound-guided paravertebral block with ropivacaine vs. bupivacaine for post-operative pain relief in children undergoing thoracotomy for patent ductus arteriosus ligation surgery. Indian J Anaesth 59:493-498.

14. Dutta V, Kumar B, Jayant A, Mishra AK (2016) Effect of Continuous Paravertebral Dexmedetomidine Administration on Intraoperative Anesthetic Drug Requirement and Post-Thoracotomy Pain Syndrome After Thoracotomy: A Randomized Controlled Trial. J Cardiothorac Vasc Anesth 31: 159-165.

15. Merkel SI, Voepel-Lewis T, Shayevitz JR, Malviya S (2003) The FLACC: A behavioral scale for scoring postoperative pain anesthesia for inguinal hernia repair. World J Surg 27: 425-429.

16. Verghese ST, Hannallah RS (2010) Acute pain management in children. J Pain Res 3: 105-123.

17. Weltz CR, Klein SM, Arbo JE, Greengrass RA (2003) Paravertebral block anesthesia for inguinal hernia repair. World J Surg 27: 425-429.

18. Tug R, Ozcengiz D, Güneş Y (2011) Single level paravertebral vs. caudal block in paediatric inguinal surgery. Anaesth intensive Care 39: 909-913.

19. Akcaboy EY, Akcaboy ZN, Gogus N (2009) Ambulatory inguinal herniorrhaphy: paravertebral block vs. spinal anesthesia. Minerva Anestesiol 75: 684-691 .

20. Esmaoglu A, Yegenoglu F, Akin A, Turk CY (2010) Dexmedetomidine added to levobupivacaine prolongs axillary brachial plexus block. Anesth Analg 111: 1548-1551.

21. Davies RG, Myles PS, Graham JM (2006) A comparison of the analgesic efficacy and side effects of paravertebral vs. epidural blockade for thoracotomy-a systematic review and meta analysis of randomized trials. Br J Anaesth 96: 418-426.

22. Naja ZM, Raf M, El Rajab M, Ziade FM, Al Tannir MA, et al. (2006) Nerve stimulator-guided paravertebral blockade combined with sevoflurane sedation vs. general anaesthesia with systemic analgesia for postherniorrhaphy pain relief in children: a prospective randomized trial. Anesthesiology 103: 600-605.

23. Naja ZM, Raf M, El Rajab M, Daoud N, Ziade FM, et al. (2006) A comparison of nerve stimulator guided paravertebral block and ilio-inguinal nerve block for analgesia after inguinal herniorrhaphy in children. Anaesthesia 61: 1064-1068.

9

Patient Susceptibility & Technical Factors Associated with Persistent Diaphragmatic Paralysis after Interscalene Nerve Block

Matthew R Kaufman[1,2,3*], **Ryan Fields**[4], **John Cece**[2], **Catarina P Martins**[2], **Kameron Rezzadeh**[2], **Andrew I Elkwood**[1,2] and **Reza Jarrahy**[3]

[1]*The Center for Treatment of Paralysis and Reconstructive Nerve Surgery, Jersey Shore University Medical Center, Neptune, New Jersey, USA*

[2]*The Institute for Advanced Reconstruction, Shrewsbury, New Jersey, USA*

[3]*Division of Plastic and Reconstructive Surgery, David Geffen UCLA Medical Center, Los Angeles, California, USA*

[4]*Department of Anesthesiology, Jersey Shore University Medical Center, Neptune, New Jersey, USA*

*****Corresponding author**: Matthew R Kaufman, The Institute for Advanced Reconstruction, 535 Sycamore Avenue, Shrewsbury, New Jersey, USA, E-mail: kaufmanmatthew@hotmail.com

Abstract

Background and objectives: Interscalene nerve blocks (ISB) have been associated with the rare complication of persistent diaphragmatic paralysis. Little is known regarding patient susceptibility or technical factors that may contribute to the development of this debilitating adverse reaction.

Methods: An observational study was performed between 2009 and 2014 to compare two groups of patients who received ISB for upper extremity surgery. Patient demographic factors, co-morbidities, and technical aspects of the nerve block were reviewed and compared in two groups: 50 consecutive patients receiving ISB without consequence at a university-based hospital and affiliated outpatient surgery center (Group I); 29

patients with persistent diaphragmatic paralysis after ISB evaluated and treated at a tertiary referral center (Group II). We analyzed the following patient factors between groups: age, sex, BMI, laterality, history of peripheral or diabetic neuropathy, prior nerve blocks, and underlying cervical spondylosis. An assessment of technical aspects of the nerve block was also performed.

Results: In Group I there was 26 females and 24 males with an average age of 55, whereas in Group II there were 4 females and 25 males with an average age of 58. There was no significant difference between groups for BMI (mean=36 *vs.* 30) or laterality (Left=38% *vs.* 31%), however there were a significantly higher proportion of males in Group II (p<0.01). No difference was demonstrated between groups for peripheral or diabetic neuropathy, whereas prior ipsilateral blocks and cervical spondylosis were significantly more prevalent in Group II (p<0.01 & p<0.01, respectively). In Group I, 86% of patients received blocks performed with either nerve stimulator (64%) or ultrasound (22%) guidance, and 10% using both modalities. This contrasts to 79% of patients in Group II whose blocks were performed using either nerve stimulator (24%) or ultrasound (55%) guidance, and 6% in combination.

Conclusion: Both patient factors and technical aspects of ISB may impact occurrence of persistent diaphragmatic paralysis. Use of ultrasound and nerve stimulator guidance can improve accuracy and reduce associated tissue inflammation, and there should be a redoubling of efforts to ensure technical expertise with these modalities in clinical practice.

Keywords: Diaphragmatic paralysis; Interscalene nerve block

Introduction

The incidence of persistent diaphragmatic paralysis after ISB is not precisely known, however has been estimated to be one percent or less [1]. Alternatively, transient paralysis of the diaphragm after ISB due to the local anesthetic effect has been widely reported [1-3]. Early reports cite incidences approaching 100%, however with modified anesthetic regimens and use of ultrasound and/or nerve stimulators, the likelihood appears to be much lower [2-4]. Regional anesthesia experts have not been able to elucidate the cause(s) of persistent diaphragmatic paralysis, yet this rare, debilitating event remains a common topic of discussion. There has been much debate concerning the patient factors

and technical variations that may lead to diaphragmatic paralysis, but without much supporting evidence to date.

Numerous pathogenic processes may cause an insult to a peripheral nerve resulting in segmental ischemia and muscular paralysis [5]. The inciting event may be a mechanical process (i.e. compression, traction, piercing), or pharmacologic toxicity, but the pathological result is often the same-loss of the myelin sheath and/or axons resulting in a conduction delay or block, and leading to persistent muscular paralysis. In the case of the diaphragm muscle, the insult may impact the 3rd through 5th cervical roots, and/or phrenic nerves. Although diaphragmatic paralysis is easily diagnosed on chest fluoroscopy with inspiration (sniff testing) or ultrasound, the ability to localize and quantitate injury to this neural system is not possible with any current radiographic imaging modalities. Clinicians must rely instead on electro diagnostic testing [diaphragm electromyography (EMG) and phrenic nerve conduction testing (NCS)] to confirm and quantify the extent of cervical root and/or phrenic nerve damage.

Although unilateral diaphragmatic paralysis is sometimes considered a condition that is relatively well-tolerated, there are often deficits in respiratory activity and physical functioning that have major consequences as reported on quality of life surveys [6]. The literature is vague regarding whether individuals with unilateral paralysis are more susceptible to co-morbid respiratory conditions such as pneumonia or sleep disordered breathing, however it is conceivable that diminution of lung expansion as a result of the elevated diaphragmatic position has a negative impact on overall respiratory well-being.

The aim of the current study is to investigate associations between ISB and persistent diaphragmatic paralysis. The observational study design includes careful evaluation of possible patient susceptibility factors, such as pre-existing cervical spondylosis or diabetic peripheral neuropathy, as well as technical aspects of the ISB (i.e. anesthetic agent, ultrasound guidance, and type of needle used). Our goal is to enhance current knowledge regarding susceptibility and causation of this adverse event following ISB to reduce or eliminate its occurrence for regional anesthesia practitioners.

Materials and Methods

The study design matched patients with persistent diaphragmatic paralysis after ISB to patients who had ISB without complication between 2009 and 2014. Groups were matched based upon receiving ISB for upper extremity surgery and during the same time period at accredited inpatient or outpatient surgical facilities. Patients were excluded if they had pre-existing diaphragmatic paralysis or a history of exertional dyspnea.

Group I consisted of 50 consecutive patients receiving ISB without consequence at a university-based hospital and affiliated outpatient surgery center in central New Jersey (Jersey Shore University Medical Center, Neptune, NJ). Group II was comprised of 29 patients diagnosed with persistent diaphragmatic paralysis after ISB that had been performed at various inpatient and outpatient centers throughout the United States. These patients were actively seeking specialized medical care for their symptomatic condition and travelled to one of our multidisciplinary referral centers for surgical treatment (Center for Treatment of Paralysis and Reconstructive Nerve Surgery, Neptune, NJ, and Phrenic Nerve Reconstruction Program, Division of Plastic & Reconstructive Surgery, UCLA Medical Center, Los Angeles, CA). Details of phrenic nerve reconstruction for treatment of persistent diaphragmatic after ISB can be found in prior publications [7-10].

Patients in Group I did not report any early or late respiratory symptomatology following ISB, therefore there was no indication to undergo any follow-up testing for diaphragmatic paralysis. All patients in Group II underwent an extensive diagnostic evaluation to confirm and quantitate the diaphragmatic paralysis. Diagnostic testing included: chest fluoroscopy (sniff testing), pulmonary function testing, maximal inspiratory pressure assessment, electrodiagnostic evaluation (phrenic NCS & diaphragmatic EMG), MRI cervical spine, and CT neck & chest. Diagnosis of persistent diaphragmatic paralysis was made when the patient exhibited complete paralysis (or paradoxical movement) on sniff testing, and abnormal (or absent) phrenic nerve conduction and diaphragmatic motor amplitudes on electrodiagnostic assessment. Furthermore, the injury had to be present for at least 8 months without any objective or subjective improvement.

Patient demographic factors and technical aspects of the nerve block were reviewed and compared. IRB approval was obtained at our host institution and the analysis was undertaken in accordance with study approval. We analyzed the following patient factors between groups: age, sex, BMI, laterality, history of peripheral or diabetic neuropathy, prior nerve blocks (on the same side), and underlying cervical spondylosis. A co-diagnosis of cervical spondylosis was based upon patient self-reporting, diagnostic findings on cervical spine MRI, and/or a history of prior cervical spine surgery.

An assessment of technical aspects of the nerve block was obtained from operative and anesthesia reports, and included: type of surgical procedure, use of ultrasound and/or a nerve stimulator, anesthetic agent and dosing, use of epinephrine, type of needle, and application of an indwelling catheter. During chart review there were noted to be inconsistencies in the comprehensiveness of recorded information provided in anesthesia reports from different institutions, therefore missing data points are indicated in the presentation of results.

Results

In Group I there were 26 (52%) females and 24 (48%) males with an average age of 55 ± 17, whereas in Group II there were 4 (14%) females and 25 (86%) males with an average age of 58 ± 10 (Table 1). Chi-square analysis revealed significance for male sex (48% *vs.* 86%), with a significantly higher proportion of males in Group II (p<0.01). There was no difference between groups for mean BMI (Group I=36 ± 8 *vs.* Group II=30 ± 4) or laterality [Left sided injury: Group I=19 (38%) *vs.* Group II=9 (31%)].

There was no statistical difference demonstrated between Groups I and II for underlying peripheral or diabetic neuropathy (14% *vs.* 31%), whereas a history of another ipsilateral nerve block prior to the ISB (0% *vs.* 21%) and cervical spondylosis (12% *vs.* 45%) were significantly more prevalent in Group II [(p<0.01) &(p<0.01), respectively].

Shoulder arthroplasty, arthroscopy, and rotator cuff repairs were the most common surgical procedures in both Groups I (64%) and II (89%). In Group I, 22% of patients underwent total shoulder replacement, whereas in Group II this procedure was performed in 7% of patients. The remaining procedures included various musculo-tendinous and bony repairs of the hand, forearm, and upper arm.

	Group I (n=50)	Group II (n=29)
Age (mean)	55.3	58.2
Sex(#) (M/F)	24/26	25/4
BMI (mean)	36.2	20
Side(#)(L/R)	19/31	9/20

Prior block (#)	0	3
Cervical Spondylosis (%)	12	45
Diabetic Neuropathy (%)	14	7
Peripheral Neuropathy (%)	0	24

Table 1: Demographic factors and co-morbid conditions in ISB cohorts.

In Group I, 86% of patients received blocks performed with either nerve stimulator (64%) or ultrasound (22%) guidance, and 10% using both modalities (Table 2). This contrasts to 79% of the 20 patients in Group II (20/29 (69%) of anesthesia reports indicated use of technological modalities) whose blocks were performed using either nerve stimulator (24%) or ultrasound (55%) guidance, and 4% in combination. A 2-sided Fisher exact test to compare Groups in the application of at least one technological modality did not demonstrate a difference (p=0.137).

In both groups the following individual or combination agents were used to perform ISB: Bupivicaine, Lidocaine, Ropivicaine, or in combination. Ropivacaine (66%) was the most common anesthetic agent used in Group I, followed by bupivacaine (34%), whereas in Group II lidocaine (45%) was used most commonly followed by ropivacaine (24%). In 70% of Group I patients and 60% of Group II patients, 30 or 40 mL anesthetic volumes were used regardless of agents(s). Epinephrine was used in 19 patients (38%) in Group I and 7 patients (24%) in Group II. In Group I all patients received ISB with a 21 or 22-gauge Tuohy needle (B. Braun, Bethlehem, PA), whereas in the 55% of Group II anesthesia reports that indicated needle size, a 22-gauge was used in 10 patients (63%), 18-gauge in 5 patients (31%), and 20-gauge in 1 patient (6%). Indwelling catheters remained in place for post-operative pain relief in 3 patients (10%) in Group II (for an average of 2.7 ± 1.5 days) and were not used in any patients (0%) in Group I.

		Group I	Group II
Technological Guidance			(69% of reports)
No guidance (%)		4 (N=2)	15 (N=3)
Ultrasound guidance (%)		22 (N=11)	55 (N=11)
Nerve Stimulator guidance (%)		64 (N=32)	24 (N=5)
Both (%)		10 (N=5)	6 (N=1)
Anesthetic agent (%)			
	Bupivicaine	34 (N=17)	4 (N=1)
	Ropivacaine	66 (N=33)	24 (N=4)
	Lidocaine	0 (N=0)	45 (N=9)
	Other	0 (N=0)	27 (N=6)
Needle gauge, (%)			(55% of reports)
	18	0 (N=0)	31 (N=5)
	20	0 (N=0)	0 (N=0)
	21	10 (N=5)	6 (N=1)
	22	90 (N=45)	63 (N=10)
Epinephrine (%)		38 (N=19)	24 (N=4)
Indwelling catheter (#)		N=0	N=3

Table 2: Technical aspects of ISB in cohorts.

Discussion

ISB is a well-established regional anesthetic technique with demonstrated value for upper extremity surgery, particularly of the shoulder [11-14]. The safety of the procedure and the extremely low risk of adverse events have been well documented in the literature [15-17]. Critical analysis of persistent diaphragmatic paralysis after ISB, a complication that occurs infrequently, can only assist in increasing the safety profile of the technique, and ensure that practitioners optimize regional anesthetic care.

There are three questions that must be addressed in analyzing the association between persistent diaphragmatic paralysis and ISB: 1. Are there patients who may be susceptible to occurrence of this adverse event?; 2. What are the technical aspects of the block that may contribute to, or prevent this from happening?; 3. What is the pathological process that leads to persistent diaphragmatic paralysis after ISB?

Although there are limitations of this observational study (i.e. non-randomized, retrospective chart review, unmatched groups), our unique position to be able to evaluate and treat relatively large numbers of patients with persistent diaphragmatic paralysis following ISB justifies assessment with the current study design. This is especially true since the literature is absent of any sort of outcomes analysis addressing this topic and the relative rarity of the disorder makes prospective analysis quite difficult.

Our observational study focused on patient demographics and co-morbid conditions that may increase susceptibility to diaphragmatic paralysis after ISB. We found there were a significantly higher proportion of males in Group II. Although it could be suggested that ISB is more technically difficult in males due to larger body habitus, we did not find an association with increased BMI. Alternatively, it could be related to the previously established notion that males have higher rates of clinical and sub-clinical nerve compression injuries due to sports and work-related trauma [16-18].

There was also a demonstrated association between cervical spondylosis and diaphragmatic paralysis after ISB. Patients deemed to have cervical spondylosis were grouped according to diagnostic MRI findings, a history of cervical spine surgery, and/or self-reported symptoms and prior treatment. The double-crush phenomenon has been widely reported in the literature for various neuropathic conditions throughout the body, but especially as it relates to a susceptibility to carpal tunnel syndrome in patients with cervical spondylosis [19-22]. Perhaps an otherwise insignificant inflammatory process occurring around the phrenic nerve during ISB in patients with cervical spondylosis is enough to result in clinical manifestation of permanent diaphragmatic paralysis. It may be suggested that clinicians consider enhanced screening and increased selectivity during pre-operative anesthesia assessment.

Previous ISB on the same side was found to be a risk factor for persistent diaphragmatic paralysis and ISB. There is the possibility of a cumulative impact on the phrenic nerve with each successive block, ultimately leading to diaphragmatic paralysis. It has been reported in the peripheral nerve literature that repetitive insults or "mini-traumas" to a nerve can be the etiology for various compression neuropathies [23-25]. Patients being considered for ISB who have had prior blocks could be sent for phrenic NCS and diaphragmatic EMG to look for sub-clinical phrenic neuropathy. A better understanding of the pathological process would assist in confirming or refuting the notion that every ISB causes at least a minimal amount of peri-neural scar following mechanical or pharmacological induced inflammation. The pathological findings observed intra-operatively during phrenic nerve reconstruction will be discussed below.

Consistent with numerous reports in the anesthesia literature, our study findings appear to support the use of ultrasound and/or nerve stimulator guidance when performing ISB [26-29]. Stundner et al. found that ultrasound-guided ISB permitted low volume injection that

resulted in less central foraminal and aberrant spread, and extrapolated the possibility of a lower risk profile. The precise localization of nerves for accurate needle placement clearly reduces the chances of multiple needle sticks, repetitive needle passes, and improper distribution of the injected solution. Nerve stimulator guidance may also provide a means to co-localize appropriate needle placement, however this device may tend to be less specific when used alone [26]. Mejia-Terrazas et al. compared ultrasound versus neurostimulation for ISB in a prospective non-randomized study and concluded ultrasound-guided ISB is the technique of choice based upon a statistically significant difference in complication rates [29-31]. Current and future studies may address the value of EMG recording during ISB as a way to determine if there is diaphragmatic activity occurring concomitant with needle passage. Jeong et al. in a prospective randomized evaluation of patients undergoing ultrasound-guided ISB with nerve stimulation thresholds, found a lower rate of intramuscular spreading of local anesthetic at 0.2 mA versus 0.5 mA [27].

Although prior studies have analyzed the anesthetic agents, dosing regimens, and use of epinephrine for ISB, our results did not demonstrate any to be a particular risk factor for persistent diaphragmatic paralysis [32-34]. Alternatively, modified dosing regimens have been shown to reduce occurrence of transient diaphragmatic paralysis as part of the short-term anesthetic effect [35]. Furthermore, it has been reported that epinephrine has the potential to act as a neurotoxic agent [36]. Whether use of epinephrine for ISB may impart any negative consequences is unclear, however surgical practitioners use local anesthesia and epinephrine routinely in proximity to peripheral nerves without impactful clinical evidence to support otherwise [37].

Additional technical factors that were analyzed for possible association with diaphragmatic paralysis included, needle size and use of indwelling catheters. Although we did not find a significant association for either, it is reasonable to consider options expected to create the least amount of peri-neural inflammation. This may include smaller needle gauges and being very selective in whom post-operative catheters are placed.

It is most difficult to address the third question regarding the exact pathological process following ISB that results in persistent diaphragmatic paralysis. Many theories abound, everything from the phrenic nerve being "pierced" by the needle, to inflammation in adjacent tissues that leads to phrenic nerve compression, and even that paralysis occurs not from ISB at all, but rather from patient positioning or a traction injury during the surgical procedure [38].

Although we may never completely know the exact mechanism, it is possible to comment on the intra-operative findings from performing phrenic nerve reconstruction on numerous patients with this condition. In the majority of patients treated, there has been a consistent finding of nerve degeneration at the C5 root contribution to the phrenic nerve along the posterior portion of the anterior scalene muscle (Figure 1).

Whereas both the proximal and distal portions along this neuraxis typically appear to be of good integrity, the involved segment is narrowed in caliber and exhibits an orange hue, a clear indication of myelin sheath loss and axonal degeneration. Commonly, there are dense fascial and vascular adhesions in the region that encompass the phrenic nerve, findings that also support a compression neuropathy (Figure 2).

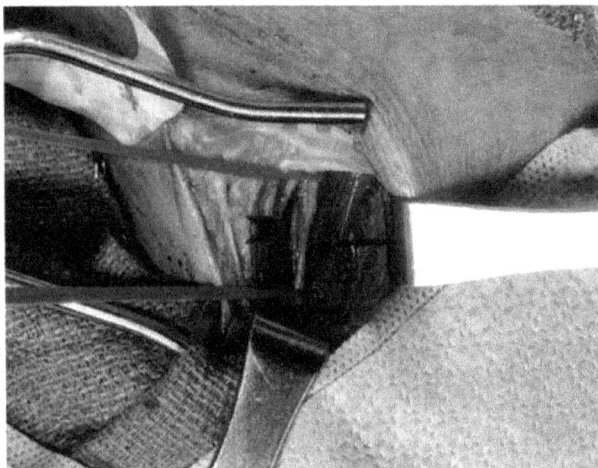

Figure 1: Atrophic segment of the phrenic nerve (arrow) at the C5 root (arrowhead) contribution along the posterior portion of the anterior scalene muscle. The proximal and distal loops are on relatively normal appearing phrenic nerve.

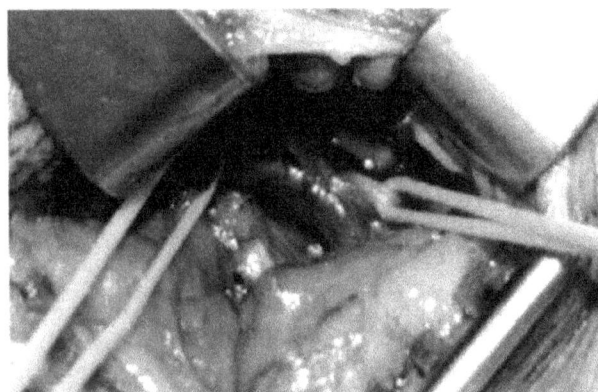

Figure 2: Perineural fibrosis and adhesions encompassing the phrenic nerve (loops proximal and distal to adhesions).

Given these findings, it certainly appears that inflammation plays a role in the nerve pathology, especially in susceptible patients. Thus, every effort should be made to limit the inflammatory process during ISB. This may include any or all of the following: ultrasound and/or nerve stimulator guidance, smaller gauge needle, maximum number of allowed needle sticks or passes, limited use of indwelling catheters, and pre-operative steroids. Future studies should compare the possible clinical benefits (versus cost) of implementing additional screening measures (i.e. MRI cervical spine, phrenic NCS & diaphragmatic EMG) for "at risk" patients.

References

1. [No authors listed] (1992) American Academy of Pediatrics Committee on Drugs: Guidelines for monitoring and management of pediatric patients during and after sedation for diagnostic and therapeutic procedures. Pediatrics 89: 1110-1115.

2. Asahi Y, Kubota K, Omichi S (2009) Dose requirements for propofol anaesthesia for dental treatment for autistic patients compared with intellectually impaired patients. Anaesth Intensive Care 37: 70-73.

3. Buggy DJ, Nicol B, Rowbotham DJ, Lambert DG (2000) Effects of intravenous anesthetic agents on glutamate release: a role for GABAA receptor-mediated inhibition. Anesthesiology 92: 1067-1073.

4. Cressey DM, Claydon P, Bhaskaran NC, Reilly CS (2001) Effect of midazolam pretreatment on induction dose requirements of propofol in combination with fentanyl in younger and older adults. Anaesthesia 56: 108-113.

5. Dalal PG, Murray D, Cox T, McAllister J, Snider R (2006) Sedation and anesthesia protocols used for magnetic resonance imaging studies in infants: provider and pharmacologic considerations. Anesth Analg 103: 863-888.

6. Daskalopoulos R, Korcok J, Farhangkhgoee P, Karmazyn M, Gelb AW, et al. (2001) Propofol protection of sodium-hydrogen exchange activity sustains glutamate uptake during oxidative stress. Anesth Analg 93: 1199-1204.

7. Eaves RC, Milner B (1993) The criterion-related validity of the Childhood Autism Rating Scale and the Autism Behavior Checklist. J Abnorm Child Psychol 21: 481-491.

8. Eggermont JJ, Don M (1986) Mechanisms of central conduction time prolongation in brain-stem auditory evoked potentials. Arch Neurol 43: 116-120.

9. Fein D, Skoff B, Mirsky AF (1981) Clinical correlates of brainstem dysfunction in autistic children. J Autism Dev Disord 11: 303-315.

10. Fodale V, Pratico C, Santamaria LB (2004) Coadministration of propofol and midazolam decreases bispectral index value as a result of synergic muscle relaxant action on the motor system. Anesthesiology 101: 799.

11. Gillberg C, Rosenhall U, Johansson E (1983) Auditory brainstem responses in childhood psychosis. J Autism Dev Disord 13: 181-195.

12. Gomot M, Giard MH, Adrien JL, Barthelemy C, Bruneau N (2002) Hypersensitivity to acoustic change in children with autism: electrophysiological evidence of left frontal cortex dysfunctioning. Psychophysiology 39: 577-584.

13. Hadjikhani N, Joseph RM, Snyder J, Tager-Flusberg H (2006) Anatomical differences in the mirror neuron system and social cognition network in autism. Cereb Cortex 16: 1276-1282.

14. Herbert MR (2005) Large brains in autism: the challenge of pervasive abnormality. Neuroscientist 11: 417-440.

15. Hosey MT, Makin A, Jones RM, Gilchrist F, Carruthers M (2004) Propofol intravenous conscious sedation for anxious children in a specialist paediatric dentistry unit. Int J Paediatr Dent 14: 2-8.

16. Just MA, Cherkassky VL, Keller TA, Kana RK, Minshew NJ (2007) Functional and anatomical cortical underconnectivity in autism: evidence from an FMRI study of an executive function task and corpus callosum morphometry. Cereb Cortex 17: 951-961.

17. Kitt E Friderici J, Kleppel R, Canarie M (2015) Procedural sedation for MRI in children with ADHD. Paediatr Anaesth 25: 1026-1032.

18. Klin A, Pauls D, Schultz R, Volkmar F (2005) Three diagnostic approaches to Asperger syndrome: implications for research. J Autism Dev Disord 35: 221-234.

19. Leitch JA, Anderson K, Gambhir S, Millar K, Robb ND, et al. (2004) A partially blinded randomised controlled trial of patient-maintained propofol sedation and operator controlled midazolam sedation in third molar extractions. Anaesthesia 59: 853-860.

20. Leung AK, Kao CP (1999) Evaluation and management of the child with speech delay. Am Fam Physician 59: 3121-3128.

21. Ma DQ, Whitehead PL, Menold MM, Martin ER, Ashley-Koch AE, et al. (2005) Identification of significant association and gene-gene interaction of GABA receptor subunit genes in autism. Am J Hum Genet 77: 377-388.

22. Matschke RG, Stenzel C, Plath P, Zilles K (1994) Maturational aspects of the human auditory pathway: anatomical and electrophysiological findings. ORL J Otorhinolaryngol Relat Spec 56: 68-72.

23. McClelland RJ, Eyre DG, Watson D, Calvert GJ, Sherrard E (1992) Central conduction time in childhood autism. Br J Psychiatry 160: 659-663.

24. Miyawaki T, Kohjitani A, Maeda S, Egusa M, Mori T, et al. (2004) Intravenous sedation for dental patients with intellectual disability. J Intellect Disabil Res 48: 764-768.

25. Norrix LW, Trepanier S, Atlas M, Kim D (2012) The auditory brainstem response: latencies obtained in children while under general anesthesia. J Am Acad Audiol 23: 57-63.

26. Paspatis GA, Charoniti I, Manolaraki M, Vardas E, Papanikolaou N, et al. (2006) Synergistic sedation with oral midazolam as a premedication and intravenous propofol versus intravenous propofol alone in upper gastrointestinal endoscopies in children: a prospective, randomized study. J Pediatr Gastroenterol Nutr 43: 195-199.

27. Rainey L, van der Walt JH (1998) The anaesthetic management of autistic children. Anaesth Intensive Care 26: 682-686.

28. Ramsay MA, Savege TM, Simpson BR, Goodwin R (1974) Controlled sedation with alphaxalone-alphadolone. Br Med J 2: 656-659.

29. Schopler E, Reichler RJ, DeVellis RF, Daly K (1980) Toward objective classification of childhood autism: Childhood Autism Rating Scale (CARS). J Autism Dev Disord 10: 91-103.

30. Sebel LE, Richardson JE, Singh SP, Bell SV, Jenkins A (2006) Additive effects of sevoflurane and propofol on gamma-aminobutyric acid receptor function. Anesthesiology 104: 1176-1183.

31. Shinohe A, Hashimoto K, Nakamura K, Tsujii M, Iwata Y, et al. (2006) Increased serum levels of glutamate in adult patients with autism. Prog Neuropsychopharmacol Biol Psychiatry 30: 1472-1477.

32. Sitar SM, Hanifi-Moghaddam P, Gelb A, Cechetto DF, Siushansian R, et al. (1999) Propofol prevents peroxide-induced inhibition of glutamate transport in cultured astrocytes. Anesthesiology 90: 1446-1453.

33. Stephens AJ, Sapsford DJ, Curzon ME (1993) Intravenous sedation for handicapped dental patients: a clinical trial of midazolam and propofol. Br Dent J 175: 20-25.

34. Wakasugi M, Hirota K, Roth SH, Ito Y (1999) The effects of general anesthetics on excitatory and inhibitory synaptic transmission in area CA1 of the rat hippocampus in vitro. Anesth Analg 88: 676-680.

35. Westphalen RI, Hemmings HC (2003) Selective depression by general anesthetics of glutamate versus GABA release from isolated cortical nerve terminals. J Pharmacol Exp Ther 304: 1188-1196.

36. Yu ZY, Wang W, Fritschy JM, Witte OW, Redecker C (2006) Changes in neocortical and hippocampal GABAA receptor subunit distribution during brain maturation and aging. Brain Res 1099: 73-81.

10

Percutaneous Nephrolithotomy under Thoracic Paravertebral Block: A Preliminary Report

Doaa G Ahmed[1]*, Diab Fuad Hetta[1] and Abdelraouf M S Abdelraouf[2]

[1]*Department of Anesthesia and Pain Management, South Egypt Cancer Institute, Assuit University, Egypt*

[2]*Department of Anaesthesia and Critical Care, Assuit University, Egypt*

*__Corresponding author:__ Doaa Gomaa Sayed, Department of Anesthesiology and Pain Management, South Egypt Cancer Institute, Assiut University, Egypt, E-mail: doaagomaa78@yahoo.com

Abstract

Background: The second look percutaneous nephrolithotomy (PCNL) is usually done under general anesthesia. Thoracic paravertebral block has been shown to provide sufficient postoperative analgesia for a variety of thoracic and upper abdominal surgeries.

Objectives: We propose a case series study for performing the second look PCNL under paravertebral block (PVB) and conscious sedation using dexmedetomidine.

Methods: 33 patients scheduled for second look PCNL received PVB at the level of T 11, 15 ml of 0.5 % of bupivacaine was injected under ultrasonographic guidance. During the procedure, the patients received conscious sedation with dexmedetomidine (initial infusion of 1 µg/kg/h, followed by a maintenance infusion of 0.2 µg/kg/h). We measured the rate of success of the anesthetic technique, the level of sedation and hemodynamics. The time to complete recovery using (MPADSS), postoperative paracetamol consumption and postoperative intensity of pain using VAS.

Results: the anesthetic technique was satisfactory in 30 patients. The median (IQ) patient's satisfaction with the anesthetic technique was 6 (6:7). The median (IQ) surgeon's satisfaction with the anesthetic technique was 7 (6:7). Complete recovery from sedation using the modified post anesthesia discharge scoring system (time to score 10) was achieved within 40 (30:52.5) min. The mean MAP and heart rate were significantly decreased in comparison to baseline value.

Conclusion: We concluded that the anesthetic technique with PVB and conscious sedation with dexmedetomidine for patients undergoing second look PCN provided sufficient sedation, adequate analgesia, minimal side effects, and rapid recovery.

Keywords: PCNL; PVB; Dexmedetomidine

Introduction

The incidence and prevalence of urolithiasis are globally increasing [1] and is considered a major healthcare concern that affects approximately 10% of the American population. [2] Percutaneous nephrolithotomy (PCNL) is currently the gold standard for treatment of patients with renal stones as it is less invasive than open surgery and is generally associated with lower morbidity and faster recovery [3].

PCNL is a percutaneous extraction of renal stone >2 cm with a nephroscope, through a small incision, in the patient's back on the side overlying the affected kidney. It is usually done under general anesthesia and sometimes neuraxial anesthesia [4-6].

Unfortunately, missed stones after PCNL are not uncommon [7]. According to the size of the remained stone, it could be managed by ESWL or if it is larger enough, it should be picked up through another session of PCNL what is called "a second look PCNL". Anesthetic management for a second look PCNL ranges from intravenous sedation for a small stone that can be extracted easily by dormia basket to general anesthesia for larger stones that needs further disintegration. Indeed, re-exposure to general anesthesia for second look PCNL especially in prone position has its own hazards [4]. While many of the issues related to positioning are resolved with neuraxial anesthesia, hypotension is still a major concern [6].

Thoracic paravertebral block has been shown to provide sufficient postoperative analgesia for a variety of thoracic and upper abdominal surgeries [8-14].

The aim of this study is to provide alternative anesthetic technique other than general and neuraxial anesthesia for patients undergoing a second look PCNL that is paravertebral block and conscious sedation using dexmedetomidine.

Methods

The ethical committee of the faculty of medicine, Assuit University approved a feasibility study in 33 patients (IRB NO; IRB0008718) who gave written informed consent for the procedure and the study.

The inclusion criteria included patients, classified as American Society of Anesthesiologists (ASA) physical status class I and II, aged 20 to 70 years and scheduled for second look PCNL for removal of residual renal stones that needs disintegration, (multiple stones or solitary stone >2 mm). The exclusion criteria included patients with mental dysfunction, morbid obesity, a history of substance abuse, chronic analgesic use, and a history of allergy to the study drugs.

During the preoperative visit, it was made very clear to all patients that any pain, discomfort, or anxiety would be dealt with, immediately by the administration, on their request, of a potent analgesic or, if they preferred, conversion to general anesthesia. Similarly, the surgeons were instructed to ask for general anesthesia if they felt that the anesthetic technique was adding to the technical difficulty of the procedure. Also, the patients were instructed how to evaluate their pain intensity using VAS (visual analogue scale) scored from 0 to 10 where 0=no pain and 10=worst pain imaginable.

On arrival to the preoperative room, an IV catheter was inserted and a baseline measurement of vital signs was recorded.

The PVB was performed under ultrasonographic guidance in the sitting position. Surgical disinfection of thoracoabdominal paravertebral area was done. A linear high-frequency transducer (10-12 MHz, Sonosite, Bothell, WA, USA) was used. The scanning process (Longitudinal out-of-plane technique) was started at 5-10 cm lateral to the spinous process of T11 to identify the rounded ribs and parietal pleura underneath. The transducer is then moved progressively more medially until the transverse processes are identified as more squared structure deeper to the ribs. Once the transverse processes were identified, skin infiltration with 2 ml of 1% lidocaine was done. A 100 mm needle (Stimuplex D, B Braun, Melsungen AG, Germany) was inserted out-of-plane to contact the transverse process of T11 and then, walked off above the transverse process 1-1.5 cm deeper searching for loss of resistance injecting 15 ml of 0.5% bupivacaine in incremental doses of 5 ml. This will result in a displacement of the parietal pleura. Test of the block was done by pinprick examination every 3 min in the ipsilateral flank area in comparison to the other side. Failure to obtain loss of pinprick sensation within 20 min was considered a failed block. After confirmation of the success of the block, the patient was transferred to the operating room, monitoring probes were attached, the patient was turned to the prone position and conscious sedation was started. To minimize variations in the technique, all the blocks were done by the same experienced investigator. Conscious sedation entailed IV administration of dexmedetomidine, infused initially over 10 min at 1 µg/kg/h, maintained at 0.2 µg/kg/h and manipulated to keep the sedation level, assessed by the modified observer of alertness and sedation (OAA/S) scale at level 3.

During the procedure, if SpO_2 was ≤ 90%, bradycardia (HR<50 beat/min), and hypotension (MAP<50 mmHg), 4 L/min of oxygen was supplemented *via* a nasal cannula, IV 0.01 mg/kg atropine was administered, and IV 6 mg ephedrine was given, respectively.

10 minutes following the beginning of dexmedetomidine infusion and after reaching the conscious sedation state, the technique of PCNL was started by cutting the nephrostomy tube at the skin level, a guide wire is inserted in the collecting system, the remaining part of nephrostomy tube is taken off, a nephroscope is passed alongside the guide wire and the process of disintegration is started.

If the patient complained of pain (VAS>3) or discomfort, we administered IV 50 µ fentanyl boluses, if the problem is not resolved,

the patient is turned supine and received general anesthesia with endotracheal intubation and we reported it as failed anesthetic technique.

After the end of the procedure, all the patients were admitted to the post-anaesthesia care unit (PACU) for one day follow up. Patients' satisfaction with sedation and analgesia was performed after recovery from sedation, also the surgeons were asked to rate their satisfaction with patient sedation at the end of surgery.

Postoperative analgesia consisted of 1 gm. Paracetamol infusion once requested by the patients. The limiting dose was 4 g/day. If the patient was still complaining of pain, 0.1 mg/kg nalbuphine was administered. All postoperative data was reported by a nurse blinded to the study protocol.

The following parameters have been assessed.

- The intensity of pain using VAS measured postoperatively at the following time points, 0 h, 2 h, 4 h, 6 h, 10 h, 16 h and 24 h.
- The vital signs including MAP and heart rate measured immediately before dexmedetomidine infusion and each five minutes till end of the procedure and postoperatively at the following time points, 30 min, 60 min and 90 min. SpO_2 less than 90% during the procedure and till 90 min postoperatively is recorded
- The level of sedation using the modified observer of alertness and sedation (OAA/S) scale, assessed every five minutes intraoperatively and at 30 min, 60 min and 90 min postoperatively.
- The level of recovery from sedation was studied using the modified post anesthesia discharge scoring system (MPADSS) [15]. Time to reach a score of 10 was reported.
- The level of satisfaction of the patients and the surgeons with the procedure assessed by Likert-like verbal rating scale, where: Extremely dissatisfied=1. Dissatisfied=2. Somewhat dissatisfied=3. Undecided=4. Somewhat satisfied=5. Satisfied=6. Extremely Satisfied=7
- The time to first analgesic request and the first 24 h analgesic consumption were recorded.

Statistical analysis

Statistical analysis was carried out on a personal computer using SPSS version 20 software. Normally distributed data was expressed as mean ± SD, where categorical and skewed data were expressed as median ± (IQ) range. Comparison of VAS pain score at each time point was compared with baseline using student's t test.

Results

33 patients were recruited for second look PCNL under PVB and conscious sedation with dexmedetomidine, the demographic data of the patients are shown in (Table 1), the procedure was successful in 30 patients, one patient is excluded due to block failure and another 2 patients are excluded due to intraoperative pain necessitating IV fentanyl administration (200 µ).

The median (IQ) patient's satisfaction with the anesthetic technique was 6 (6:7). The median (IQ) surgeon's satisfaction with the anesthetic technique was 7 (6:7), (Table 2). The level of sedation assessed by OAA/S score was maintained at the level 3 most of the time during the procedure and returned to level 5 within 30 min postoperatively (Figure 1).

Variable	Value
Age (year)	36 ± 7
Sex, M/F	18/12
BMI (kg/m2)	25 (20-30)
ASA grade, I/II	27/3

BMI: Body Mass Index; ASA: American Society of Anesthesiologists; M/F: Male/Female

Table 1: Demographic data and patients characteristics.

Variable		Value
Operative duration (min) (mean ± SD)		46 ± 5.5 (35-50)
Failed anesthetic technique (n)		3
	Failed block (n)	1
	Patient received fentanyl (n)	2
	Patient received general anesthesia (n)	0
Patient satisfaction score, median (IQ)		6 (6:7)
Surgeon satisfaction score, median (IQ)		7 (6:7)
Time to aldrete score 10, (min), median (IQ)		40 (30:52.5)

Table 2: Procedure characteristics and overall satisfaction.

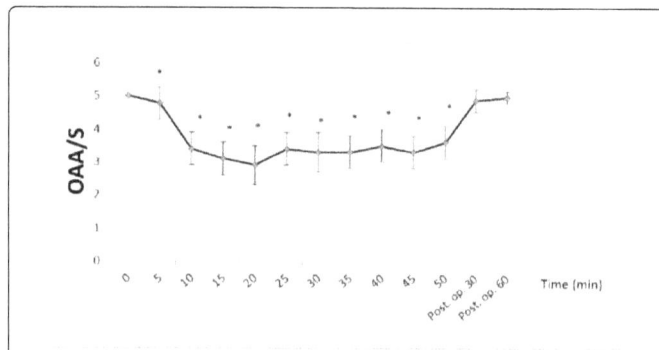

Figure 1: A line graph of Observer's Assessment Alertness/Sedation (OAA/S) values at baseline and during PCNL procedure. Data are expressed as mean ± SD. *=P<0.05, considered statistically significant in comparison to the base line value using t-test.

Complete recovery from sedation (time to score 10) was achieved within 40 (30:52.5) min (Table 2). The mean MAP was significantly decreased in comparison to baseline value starting from 5 min after initial infusion of dexmedetomidine till the end of the procedure while no significant reduction was observed at the following time points 30, 60 and 90 min postoperatively (Figure 2).

None of the patients developed severe hypotension (mean BP<50 mmHg) necessitating treatment. The mean heart rate was significantly decreased in comparison to baseline value starting from 5 min after

initial infusion of dexmedetomidine till 30 min postoperatively, while no significant reduction was observed at the following time points 60 and 90 min postoperatively (Figure 2).

Two patients developed bradycardia and successfully treated with atropine. Two patients developed oxygen desaturation (SpO$_2$<90%) and successfully managed with nasal oxygen administration (Table 3). The patients required analgesic (paracetamol) in the first 24 h postoperatively were 8 (26.7 %) (Table 4).

Variable	Value
Hypotension (mean BP<50) (n) %	0`
Bradycardia (pulse<50) (n) %	2 (6.67)
Oxygen desaturation (SpO2<90%) (n) %	2 (6.67)
Dry mouth (n) %	6 (20%)
Nausea (n) %	3 (10 %)
Vomiting (n) %	1 (3.33%)

Table 3: Adverse events.

Variable		Value
VAS 0 h		1 (0:1)
VAS 2 h		1 (1:2)
VAS 4 h		2 (1:2)
VAS 6 h		2 (1:2)
VAS 10 h		2 (2:2)
VAS 16 h		2 (1:3)
VAS 24 h		2 (2:3)
Patients required analgesic in 24 h (n)		8/30 (26.7 %)
	Patients consumed paracetamol, 1 gm (n)	7
	Patients consumed paracetamol, 2 gm (n)	1
	Patients consumed nalbuphine (n)	0
Time to first analgesic request (h)		15 ± 3.9 (6-18)

Table 4: Postoperative analgesia.

Discussion

The present study showed that anesthesia with thoracic PVB and conscious sedation for patients undergoing a second look PCNL is a reasonable and a safe alternative to general or neuraxial anesthesia.

In this study, we enrolled the patients scheduled for a second look PCNL as the primary PCNL necessitates cystoscopy for ureteric catheterization, which could not be covered by unilateral PVB. Thoracic PVB has been introduced in anesthesia practice for postoperative analgesia. Few case reports described it as a sole anesthetic technique for patients with multiple comorbidities undergoing mastectomy (Figure 2) [16,17].

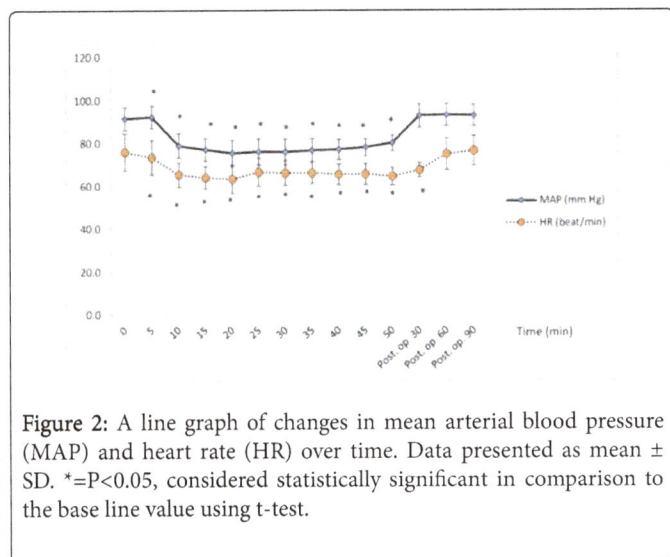

Figure 2: A line graph of changes in mean arterial blood pressure (MAP) and heart rate (HR) over time. Data presented as mean ± SD. *=P<0.05, considered statistically significant in comparison to the base line value using t-test.

Thoracic paravertebral block has been shown to be a proven technique to provide sufficient postoperative analgesia for a variety of thoracic and upper abdominal surgeries [8-11].

Although PCNL can be done under spinal or epidural anesthesia, they carry their own drawbacks (which can be avoided by using PVB) that include, hypotension especially after positioning the patient prone (due to sympathetic blockade) which necessitates fluid administration added to the irrigation fluids with subsequent electrolyte imbalance and subsequent increased perioperative shivering, the surgeon may not feel comfortable in making skin punctures, especially those close to the 11th rib, patient discomfort increases with increased duration of the procedure and they carry the risks of post-dural puncture headache (PDPH) and neurological complications [6].

The thoracic paravertebral space has been illustrated as a wedge-shaped area, the parietal pleura resembles its anterior boundary and the postero-lateral aspect of the vertebra, the intervertebral foramen, and the intervertebral disc resemble its medial boundary, posteriorly it is bounded by the superior costotransverse ligament and inferiorly by the origin of the psoas major muscle limiting the caudal extension of local anesthetic [18-20].

In the present study, we performed PVB under ultrasonographic guidance as the classic, blind landmark technique [21] has an overall failure rate of 10% and pleural puncture of 1.1%. [22] We reported only one case of failed block that could be attributed to injection anterior to endothoracic fascia which is not visible by ultrasonography making contact with injected local anesthetic is unlikely.

We administered 15 ml of 0.5% bupivacaine as a single injection at the level of T 11 and were successful in nearly all cases. Cheema and colleagues injected 15 ml of bupivacaine 0.5% in thoracic PVB and resulted in somatic block of at least five dermatomes and a sympathetic block of eight dermatomes [13], thus, we believe that multilevel injections would unnecessarily expose patients to additional risks related to multiple punctures.

The pain signals of renal origin travel through afferent Aδ and C sympathetic fibers on the adventitia of the renal arteries, reaching the renal and intermesenteric plexus, then pass through the lowest splanchnic nerve, to enter the spinal cord *via* T11 - L2 dorsal roots and finally relay on the medial medullary reticular formation [23].

The mechanism of action of anesthesia and analgesia produced by PVB is most probably due to direct penetration of LA into the spinal nerves contained within the PV space, where they lack their coverings, except of a thin layer which is easily and efficiently blocked [24]. Also, block of thoracic sympathetic ganglia relieves visceral pain arising from the kidney.

More than two thirds of our patients do not require supplemental postoperative analgesia at all, reflecting the efficiency of PVB facilitated by IV dexmedetomidine administration. It deserves mentioning, PCNL is a moderately painful procedure as it is performed percutaneously (no major tissue destruction).

Our choice of dexmedetomidine as a conscious sedative is due to its unique sedation without affection of respiration [25], which is of specific importance for operations in the prone position, in addition to its analgesic-sparing effect, which markedly reduced perioperative opioid consumption [26]. In the present study, only two patients developed oxygen desaturation less than 90% and corrected easily by supplemental oxygen administration through a nasal cannula.

The reduction in hemodynamics in comparison to the baseline values observed in the current study was in concordance with previous studies used dexmedetomidine [27]. Only two cases developed bradycardia and readily reversed with atropine. This is explained by the activation of presynaptic α2-adrenoceptors on sympathetic nerves and in the central nervous system leading to a reduction of sympathetic outflow [28].

Future studies using PVB and conscious sedation with dexmedetomidine for more painful surgery, like open nephrolithotomy or nephrectomy are suggested.

The study is limited by the small sample size, the observation period is limited only to 24 h postoperatively and no comparison has yet been made with other regional or general anesthetic technique for such procedure.

Conclusion

We concluded that the anesthetic technique with PVB and conscious sedation with dexmedetomidine for patients undergoing second look PCN provided sufficient sedation, adequate analgesia, minimal side effects, and rapid recovery.

Funding

None

References

1. Knoll T, Schubert AB, Fahlenkamp D, Leusmann DB, Wendt-Nordahl G, et al. (2011) Urolithiasis through the ages: data on more than 200,000 urinary stone analyses. J Urol 185: 1304-1311.

2. Scales CJ, Smith AC, Hanley JM, Saigal CS (2012) Prevalence of kidney stones in the United States. Eur Urol 62: 160-165.

3. Antonelli JA, Pearle MS (2013) Advances in percutaneous nephrolithotomy. Urol Clin North Am 40: 99-113.

4. Movasseghi G, Hassani V, Mohaghegh MR, Safaeian R, Safari S, et al. (2014) Comparison between spinal and general anesthesia in percutaneous nephrolithotomy. Anesth Pain Med 4: e13871.

5. Cicek T, Gonulalan U, Dogan R, Kosan M, Istanbulluoglu O, et al. (2014) Spinal anesthesia is an efficient and safe anesthetic method for percutaneous nephrolithotomy. Urology 83: 50-55.

6. Mehrabi S, Karimzadeh Shirazi K (2010) Results and complications of spinal anesthesia in percutaneous nephrolithotomy. Urol J 7: 22-25.

7. Antonelli JA, Pearle MS (2013) Advances in percutaneous nephrolithotomy. Urol Clin North Am 40: 99-113.

8. Richardson J, Sabanathan S, Jones J, Shah RD, Cheema S, et al. (1999) A prospective, randomized comparison of preoperative and continuous balanced epidural or paravertebral bupivacaine on post-thoracotomy pain, pulmonary function and stress responses. Br J Anaesth 83: 387-392.

9. Davies RG, Myles PS, Graham JM (2006) A comparison of the analgesic efficacy and side-effects of paravertebral vs. epidural blockade for thoracotomy-a systematic review and meta-analysis of randomized trials. Br J Anaesth 96: 418-426.

10. Baik JS, Oh AY, Cho CW, Shin HJ, Han SH, et al. (2014) Thoracic paravertebral block for nephrectomy: a randomized, controlled, observer-blinded study. Pain Med 15: 850-856.

11. Klein SM, Bergh A, Steele SM, Georgiade GS, Greengrass RA (2000) Thoracic paravertebral block for breast surgery. Anesth Analg 90: 1402-1405.

12. Saito T, Gallagher ET, Cutler S, Tanuma K, Yamada K, et al. (1996) Extended unilateral anesthesia. New technique or paravertebral anesthesia? Reg Anesth 21: 304-307.

13. Cheema SP, Ilsley D, Richardson J, Sabanathan S (1995) A thermographic study of paravertebral analgesia. Anaesthesia 50: 118-121.

14. Gilbert J, Hultman J (1989) Thoracic paravertebral block: a method of pain control. Acta Anaesthesiol Scand 33: 142-145.

15. Chung F (1995) Discharge criteria-a new trend. Can J Anaesth 42: 1056-1058.

16. Oguz S, Kucuk C, Eskicirak E, Akaltan A, Kuru N, et al. (2007) Thoracic paravertebral block for breast surgery in a patient with myasthenia gravis. J Anesth 21: 449.

17. Mozanski MM, Rustecki B, Kalicki B, Jung A (2015) Thermal imaging evaluation of paravertebral block for mastectomy in high risk patient: case report. J Clin Monit Comput 29: 297-299.

18. Cowie B, McGlade D, Ivanusic J, Barrington MJ (2010) Ultrasound-guided thoracic paravertebral blockade: a cadaveric study. Anesth Analg 110: 1735-1739.

19. Richardson J, Lonnqvist PA (1998) Thoracic paravertebral block. Br J Anaesth 81: 230-238.

20. Lonnqvist PA, Hildingsson U (1992) The caudal boundary of the thoracic paravertebral space. A study in human cadavers. Anaesthesia 47: 1051-1052.

21. Eason MJ, Wyatt R (1979) Paravertebral thoracic block-a reappraisal. Anaesthesia 34: 638-642.

22. Lonnqvist PA, MacKenzie J, Soni AK, Conacher ID (1995) Paravertebral blockade. Failure rate and complications. Anaesthesia 50: 813-815.

23. Saito T, Den S, Cheema SPS, Tanuma K, Carney E, et al. (2001) A single-injection, multisegmental paravertebral block extension of somatosensory and sympathetic block in volunteers. Acta Anaesthesiol Scand 45: 30-33.

24. Ammons WS (1992) Bowditch Lecture. Renal afferent inputs to ascending spinal pathways. Am J Physiol 262: R165-176.

25. Kenan Kaygusuz k, Gokce G, Gursoy S, Ayan S, Mimaroglu C, et al. (2008) A comparison of sedation with dexmedetomidine or propofol during shockwave lithotripsy: A randomized controlled trial. Anesth Analg 106: 114-119.

26. Karmakar MK (2001) Thoracic paravertebral block. Anesthesiology 95: 771-780.

27. Herr DL, Sum-Ping STJ, England M (2003) ICU sedation after coronary artery bypass graft surgery: dexmedetomidine-based versus propofol-based sedation regimens. J Cardiothorac Vasc Anesth 17: 576-184.

28. Hoy SM, Keating GM (2011) Dexmedetomidine: a review of its use for sedation in mechanically ventilated patients in an intensive care setting and for procedural sedation. Drugs 71: 1481-1501.

11

POSSUM and P-POSSUM: Predictors of Morbidity and Mortality in Laparoscopic Roux-En-Y Gastric Bypass?

Daniela Pinho[1], Sílvia Pinho[1], Marta Carvalho[1], Maria Soares[1], Carla Cavaleiro[1] and Humberto S Machado[1,2*]

[1]Servico de Anesthesiologia, Centro Hospitalar do Porto, Portugal

[2]Instituto de Ciências Biomédicas Abel Salazar, Portugal

*Corresponding author: Humberto S Machado, Serviço de Anesthesiologia, Centro Hospitalar do Porto, Portugal Largo Prof. Abel Salazar, 4099-001 Porto, Portugal, E-mail: hjs.machado@gmail.com

Abstract

Background: Evidence to support the use of Physiological and Operative Severity Score for the enumeration of Mortality and morbidity (POSSUM) and Portsmouth-POSSUM (P-POSSUM) to predict outcomes in bariatric surgery is sparse.

Objectives: The aim of this study is prospectively evaluate their usefulness in laparoscopic gastric bypass.

Setting: University Hospital

Methods: All patients undergoing primary laparoscopic gastric bypass between November/14 and September/15 in our institution were included. POSSUM and P-POSSUM scores were applied preoperatively. The observed to expect ratios for morbidity and mortality at 30 days after surgery were calculated. Chi-square and binomial tests were used to compare observed and expected outcomes. A p-value <0.05 was considered significant.

Results: Ninety-four patients (76 female) were included, mean age of 45.5years, 66 patients were ASA 2. Mean BMI was 43.9Kg/m^2. Estimated morbidity by POSSUM score was 24.1%. Estimated mortality was 4.4% by POSSUM, 1.0% by P-POSSUM. Observed morbidity was 23.4%. No patient died. Both scores resulted in over predicted outcomes. In contrast to P-POSSUM, POSSUM expected outcomes were statistically different from the ones observed.

Conclusion: POSSUM was not a good predictor of morbidity and mortality in the sample. The use of these scores in bariatric surgery has to be careful. These results should be assessed further in larger, multicenter, studies.

Keywords: Obesity; Morbidity; POSSUM; P-POSSUM; Laparoscopic Gastric Bypass

Introduction

Obesity is currently considered a serious public health problem. In 2008, the World Health Organization (WHO) estimated that, globally, there were more than 1.4 billion overweight adults, which represents more than 10% of the world population [1]. Worldwide there has been a significant increase in the number of obese patients undergoing bariatric surgical interventions.

Laparoscopic Roux-en-Y gastric bypass (LRYGB) has a very low incidence of mortality. Although it presents a low morbidity incidence, the large number of surgeries performed every year makes this outcome an important issue to take into account in anesthetic and surgical planning. Young et al. found a 30 day mortality of 0.15% and an incidence of serious morbidity of 5.8% in a review of 19 172 patients, submitted to laparoscopic gastric bypass [2].

Preoperative prediction of the risk of complications is a key instrument for the best intraoperative and immediate postoperative anesthetic planning. This can also be used to audit the quality of care provided to patients.

In a recent systematic review, Moonesinghe et al. showed that, of 34 postoperative risk stratification tools, POSSUM score (Physiological and Operative Severity Score for the Enumeration of Mortality and morbidity) is one of the most credible to predict morbidity and mortality in the postoperative period [3].

POSSUM score, described by Copeland et al. (1991), is a system based on 12 physiological (age, Glasgow Coma Score, hemoglobin concentration, white cell count, serum sodium, potassium and urea concentrations, heart rate, systolic blood pressure, respiratory and cardiac co-morbidities, electrocardiographic abnormalities) and six operative variables (operative severity, degree of cancer spread, peritoneal soiling, number of procedures required, blood loss and urgency of surgery) that estimate the risk of mortality and morbidity at 30 days after surgery (Table 1) [4].

This score differs from others risk stratification tools because it also includes variables related to the surgical procedure. Each variable is sub-divided into three or four levels with different severities, weighted to a value of 1, 2, 4 or 8. The physiological parameters are taken at the time of surgery. The inclusion of operative values precludes its use in the preoperative setting.

Physiological Parameters	Operative parameters
Age	Operative magnitude, number of procedures, timing of operation
Cardiac and respiratory signs, electrocardiographic findings	Blood loss
Systolic arterial pressure, heart rate	Peritoneal contamination
Glasgow Coma Scale	Presence of malignancy
Urea, sodium, potassium	
Hemoglobin, white cell count	
POSSUM - Physiological and Operative Severity Score for the enUmeration of Mortality and morbidity; P-POSSUM - Porthmouth-POSSUM.	

Table 1: Variables included in the determination of morbidity and mortality by scores POSSUM and P- POSSUM.

Several studies have shown that POSSUM overestimates morbidity mainly in low-risk patients [5-7]. P-POSSUM (Portsmouth-POSSUM) uses the same variables but estimates the risk of postoperative mortality through a linear regression model, increasing its predictive value [7-9]. However, it is not validated to estimate morbidity and has some limitations like the underestimation of mortality in the elderly and in emergent procedures [5]. Both scores were already validated for colorectal (CR-POSSUM), vascular (V-POSSUM) and gastroesophageal (O-POSSUM) surgeries [10].

There is a small number of studies looking at risk assessment scores for bariatric surgery, and all of them have important limitations regarding the way in which POSSUM and P-POSSUM were applied and their sample size, raising questions about their external validity in the current bariatric practice [11,12].

Only one study was published about the usefulness of these scores in gastric bypass surgery [13]. It was a retrospective study in which POSSUM and P-POSSUM scores were applied to patients undergoing laparoscopic gastric bypass or sleeve gastrectomy. The investigators concluded that both scores overestimated 30 day morbidity and mortality. However the study was retrospective, with the physiologic variables collected few weeks before surgery rather than on the day of the procedure. It also evaluated two procedures with different operative magnitudes and as such, with distinct incidence of postoperative complications.

The purpose of this study was to prospectively assess the usefulness of POSSUM and P-POSSUM scores in morbidity and mortality prediction at 30 days after surgery, in patients undergoing elective laparoscopic gastric bypass, in our hospital.

Methods

After Hospital Ethics Committee approval, all patients scheduled for elective LRYGB from November 2014 to September 2015 were enrolled in the study. In our hospital, laparoscopic gastric bypass is usually performed for patients with a body mass index (BMI) ≥ 40 kg/m^2 or ≥ 35 kg/m^2 in association with obesity-associated comorbidities. The great majority of patients are maintained with a balanced general anesthesia with remifentanil, desflurane and rocuronium. Demographic data and physiological parameters were recorded the day before surgery. The perioperative surgical parameters were recorded by the anesthetist in the anesthesia sheet. Blood loss was evaluated considering the volume of blood in surgical aspirator and the weight of surgical dressings. According to other authors, LRYGB were graded as a "major +" surgery [13]. The Clavien-Dindo classification was used for the stratification of postoperative morbidity events [14,15]. It is described in Table 2.

Grade	Complications definition
I	Any deviation from the normal postoperative course without the need for pharmacological treatment or surgical, endoscopic and radiological interventions. Allowed therapeutic regimens are: drugs as antiemetics, antipyretics, analgesics, diuretics and electrolytes and physiotherapy. This grade also includes wound infections opened at the bedside.
II	Requiring pharmacological treatment with drugs other than such allowed for grade I complications. Blood transfusions and total parenteral nutrition are included.
III	Requiring surgical, endoscopic or radiological intervention.
IIIa	Intervention not under general anesthesia.
IIIb	Intervention under general anesthesia.
IV	Life-threatening complication (including CNS complications)‡ requiring IC/ICU-management.
IVa	Single organ dysfunction (including dialysis).
IVb	Multi-organ dysfunction.
V	Patient death.
Suffix "d"	If the patients suffer from a complication at the time of discharge, the suffix "d" (for 'disability') is added to the respective grade of complication. This label indicates the need for a follow-up to fully evaluate the complication.

Table 2: Clavien-Dindo Classification of post-operative morbidity (adapted from) [14,15].

POSSUM equations for morbidity (ln (R/1-R)=5.19+0.16 PS+0.19 OS) and mortality (ln (R/1R)=7.04+0.13 PS+0.16 OS) were applied for each patient. Estimated mortality was also calculated by the equation of P-POSSUM score (ln (R/1-R)=-9.065+0.1692 PS+0.155 OS). In these equations PS and OS represent the physiological and operative total scores, respectively, and R is the probability of event occurrence.

Patients were stratified into estimated mortality (A,B,C,D) and morbidity risk groups (I,II,III,IV).

The mean estimated morbidity (ME) and mortality (MTE) were calculated for each risk group. With this value the estimated number of cases of morbidity and mortality for each group (n1) was calculated. The ratio of observed and estimated cases (O/E) for each risk group was determined. Considering that O/E=1, the predictive ability of the score is good if O/E<1 its predictive ability is low and if O/E>1 the score overestimates the outcome.

Continuous variables were presented as mean ± standard deviation (SD). Results related to the morbidity and mortality is shown in absolute value and/or in percentage.

Chi-square test or Fisher exact test were used as a measure of calibration or goodness of fit to assess if a relationship could be found between the observed and the predicted outcomes. As these p-values do not show if the score is accurate to predict if the expected low or high risk groups are the ones that indeed have the lowest or the highest observed outcomes, respectively, we performed a non-parametric binomial test to see whether the values of the observed outcomes were significantly different from the expected ones for each group. A p-value of less than 0.05 was taken to be significant.

Statistical analysis was performed using SPSS 21˚ IBM˚ software.

Results

A total of 94 patients, of whom 76 (81%) were females, were included in the study. There were no conversions from laparoscopic to open surgery, and all the patients were submitted only to one procedure-LRYGB.

Mean age was 45.5 ± 10.1 (range 21 to 64 years). According to the American Society of Anesthesiologists (ASA) physical status classification, 66 patients (70.2%) were ASA 2 and the remaining was ASA 3. The mean ± SD of BMI was 43.9 ± 6.7 Kg/m². Mean length of stay after surgery was two days.

According to Clavien-Dindo Classification of surgical complications, at 30 days after surgery there were 22 patients with postoperative complications (23.4% of the sample), of which 12 were grade I (persistent postoperative vomiting postponing discharge), eight were grade II (two cases of surgical wound infection, 1 of dysrythmia, 2 of respiratory insufficiency with need of noninvasive ventilation, 1 of digestive hemorrhage with need of transfusion, 1 patient with respiratory tract infection and another with acute kidney injury with dehydration) and two were a high grade complication (Clavien-Dindo IIIb - gastrointestinal suture dehiscence needing urgent surgical repair). No patient died during follow-up period.

The mean ± SD of physiological score was 14.2 ± 1.7 (range 12 to 20). All the patients had a score of 13 in operative variables.

Mean (range) estimated morbidity by POSSUM score for the sample was 29.4% (17.9-41.4%). Mean (range) estimated mortality was 4.4% (3.2-8.6%) by POSSUM and 1.0% (0.7-2.5%) by P-POSSUM equations.

Table 3 shows the results obtained by the use of POSSUM exponential analysis to estimate morbidity for each risk group. Eighty-five patients (90.4%) had an estimated morbidity lower than 30%. Three groups had an O/E ratio<1 which means that the score over predicted morbidity in the entire sample.

Risk group (expected morbidity - %)	No. of patients (n)	Mean predicted risk of morbidity (%)	No. of expected cases (E)[a]	No. of observed cases (E)	Clavien-Dindo classification of complications (n)	O/E ratio	p-value[b]
I (5.47*-20)	9	17.9	1.6	1	Grade I: 1	0.62	0.33
II (20-30)	76	23.3	17.7	17	Grade I: 10	0.96	0.11
					Grade II: 6		
					Grade III: 1		
III (30-40)	6	35.2	2.1	3	Grade I: 1	1.42	0.24
					Grade II: 2		
					Grade III: 1		
IV (40-100)	3	41.4	1.2	1	Grade I:1	0.81	0.43
Total (5.47-100)	94	29.4	27.6	22	Grade I: 12	0.97	0.04
					Grade II: 7		
					Grade III: 2		

Abbreviations: POSSUM: Physiological and Operative Severity Score for the enUmeration of Mortality and morbidity; No: Number; n: Absolute Frequency; O: Observed Cases; E: Expected Cases; O/E: Observed to Expected Morbidity Ratio. *Minimum expected morbidity by POSSUM is 5.47%.
[a] Expected morbidity was calculated by multiplying the effective patient number per risk group by the expected percentage of morbidity by POSSUM. [b] P-value obtained by binomial test.

Table 3: Group-specific comparisons of expected and observed morbidity by POSSUM.

This does not happened in group III, in which there were more complications than expected. Using Chi-square test for the entire sample it turns out that there was a statistically significant difference between estimated morbidity and the observed outcome (p=0.0235). So in our sample, observed morbidity was significantly different from the one expected by POSSUM score. This result is supported by the low probabilities obtained when comparing the observed and expected morbidity for each risk group using binomial test.

Table 4 shows the analysis of POSSUM estimated mortality.

Risk group (expected mortality- %)	No. (nP)	Mean predicted risk of mortality (%)	No. of expected cases (E)[a]	No. of observed cases (O)	O/E ratio	p-value[b]
A (1.1*-4)	36	3.58	1.29	0	0	0.27
B (4-6)	49	4.46	2.23	0	0	0.11
C (6-8)	8	6.84	0.55	0	0	0.57
D (8-100)	1	8.6	0.09	0	0	0.91
Total	94	5.87	4.14	0	0	0.07

POSSUM: Physiological and Operative Severity Score for the enUmeration of Mortality and Morbidity; No: Number; nP : Absolute Frequency; O/E: Observed to Expected mortality ratio; *Minimum expected mortality by POSSUM is 1.1%. [a]: Expected mortality was calculated by multiplying the effective patient number per risk group by the expected percentage of mortality by POSSUM; [b]: p-value obtained by binomial test.

Table 4: Group-specific comparisons of expected and observed mortality by POSSUM.

As could be expected, knowing the very low incidence of mortality described in LRYGB, the majority of patients had a low expected mortality. Indeed, in 79 patients POSSUM score for mortality was lower than 5%. A total of 4 deaths were predicted by POSSUM score. In our sample there were no deaths. So, POSSUM over predicted mortality in the sample. As with morbidity, POSSUM was not a good predictor of mortality (p=0.07). The same results were obtained analyzing each risk group with binomial test, except in the group whose expected mortality was 8-100%. However this group had only one patient.

Table 5 shows the analysis of POSSUM estimated mortality. In our sample, expected mortality for each risk group do not significantly differ from the one observed (p=0.33). In our sample mortality prediction by P-POSSUM seems to be more close to the actual one. The expected number of deaths in our sample by P-POSSUM was lower than one patient.

Risk group (expected mortality - %)	No.(nP-P)	Mean predicted risk of mortality (%)	No. of expected cases (E)[a]	No. of observed cases (O)	O/E ratio	p-value[b]
A (0.2*-1)	62	0.83	0.51	0	0	0.95
B (1-2)	29	1.27	0.37	0	0	0.69
C (2-100)	3	2.23	0.07	0	0	0.93
Total	57	1.05	0.6	0	0	0.36

P-POSSUM: Portsmouth-POSSUM; No: number; nP-p: absolute frequency; O/E: Observed to Expected mortality ratio; *Minimum expected mortality by POSSUM is 0.2%. [a] :Expected mortality was calculated by multiplying the effective patient number per risk group by the expected percentage of mortality by P-POSSUM; [b]: p-value obtained by binomial test.

Table 5: Group-specific comparisons of expected and observed mortality by P-POSSUM.

However, analysis of the usefulness of the scores to predict mortality is limited due to the absence of deaths and to the very low incidence of mortality expected for LRYGB.

Discussion

Morbidity and mortality rates found in our sample are within the ranges described for LRYGB.

POSSUM score was not a good predictor of 30 day morbidity and mortality in the sample. In contrast, P-POSSUM expected mortality was not statistically different from the one observed. As expected, mortality rate predicted by POSSUM was larger than the one predicted by P-POSSUM. Still, given the fact that there were no deaths in the sample (which is consistent with what is described for LRYGB), it was not possible to detect significant differences in the performance of the two scores to predict mortality.

POSSUM and P-POSSUM scores are not specific for a specific surgical procedure, with no discrimination of potential variables specific to certain surgical contexts, POSSUM and P-POSSUM scores have proven useful across different surgical specialties [5,7,16,17]. Like other scores their use in clinical practice requires time and they do not allow for an accurate preoperative risk estimation because they are dependent on operative variables that can only be obtained during and after surgery. So they just permit to do a prediction based on the presumptive values of operative values. However the impact of intraoperative variables in the patient outcome is unquestionable. Besides, they can be used as indirect indicators of the quality of health care by allowing comparison of the outcomes expected and observed in the institution for a specific surgical procedure for which those scores they are validated.

The results of POSSUM analysis are in agreement with those obtained recently by Charalampakis et al. who found a statistically significant difference between the expected compared to the observed complications. In the study both scores over predicted the outcomes [13]. In our study P-POSSUM mortality was not different from the one observed in the sample. This result is not in accordance with the conclusions of Charalampakis. The median expected mortality by P-POSSUM in our sample is $1.0 \pm 0.34\%$. Literature describes a lower incidence of deaths, around 0.15% [2,18]. So P-POSSUM ability to predict mortality has to be further investigated, preferentially by a multicentric study.

Our study is pioneer because it was done only in LRYGB patients, with assessment of POSSUM and P-POSSUM variables through direct reporting from the patient clinical evaluation in perioperative setting, as described by Copeland in his original work. There were no estimates of any variable. As recently described by Young et al., LRYGB has a higher risk-adjusted 30-day serious morbidity compared to laparoscopic sleeve gastrectomy [2]. As such, the inclusion of these two different surgical procedures with different expected morbidity can influence the assessment of the predictive ability of the scores, as 24% of patients had sleeve gastrectomy in the study of Charalampakis. However that study had a higher number of patients, so its results had to be taken into account. Another important difference that has to be considered is the lower mean BMI found in our sample (45 versus 51.8 kg/m^2). ASA classification was not described in the study but it also could be another factor influencing outcome.

POSSUM and P-POSSUM scores lack some specificity for surgeries in bariatric patients. For example they do not take into account body mass index, which has been shown to correlate with morbidity and mortality after bariatric surgery [2]. Also they include some variables that are not very important in LGRYB, like blood loss (in our patients it was always lower than 100 mL), emergency of the procedure and Glasgow Coma Scale. Obesity Surgery Mortality Risk Score (OS-MRS), Longitudinal Assessment of Bariatric Surgery consortium risk stratification system and Metabolic Acuity Score and a nomogram include some obesity specific variables and comorbidities in their equations. Only OS-MRS was validated to predict mortality by multiple centers but it is not validated to estimate morbidity, which is more relevant to predict because of its higher incidence in LRYGB. In a previous study we evaluated the performance of OS-MRS as a predictor of postoperative complications in obese patients submitted to LRYGB and we had evidence that it could be a good tool to use with that goal [19].

Conclusion

This study denotes that POSSUM score does not fit to predict morbidity and mortality in LRYGB patients. The usefulness of P-POSSUM has to be confirmed in other multicenter and larger studies. It seems that, in laparoscopic bariatric surgery, there is the need to use specific scores, which take into account, specific features of the patients (like body mass index, previous medical history, and physical status) and of the procedure. Other multicenter studies, with a higher number of patients are needed to confirm our results. Another suggestion of research could be to compare other assessment methods of postoperative morbidity and mortality, like OS-MRS, with POSSUM and P-POSSUM to assess the ability to predict those variables.

References

1. Fact sheet nº 311 WHO–March2013.Retrieved June 11, 2015.

2. Young MT, Gebhart A, Phelan MJ, Nguyen NT (2015) Use and Outcomes of Laparoscopic Sleeve Gastrectomy vs Laparoscopic Gastric Bypass: Analysis of the American College of Surgeons NSQIP. J Am Coll Surg 220: 880-885.

3. Moonesinghe SR, Mythen MG, Das P, Rowan KM, Grocott MP (2013) Risk Stratification Tools for Predicting Morbidity and Mortality in Adult Patients Undergoing Major Surgery Qualitative Systematic Review. Anesthesiology 119: 959-981.

4. Copeland GP, Jones D, Walters M (1991) POSSUM: a scoring system for surgical audit. Br J Surg 78: 355-360.

5. Prytherch DR, Whiteley MS, Higgins B, Weaver PC, Prout WG, et al. (1998) POSSUM and Portsmouth POSSUM for predicting mortality. Physiological and Operative Severity Score for the enUmeration of Mortality and morbidity. Br J Surg 85: 1217-1220.

6. Teeuwen PH, Bremers AJ, Groenewoud JM, van Laarhoven CJ, Bleichrodt RP (2011) Predictive value of POSSUM and ACPGBI scoring in mortality and morbidity of colorectal resection: a case-control study. J Gastrointest Surg 15: 294-303.

7. Menon KV, Farouk R (2002) An analysis of the accuracy of P-POSSUM scoring for mortality risk assessment after surgery for colorectal cancer. Colorectal Dis 4: 197-200.

8. Canet J, Gallart L, Gomar C, Paluzie G, Valles J, et al. (2010) Prediction of Postoperative Pulmonary Complications in a Population-based Surgical Cohort. Anesthesiology 113:1338-1350.

9. Gawande AA, Kwaan MR, Regenbogen SE, Lipsitz SA, Zinner MJ (2007) An Apgar score for surgery. J Am Coll Surg 204: 201-208.

10. Prytherch DR, Whiteley MS, Higgins B, Weaver PC, Prout WG, et al. (1998) POSSUM and Portsmouth POSSUM for predicting mortality. Physiological and Operative Severity Score for the enUmeration of Mortality and morbidity. Br J Surg 85: 1217-1220.

11. Sabench Pereferrer F, Hernandez Gonzalez M, Abello Salas M, Domènech Calvet J, Blanco Blasco S, et al. (2005) Morbid obesity: postsurgical predictive factors and prioritization of the waiting list. Rev Esp Enferm Dig 97: 161-169.

12. Cagigas JC, Escalante CF, Ingelmo A, Hernandez-Estefania R, Hernanz F, et al. (1999) Application of the POSSUM system in bariatric surgery. Obes Surg 9: 279-281.

13. Charalampakis V, Wiglesworth A, Formela L, Senapati S, Akhtar K, et al. (2014) POSSUM and p-POSSUM overestimate morbidity and mortality in laparoscopic bariatric surgery. Surg Obes Rel Dis 10: 1147-1153.

14. Dindo D, Demartines N, Clavien PA (2004) Classification of surgical complications: a new proposal with evaluation in a cohort of 6336 patients and results of a survey. Ann Surg 240: 205-213.

15. Clavien PA, Barkun J, de Oliveira ML, Vauthey JN, Dindo D, et al. (2009) The Clavien-Dindo classification of surgical complications: five-year experience. Ann Surg 250: 187-196.

16. Teeuwen PH, Bremers AJ, Groenewoud JM, van Laarhoven CJ, Bleichrodt RP (2011) Predictive value of POSSUM and ACPGBI scoring in mortality and morbidity of colorectal resection: a case-control study. J Gastrointest Surg 15: 294-303.

17. Constantinides VA, Tekkis PP, Senapati A (2006) Comparison of POSSUM scoring systems and the surgical risk scale in patients undergoing surgery for complicated diverticular disease. Dis Colon Rectum 49: 1322-1331.

18. Khan MA, Grinberg R, Johnson S, Afthinos JN, Gibbs KE (2013) Perioperative risk factors for 30-day mortality after bariatric surgery: is functional status important? Surg Endosc 27: 1772-1777.

19. Pinho S, Carvalho M, Soares M, Pinho D, Cavaleiro C, et al. (2015) Obesity Surgery Mortality Risk Score: can we go beyond mortality prediction?. J Anesth Clin Res 6:9.

12

Predictive Factors of Apgar Scores below 7 in Newborns: Can we Change the Route of Current Events?

Tiffany Leite Costa[1], **Angela Mota**[2], **Sonia Duarte**[2], **Marta Araujo**[2], **Patricia Ramos**[2], **Humberto S Machado**[1,2*] and **Paulo Lemos**[2]

[1]*Instituto de Ciencias Biomedicas Abel Salazar, Universidade do Porto, Portugal*

[2]*Serviço de Anestesiologia, Centro Hospitalar do Porto, Portugal*

***Corresponding author: Humberto S Machado**, Servico de Anestesiologia, Centro Hospitalar do Porto, Largo Professor Abel Salazar, 4099-001 Porto, Portugal; E-mail: hjs.machado@gmail.com

Abstract

Introduction: The Apgar score is a useful and immediate tool used in the assessment of newborns. The factors that influence its final score may be related with labor, mother or infant itself. The impact of epidural analgesia in the Apgar score is still controversial and not fully understood. One of the limitations while attributing this score is inter-observer variability.

Objectives: The objective of this study was to determine possible predictive risk factors of low Apgar scores at 5 minutes, namely the influence of maternal factors, labor and newborn characteristics, as well as the effect of different analgesic concentrations used in epidural analgesia.

Methods: This was a cross-sectional, institutional study conducted during two consecutive years-2014 and 2015, in Centro Materno Infantil do Norte, Portugal. Anesthesiology Department database was used to collect all the relevant information.

Results: 3085 deliveries were included in the study. A significant higher number of deliveries with lower Apgar scores in 2015 compared to 2014 were noticed; furthermore a similar result was found when a certain hospital team of obstetricians was on duty (Team 4), when compared with other similar teams.

Conclusion: Statistically significant differences on the Apgar indexes were found between delivery teams. Inter-observer variability on Apgar classification might explain these results. Low concentrations of local anesthetic combined with opioid in an initial moment of labor do not seem to influence Apgar scores at birth. No other factor was considered predictive of low Apgar scores.

Keywords: Apgar; Neonatal; Outcome; Variability; Analgesics; Opioids; Labor epidural analgesia

Background and Objectives

The first minutes after birth are crucial for newborn's adaptation to extra-uterine life. During this period, reliable and objective tools are required to assess its clinical state. Ever since it was described in the late fifties by Virginia Apgar, this score has been attributed virtually to every infant in western countries. It is an easy, immediate, standardized method of classification and a predictor of neonatal morbidity and mortality [1-4]. A total of seven points or more is considered normal while an Apgar score (AS) below three, combined with a low umbilical cord pH, is associated with perinatal asphyxia in children without malformations and increases the risk of cerebral paralysis 20-100 times compared to 5th minute AS scores equal or above seven (AS5th $\geq$ 7) [5-9]. Nevertheless, the vast majority of children with AS5th<7 will be healthy at birth and later in life [5,8].

However, despite its undeniable usefulness in infant's clinical primary appraisement, attributing an Apgar score is not free of limitations. Given the main parameters accounted for, the AS can be objective in some of them (heart rate, respiration), and subjective in others (muscle tone, irritability); thus, variability among observers needs to be noted. Recent studies tried to evaluate subjectivity between neonatologists using questionnaires and videos, and inconsistencies were evident regardless of newborns' clinical states [9-11].

Previously described factors associated with AS5th<7 include extremes in gestational age and birth weight, male sex and maternal obesity [1,3,4,12-14]. Additionally, maternal age, smoking habits, both low socioeconomic status and educational level, mode of delivery and previous caesarean appear linked to lower AS in some studies [1,3,15-17]. Prolongation of second stage of labor may justify the reason why nuliparity and epidural analgesia (EA) emerge as potential causes of AS5th<7 in several researches [1,3,13,16,18,19].

The influence epidural analgesia on sustaining the progression of labor and the possibility of increasing instrumental delivery are still controversial topics. Besides, the role played by EA in ambulation and maintenance of physiological bear down reflex is yet to be understood [20-24]. Some studies suggest that administering lower doses of local anesthetics along with an adjuvant opioid may bring benefits on neonatal outcome when compared with higher doses where such combination was not used [25], nonetheless, other studies advocate otherwise [26,27].

The main aim of this study was to investigate if there were any variables regarding the mother, the delivery, or the newborn that negatively influence AS, comparing analgesic technics that use high local anesthetic (LA) concentrations with those where low LA concentrations and an opioid where applied.

Methods

Study population, design and criteria

This was a cross-sectional, institutional study conducted in Centro Materno Infantil do Norte (CMIN), part of Centro Hospitalar do Porto (CHP), after approval by institutional ethics committee. CHP is a central, university and tertiary level hospital.

Data regarding deliveries that occurred between January 2014 and December 2015 was collected from the anesthesia records in patients' clinical files.

Information concerning maternal age, height, weight and parity was listed. Data included in clinical records on the birth comprised year, the obstetrician team that performed the delivery, type of delivery, time of delivery, beginning of labor, and duration of labor under EA was also collect.

Additionally, newborn's gestational age, sex, weight and 1st and 5th minute Apgar scores, were registered. Anesthesia administration features like technique (subarachnoid, intravenous or epidural), mode of administration (bolus, continuous perfusion or PCEA), used drugs, time of administration, and ambulation after EA and cervix dilatation when EA was instituted, were also listed into the database and subsequently collected for the study.

Given the similar statistical distribution, missing values on ambulation were considered as those where women did not ambulate.

To diminish the possibility of potential bias, all cesarean sections, twins deliveries, stillbirths and women submitted to intravenous or subarachnoid analgesia were not included in the analysis.

Concerning the classification of categorical variables previously mentioned, the obstetrician team of delivery was named from 1 to 8; the parity in primiparous or multiparous; the mode of delivery in eutocic or instrumental; the beginning of labor in spontaneous or induced; the duration of labor in <5 h, 5-10 h, 10-15 h and >15 h and the cervix dilatation in <3 cm or ≥ 3 cm.

The different types of anesthetics used were grouped according with concentration and combination with opioid. Regimens using 0.2% ropivacaine in either bolus or continuous perfusion (or combination of both) were considered as high concentrations. At the same time, both bolus administrations of 0.15% ropivacaine+5 μg sufentanil and either continuous perfusion or PCEA with 0.1% ropivacaine+0.25 μg/ml sufentanil (or a combination of the three) were considered as low concentrations. Other modes of administration when a combination of high and low doses was used were not the analyzed.

Continuous variables were represented using mean and standard deviation and analyzed with the Student's t-Test for independent samples. Categorical variables were presented in percentage and analyzed using Chi-Square test. After the individual analysis, a binary logistic regression was performed and both Odds Ratio and 95% Confidence Intervals were displayed. A $p<0.005$ was considered statistically relevant.

Statistical analysis was performed with SPSS Statistics, 22° (IBM°, EUA) for Windows software.

Results

3914 cases were analyzed. Apgar score data was present in 3737 deliveries. After exclusion criteria, stillbirths (n=17) and twins (n=76) were eliminated from the analysis. Simultaneously, cesarean sections (n=547) and women submitted to intravenous or subarachnoid analgesia were excluded (n=32 and n=28). Once these exclusions were made, the final sample included 3085 births, corresponding to 78.8% of the sample. Out of these, 104 newborns were classified AS5th<7, representing 3.4% of infants.

Mean women age included in the study was 30 years old, and their average BMI was 29.1 kg/m². The remaining anthropometric data (weight and height) are represented on Table 1, which also includes the newborns' mean gestational age (38.3 weeks) and their approximate mean weight (3158 g).

Parameters	AS5th<7		AS5th ≥ 7		Total		p
	n	Mean (SD)	n	Mean (SD)	n	Mean (SD)	
Women							
Age(years)	97	29.9 (7.6)	2817	29.9 (6.2)	2914	29.9 (6.3)	0.928
Weight (kg)	100	78.5 (13.3)	2845	77.4 (12.8)	2945	77.4 (12.8)	0.402
Height (cm)	97	162.8 (7.5)	2815	163.2 (6.2)	2912	163.2 (6.2)	0.562
BMI (kg/m²)	95	29.7 (4.9)	2742	29.1 (4.5)	2837	29.1 (4.5)	0.204
Infants							
Gestational Age	92	38.2 (2.7)	2679	38.3 (2.5)	2771	38.3 (2.5)	0.676
Weight (g)	98	3131 (453.4)	2887	3159 (480.9)	2985	3158 (479.9)	0.574

Table 1: Descriptive data-Continuous Variables. Differences between groups analyzed with Student's t-Test.

Considering the categorical variables analyzed, 58.8% of women were primiparous; 51.1% of infants were males; 69% of deliveries were eutocic and 82.2% occurred spontaneously. Regarding analgesia, 95% of epidurals were administered when cervix dilation was ≥ 3 cm, 66% performed with low concentrations combined with opioid. 96.9% of women did not ambulate after EA and 53.3% of deliveries lasted between 1 and 5 hours under epidural analgesia (Table 2).

Parameters	AS5th<7		AS5th ≥ 7		Total		p
	n	%	n	%	n	%	
Parity							
Primiparous	59	58.4	1716	58.4	1775	58.8	0.937
Multiparous	42	41.6	1202	41.6	1244	41.2	
Infant's sex							
Male	52	50.5	1512	51.1	1564	51.1	0.897
Female	51	49.5	1445	48.9	1496	48.9	
Year							
2014	39	37.5	1535	51.5	1574	51	0.005***
2015	65	62.5	1446	48.5	1511	49	
Team							
Team 1	14	15.4	420	16.4	434	16.4	0.016***
Team 2	8	8.8	297	11.6	305	11.5	
Team 3	6	6.6	287	11.2	293	11.1	
Team 4	24	26.4	320	12.5	344	13	
Team 5	8	8.8	310	12.1	318	12	
Team 6	10	11	271	10.6	281	10.6	
Team 7	8	8.8	317	12.4	325	12.3	
Team 8	13	14.3	338	13.2	351	13.2	
Beginning of Labour							
Spontaneous	74	83.1	2059	82.3	2133	82.3	0.836
Induced	15	16.9	443	17.7	458	17.7	
Type of delivery							
Eutocic	73	73	2006	68.9	2079	69	0.382
Instrumented	27	27	906	31.1	933	31	
Dilatation							
<3 cm	6	7.2	104	4.1	110	4.2	0.165
≥ 3 cm	77	92.8	2423	95.9	2500	95.8	
Type of EA							
Low+opioid	64	71.1	1700	66.7	1764	66.6	0.387
High concentrations	26	28.9	847	33.3	873	33.4	
Ambulation							
No	99	95.2	2889	96.9	2988	96.9	0.323

Yes	5	4.8	92	3.1	97	3.1	
Time under EA							
<1 h	3	3.8	144	6.2	147	6.2	
1-5 h	50	63.3	1237	53.5	1287	53.3	
5-10 h	18	22.8	669	28.9	687	28.7	0.505
10-15 h	5	6.3	180	7.8	185	7.7	
≥ 15 h	3	3.8	81	3.5	84	3.5	
***Statistically significant difference							

Table 2: Descriptive data-Categorical Variables. Differences between groups analysed with Chi-square test.

The remaining categorical variables and their association with AS5th<7 are also displayed on Table 2. Both the obstetrician team that performs the delivery and year of delivery were found to be statistically significant (p=0.016 and p=0.005, respectively). Obstetrician team #4 showed a higher percentage of infants with AS5th<7 (26.4%), when compared with other teams (7-15%). Moreover, an overall higher percentage of deliveries with low Apgar scores were obtained in 2015 (62.6%) when compared with 2014 (37.5%).

No differences were found between groups in regarding maternal age, weight, height or BMI, nor in infant's gestational age or birth weight (Table 1).

Likewise, no statistically significant differences were found regarding parity, gender, beginning of labor, type of labor, cervix dilatation, type of analgesia, ambulation after neither EA nor time under EA (Table 2).

Regarding the fact that Obstetrician Team 4 showed lower Apgar scores when compared to other teams (Figure 1), this variable was grouped (Team 4), and compared with the remaining Teams. Table 3 shows the results of univariable and multivariable logistic regression analysis, between Team 4 and all the other Teams, along with other variables. On univariable method both the variable Team 4 and the variable 2015 presented higher association with AS5th<7 (OR=1.77 and 2.71; p=0.006 and p<0.001. respectively).

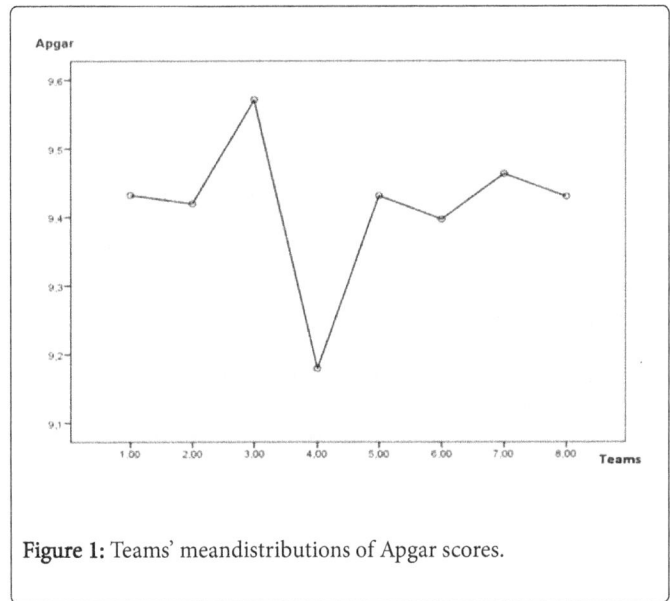

Figure 1: Teams' meandistributions of Apgar scores.

However, on multivariable regression, only Team 4 exhibit lower Apgar scores (OR=2.07 and p=0.043). According to this method, no other factor was considered statistically significant (Table 3).

Parameters	Univariable			Multivariable		
	OR	95 % C.I.	p	OR	95 % C.I.	p
Age (years)	1.01	0.97-1.03	0.928	0.99	0.95-1.05	0.959
Weight (kg)	1.01	0.99-1.02	0.402			
Height (cm)	0.99	0.96-1.02	0.526			
BMI (kg/m^2)	1.03	0.99-1.07	0.204	1.02	0.96-1.08	0.602
Primiparous *vs.* Multiparous	0.98	0.66-1.47	0.937	0.85	0.46-1.57	0.598
Gestational Age	0.98	0.91-1.06	0.676	1.08	0.94-1.24	0.304
Infant's weight (g)	1	0.99-1.00	0.574	1	0.99-1.00	0.071
Males *vs.* Females	0.97	0.66-1.44	0.897			

2015 *vs.* 2014	1.77	1.18-2.65	0.006*	1.52	0.84-2.75	0.164
Team 4 *vs.* Others	2.51	1.55-4.06	<0.001*	2.07	1.02-4.19	0.043**
Induced *vs.* Spontaneous	0.94	0.53-1.66	0.836			
Instrumented *vs.* Eutocic	0.82	0.52-1.28	0.383	0.94	0.49-1.81	0.856
<3cm *vs.* ≥ cm	1.82	0.77-4.26	0.171	1.9	0.65-5.56	0.281
High *vs.* Low+opioid	0.82	0.51-1.30	0.388	1.4	0.76-2.57	0.281
No ambulation *vs.* Yes	0.63	0.25-1.59	0.327	0.58	0.13-2.51	0.463
Time under EA (*vs.*<1h):						
1-5 h	1.94	0.60-6.30	0.27			
5-10 h	1.29	0.38-4.44	0.685			
10-15 h	1.33	0.31-5.67	0.697			
15 h	1.78	0.35-9.01	0.487			
*Statistically significant difference-univariable method, **Statistically significant difference-multivariable method.						

Table 3: Univariable and multivariable logistic regression.

Given that any cases with missing data in any of the variables were automatically excluded on multivariable regression, the sample included on this analysis consisted in 1489 cases, out of these; only 48 infants had low 5th minute Apgar scores.

In order to better elucidate what changed from 2014 to 2015 that could explain the differences found on Apgar scores, some variables were further analyzed between years (type of analgesia, cervix dilation when EA, duration of labor under EA, ambulation, type of labor and beginning of labor) (Table 4). Considering this analysis, only type of analgesia and cervix dilation differed significantly between years (p<0.001). Lower doses of analgesic combined with opioid and earlier epidurals were administered in 2015.

Parameters	2015		2014		Total		p
	n	%	n	%	n	%	
High concentrations	391	29.6	482	36.6	873	33.1	<0.001*
Low+opioid	929	70.4	835	63.4	1764	66.9	
≥ 3cm	1061	93.3	1439	97.7	2500	95.8	<0.001*
<3cm	76	6.7	34	2.3	110	4.2	
Eutocic	1026	69.5	1053	68.6	2079	69	0.609
Instrumented	451	30.5	482	31.4	933	31	
Spontaneous	1063	83.2	1070	81.5	2133	82.3	0.261
Induced	215	16.8	243	18.5	458	17.7	
<1 h	65	5.5	82	6.8	147	6.2	0.21
1-5 h	632	53.7	655	54	1287	53.8	
10-May	332	28.2	355	29.3	687	28.7	
15-Oct	99	8.4	86	7.1	185	7.7	

>15	49	4.2	35	2.9	84	3.5	
No ambulation	1462	96.8	1526	97	2988	96.9	0.758
Yes	49	3.2	48	3	97	3.1	
*Statistically significant difference							

Table 4: Descriptive data amongst years. Differences analysed with Chi-Square test.

In order to investigate if the causes of 2015's lower Apgar values rely on the bigger number of early EA or lower concentrations administered, year, type of analgesia and cervix dilation were sequentially introduced on a multivariable regression (Table 5). Differences on Apgar scores between years stopped being statistically significant (p=0.089).

Parameters	Univariable			Multivariable		
	OR	95% C.I.	p	OR	95% C.I.	p
2015 *vs.* 2014	1.77	1.18-2.65	0.006*	1.51	0.94-2.45	0.089
High *vs.* Low +opioid	0.82	0.51-1.30	0.388	1	0.60-1.67	0.955
<3cm *vs.* ≥ 3cm	1.82	0.77-4.26	0.171	1.86	0.78-4.43	0.162
*Statistically significant difference-univariable method, **Statistically significant difference-multivariable method.						

Table 5: Logistic regression-year, type of EA and cervix dilatation.

Discussion

Identifying modifiable risks factors that negatively influence Apgar scores is of major interest to improve perinatal medical care and clinical outcome.

The fact that even after exclusion of cesarean sections and twins, global prevalence of low Apgar scores found in this study represents 3.8% of deliveries is an important feature. This value is substantially higher than the ones described in studies performed by other developed European countries, some of which did not include these exclusion criteria [2,19].

On individual analysis, year and team that performed the delivery had a statistically significant impact on the occurrence of deliveries with AS5th<7 ($p=0.006$ and $p<0.001$, respectively), whereas on multivariate method, only Team 4 presented lower 5th minute Apgar scores ($p=0.043$). According to this regression, year of delivery did not exhibit a statistically significant result ($p=0.164$). Nonetheless, given that the sample was considerably reduced after exclusion of missing cases, caution is required when interpreting multivariable logistic regression.

When both years were compared in terms of obstetrical and anaesthetic variables surprisingly lower doses of analgesic combined with opioid and earlier epidurals (in terms of cervix dilatation) were administered in the year with lower Apgar scores (2015). These results do not match with what is postulated by recent literature that advises precocious administrations as soon as requested by women and lower doses of analgesics combined with opioid to reduce the amount of motor blockade. When those variables were inserted sequentially in the multivariate model, differences on Apgar scores between years were no longer relevant ($p=0.089$). Despite more precocious epidurals and lower concentrations were used since 2014, this result means they are not the probable cause of 2015's Apgar scores drop.

According to this analysis, other factors might be influencing Apgar scores in 2015 other than analgesic concentration and cervix dilation when EA was administered. However, detailed analysis of those factors is beyond the scope of this investigation

As already stated, the team that conducts the delivery remains statistically relevant after multivariable logistic regression ($p=0.043$). Many factors concerning infant's state or delivery itself can contribute to this result.

A possible explanation relies on inter-observer variability while attributing AS. Elements of the score (tone, color, reflex and irritability) can be subjective and partially dependent on infant's physiologic maturity [5]. Studies reveal that these differences are more prominent in preterm infants and are accentuated in those who require resuscitative measures [10,28]. This means that an otherwise healthy newborn, even without evidence of asphyxia, could have a lower Apgar score only due to prematurity, once tonus and irritability are both physiologically reduced on these individuals [29,30].

To circumvent this problem, a group of investigators created a new AS named Expanded-Apgar (Figure 2). According to the rules of this new Apgar, maximum score can be allocated to either a healthy term or preterm infant without any problems in postnatal adaptation, but also to infants receiving resuscitative or supportive interventions with an adequate response (good chest expansion during ventilation or pink color due to supplemental O_2). Additionally, a score is also attributed to the supportive interventions and resuscitative measures applied [31]. Some studies found a better correlation with perinatal asphyxia using expanded score compared to the conventional scoring system [32, 33].

Apgar Score Gestational age__________weeks

Sign	0	1	2	1 minute	5 minute	10 minute	15 minute	20 minute
Color	Blue or Pale	Acrocyanotic	Completely Pink					
Heart rate	Absent	<100 minute	>100 minute					
Reflex irritability	No Response	Grimace	Cry or Active Withdrawal					
Muscle tone	Limp	Some Flexion	Active Motion					
Respiration	Absent	Weak Cry; Hypoventilation	Good, Crying					
			Total					

Comments:

Resuscitation					
Minutes	1	5	10	15	20
Oxygen					
PPV/NCPAP					
ETT					
Chest Compressions					
Epinephrine					

Figure 2: Expanded-Apgar Score.

These modifications can enlighten dubious points of the score, but cannot avoid variability amongst observers. A recent study found possible solutions to unravel this problem. Significant differences on scores' consistency before and after a simple clarification of some parameters were found, especially on the points with higher degrees of variability–preterm or infants submitted to resuscitative measures [28].

The fact that no other maternal, newborn or delivery variables were related with low Apgar scores is another relevant result of this study.

Association between prematurity and low birth weight with inferior neonatal outcome is described in several publications [1,3,14,34]. Lack of lung maturation and the need for artificial ventilation can be pointed as explanations why premature infants receive lower Apgar scores. In those studies, attribution of a lower index just because of prematurity was not accounted for and possible inter-observer inconsistencies were discarded.

Despite the fact that maternal obesity has been linked to adverse perinatal events and mortality in several publications, such result was not found on this investigation [1,3,4,14]. The sample analyzed in this study had a high prevalence of obese mothers and the mean BMI was in pre-obesity range (29.9 kg/m^2). This result can be due to the multifactorial character of this variable. Maternal age, parity, socioeconomic status and educational level were already pointed as possible confounders.

Relation amongst extremes in maternal age and adverse neonatal events was already demonstrated, nevertheless, some controversial still subsists regarding this matter. Other socioeconomic factors such as a higher educational level in women older than 41 years old can mitigate the risk of possible neonatal complications [1,4,14,35-37].

Regarding parity, several bibliographic contradictions are found. Some studies report nuliparity as risk factor due to extension of second stage of labor, while others determine that having more than 6 live births increases the risk of breech delivery [34,38].

This study reveals limitations common to many retrospective studies. The initial sample was representative of two consecutive years, however, due to missing cases, after logistic regression the number of cases decreases to 1480. In order to avoid this problem, both an increase in the sample and a better anesthetic record keeping are required.

Conclusion

The relevance of this study relies on the fact that both the team that conducts the delivery (Team 4) and year 2015 presented significantly lower Apgar scores on individual analysis. This link was kept by the variable Team after multivariable logistic analysis, which indicates that it influences the occurrence of deliveries with lower Apgar scores regardless of other variables. The underlining motives of the differences obtained among teams are beyond the scope of this study.

The fact that a higher number of AS5th<7 was observed in 2015 does not seem to be related with increment in number of EA performed earlier and with lower anesthetic concentrations combined with opioid.

Further studies specifically designed to account for demographic, obstetric and analgesic differences among years are required to clarify this subject.

References

1. Straube S, Voigt M, Jorch G, Hallier E, Briese V, et al. (2010) Investigation of the association of Apgar score with maternal socio-economic and biological factors: an analysis of German perinatal statistics. Arch Gynecol Obstet 282: 135-141.

2. Saraiva A, Duarte S, Lagarto F, Figueira H, Nunes CS, et al. (2015) Is Epidural Analgesia a Predictor of Low Newborn Apgar? A Hospital-Based Observational Study. J Anesth Clin Res 6: 565.

3. Svenvik ML, Blomberg MB (2015) Preterm Birth: A Prominent Risk Factor for Low Apgar Scores. Biomed Res Int 2015: 978079.

4. Persson M, Johansson S, Villamor E, Cnattingius S (2014) Maternal overweight and obesity and risks of severe birth-asphyxia-related complications in term infants: a population-based cohort study in Sweden. PLoS Med 11: e1001648.

5. [Authors not listed] (2015) The Apgar Score. Pediatrics 136: 819-22.

6. Carter BS, AD Haverkamp, GB Merenstein (1993) The definition of acute perinatal asphyxia. Clin Perinatol 20: 287-304.

7. Hogan L, Ingemarsson I, Thorngren-Jerneck K, Herbst A (2007) How often is a low 5-min Apgar score in term newborns due to asphyxia?. Eur J Obstet Gynecol Reprod Biol 130: 169-175.

8. Ehrenstein V (2009) Association of Apgar scores with death and neurologic disability. Clin Epidemiol 1: 45-53.

9. Moster D, Lie RT, Irgens LM, Bjerkedal T, Markestad T (2001) The association of Apgar score with subsequent death and cerebral palsy: A population-based study in term infants. J Pediatr 138: 798-803.

10. Bashambu MT, Whitehead H, Hibbs AM, Martin RJ, Bhola M (2012) Evaluation of interobserver agreement of apgar scoring in preterm infants. Pediatric 130: e982-7.

11. Lopriore E, Frederiek van Burk G, Walther FG, de Beaufort AJ (2004) Correct use of the Apgar score for resuscitated and intubated newborn babies: questionnaire study. Bmj 329: 143-144.

12. Berglund S, Grunewald C, Pettersson H, Cnattingius S (2010) Risk factors for asphyxia associated with substandard care during labor. Acta Obstet Gynecol Scand 89: 39-48.

13. Andrejevic A, Cvetkovic S, Vitosevic Z, Andrejevic L, Relic G (2011) Multiparity, perinatal morbidity and mortality. Clin Exp Obstet Gynecol 38: 71-75.

14. Chen M, McNiff C, Madan J, Goodman E, Davis JM, et al. (2010) Maternal obesity and neonatal Apgar scores. J Matern Fetal Neonatal Med 23: 89-95.

15. De Zorzi Pde M, Madi JM, Rombaldi RL, De Araújo BF, Zatti H, et al. (2012) Perinatal factors associated with pH<7.1 in umbilical artery and Apgar 5 min <7.0 in term newborn. Rev Bras Ginecol Obstet 34: 381-385.

16. Hingson R, Gould JB, Morelock S, Kayne H, Heeren T, et al. (1982) Maternal cigarette smoking, psychoactive substance use, and infant Apgar scores. Am J Obstet Gynecol 144: 959-966.

17. Odd DE, Doyle P, Gunnell D, Lewis G, Whitelaw A, et al. (2008) Risk of low Apgar score and socioeconomic position: a study of Swedish male births. Acta Paediatr 97: 1275-1280.

18. Salustiano EM, Campos JA, Ibidi SM, Ruano R, Zugaib M (2012) Low Apgar scores at 5 minutes in a low risk population: maternal and obstetrical factors and postnatal outcome. Rev Assoc Med Bras (1992) 58: 587-593.

19. Altman M, Sandström A, Petersson G, Frisell T, Cnattingius S, et al. (2015) Prolonged second stage of labor is associated with low Apgar score. Eur J Epidemiol 30: 1209-1215.

20. Comparative Obstetric Mobile Epidural Trial (COMET) Study Group UK (2001) Effect of low-dose mobile versus traditional epidural techniques on mode of delivery: a randomised controlled trial. Lancet 358: 19-23.

21. Anim-Somuah M, Smyth RM, Jones L (2011) Epidural versus nonepidural or no analgesia in labour. Cochrane Database Syst Rev 12: Cd000331.

22. Leighton BL, Halpern SH (2002) The effects of epidural analgesia on labor, maternal, and neonatal outcomes: a systematic review. Am J Obstet Gynecol 186: S69-77.

23. Sng BL, Leong WL, Zeng Y, Siddiqui FJ, Assam PN, et al. (2014) Early versus late initiation of epidural analgesia for labour. Cochrane Database Syst Rev : CD007238.

24. Wilson MJ, MacArthur C, Cooper GM, Shennan A; COMET Study Group UK (2009) Ambulation in labour and delivery mode: a randomised controlled trial of high-dose vs mobile epidural analgesia. Anaesthesia 64: 266-272.

25. Sultan P, Murphy C, Halpern S, Carvalho B (2013) The effect of low concentrations versus high concentrations of local anesthetics for labour analgesia on obstetric and anesthetic outcomes: a meta-analysis. Can J Anaesth 60: 840-854.

26. Gizzo S, Noventa M, Fagherazzi S, Lamparell L, Ancona E, et al, (2014) Update on best available options in obstetrics anaesthesia: perinatal outcomes, side effects and maternal satisfaction. Fifteen years systematic literature review. Arch Gynecol Obstet 290: 21-34.

27. Lee BB, Ngan Kee WD, Lau WM, Wong AS (2002) Epidural infusions for labor analgesia: a comparison of 0.2% ropivacaine, 0.1% ropivacaine, and 0.1% ropivacaine with fentanyl. Reg Anesth Pain Med 27: 31-36.

28. Gupta S, Natarajan G, Gupta D, Karnati S, Dwaihy M, et al. (2016) Variability in Apgar Score Assignment among Clinicians: Role of a Simple Clarification. Am J Perinatol .

29. Catlin EA, Carpenter MW, Brann BS 4th, Mayfield SR, Shaul PW, et al. (1986) The Apgar score revisited: influence of gestational age. J Pediatr 109: 865-868.

30. Hegyi T, Carbone T, Anwar M, Ostfeld B, Hiatt M, et al. (1998) The apgar score and its components in the preterm infant. Pediatrics 101: 77-81.

31. Rüdiger M, Braun N, Aranda J, Aguar M, Bergert R, et al. (2015) Neonatal assessment in the delivery room--Trial to Evaluate a Specified Type of Apgar (TEST-Apgar). BMC Pediatr 15: 18.

32. [Author not listed] (2006) Committee on Obstetric Practice, ACOG; American Academy of Pediatrics; Committee on Fetus and Newborn, ACOG (2006) ACOG Committee Opinion. The Apgar score. Obstet Gynecol 107: 1209-1212.

33. Dalili H, Nili F, Sheikh M, Hardani AK, Shariat M, et al. (2015) Comparison of the four proposed Apgar scoring systems in the assessment of birth asphyxia and adverse early neurologic outcomes. PLoS One 10: e0122116.

34. Hasegawa J, Farina A, Turchi G, Hasegawa Y, Zanello M, et al. (2013) Effects of epidural analgesia on labor length, instrumental delivery, and neonatal short-term outcome. J Anesth 27: 43-47.

35. Almeida NK, Almeida RM, Pedreira CE (2015) Adverse perinatal outcomes for advanced maternal age: a cross-sectional study of Brazilian births. J Pediatr (Rio J) 91: 493-498.

36. Aviram A, Raban O, Melamed N, Hadar E, Wiznitzer A, et al. (2013) The association between young maternal age and pregnancy outcome. J Matern Fetal Neonatal Med 26: 1554-1558.

13

Premedication with Nasal Sedation as an Aid for Behaviour Management in Dental Procedures for Children

Aktham Shoukry[1*], Assem Moharram[1], Osama Shahawy[2], Abla Aly[3], Heba Morgan[3] and Fayrouz Soliman[3]

[1]Department of Intensive Care and Pain Management, Faculty of Medicine, Ain Shams University, Anesthesia, Cairo, Egypt

[2]Department of Pediatric Dentistry, Faculty of Oral and Dental Medicine, Cairo University, Cairo, Egypt

[3]Department of Pediatric Dentistry, Faculty of Oral and Dental Medicine, Future University, Cairo, Egypt

[*]**Corresponding author:** Aktham Adel shoukry, Department of Intensive Care and Pain Management, Faculty of Medicine, Ain Shams University, Anesthesia, Cairo, Egypt, E-mail: Aktham.shoukry@med.asu.edu.eg

Abstract

Background: In recent times major advancements in techniques, technologies and materials have resulted in benefits in the everyday clinical practice of dentistry, despite these gains, anxiety related to dental treatments in children is a problem suffered by many patients worldwide, and it remains a significant challenge in providing dental care.

Patients and methods: One hundred children, aged 5-8 years, presenting for simple extraction procedures were selected to participate in the study and randomly divided into two groups (50 patients each). Control group (the C group): were treated by conventional treatment (non-pharmacological behaviour management) while sedation group (the S group) were premeditated by intranasal sedation (3 mg/kg Ketamine and 0.5 mg/kg Midazolam). Perioperative sedative effects, pain, anxiety level changes were assessed, also Time of procedural were recorded.

Results: Children premeditated with intranasal sedation (S group) achieved significantly lower sedation levels (p=0.042), pain score (p=0.032), lower anxiety levels (p=0.036), and easier child-parent separation (p=0.029) than C group also, The S group showed decrease in the mean of the total time of procedural 20 minute ± 3.7 versus 25 min ± 2.8 in C group and this decrease was statistically significant in comparison with the C group (p<0.05).

Conclusion: Intranasal sedation using ketamine and midazolam was associated with lower sedation levels, lower anxiety levels, and easier child-parent separation at the time of transferring patients to the operating room than children who were not sedated. Moreover the time needed to perform a simple extraction under intranasal sedation is significantly less than that of regular chair side procedure, which suggests possible balanced cost benefit.

Keywords: Dental; Anxiety; Children; Ketamine; Midazolam; Sedation

Introduction

In recent times major advancements in techniques, technologies and materials have resulted in benefits in the everyday clinical practice of dentistry. Despite these gains, anxiety related to dental treatments in children is a problem suffered by many patients worldwide, and it remains a significant challenge in providing dental care [1]. The prevalence of dental anxiety is 5-20% in most of the populations which is seen more in children and this tends to decrease as age advances [2,3].

Dental anxiety is defined as a feeling of apprehension about dental treatment that is not necessarily connected to a specific external stimulus [4]. According to Chadwick and Hosey, anxiety is common in children and the symptoms of anxiety are dependent on the age of the child. Toddlers exhibit anxiety by crying, while older children manifest anxiety in other ways. Common anxieties among children include fearing the unknown and being worried about a lack of control both of which can occur with dental examination and treatment [5].

Many non-pharmacological behaviour management techniques have been introduced to manage anxious children such as Tell-show-do, behaviour shaping and positive reinforcement and modeling techniques [6].

Procedural sedation is frequently used for both diagnostic and therapeutic procedures, whether urgent or elective. It provides safe and effective relieve of pain and distress associated with dental procedures .It involves the use of one or more sedative and analgesic agents to relieve pain , anxiety and to control motor activity in patients undergoing diagnostic and therapeutic procedures [7].

The pre-anesthetic management of children can be a challenge for the anesthesiologist. Premedication should provide effective anxiolytics and conscious sedation to improve the conditions for parental separation [8].

Midazolam and Ketamine have been used as premedicants for children by different routes. The IM route is painful and therefore rarely used in pediatric patients. Rectal and oral application of midazolam [9,10] and ketamine [11] are widely used. With an onset time between 15 and 30 minutes, [11-13] they show a rather slow onset of sedation, and first pass hepatic metabolism which results in a low and unpredictable systemic availability [14,15]. Furthermore, both routes can be used successfully only in children who generally accept premedication, otherwise either spitting out (oral route) or immediate defecation (rectal route) may result [8]. The intranasal route is preferable since it obviates the need for intravenous access, is easily accessible and allows a more rapid rate of absorption compared to the oral route [16,17].

Intranasal Midazolam for premedication in preschool children was first described and advocated by Wilton and colleagues [18] ketamine as a premedicant has been successfully administered via nasal route as well [19,20]. Combinations of Midazolam and Ketamine given orally [21,22] or rectally [12] have been shown to result in better premedication than either drug alone. Audenaert and colleagues investigated the cardiac effects of different pediatric premedication regimes and recommended the combination of intranasally administrated Ketamine 5 mg.kg and Midazolam 0.2 mg/kg [23].

S-ketamine, one of the two ketamine isomers is now available. It has twice the anaesthetic potency of racemic ketamine [24]. Thus, a 50% reduction of the dosage is possible to achieve comparable results. Because of faster elimination of s-Ketamine, better control of anaesthesia will be provided [25]. Furthermore, it produces less psycho mimetic side effects than r-Ketamine [26], the other enantiomer of racemic ketamine [27].

Ketamine differs from other sedatives and analgesics in that it does not display a dose-response continuum. Instead, there is a dissociative threshold where, when reached, administration of additional ketamine does not result in a deeper state of sedation. Also, Ketamine have some advantages of preservation of respiratory reflexes and an intrinsic positive inotropic effect. It is an excellent analgesic, sedative and amnesic agent [28,29].

Midazolam-Ketamine combination has been used for different pediatric procedures for its anxiolytic and analgesic effects, in order to obtain more analgesia, less hypotension, the use of lower doses of drugs and, consequently a lower risk of respiratory depression [30].

The effects of intranasal administered s-Ketamine and Midazolam for pediatric premedication remain unclear [8].

Aim of study

This study was conducted to evaluate the perioperative sedative effects, anxiety level changes and the ease of child-parent separation (as a primary end-point) and to evaluate succeed of the first attempt for simple tooth extraction and the time needed to achieve the whole procedural (as a second end point).

Patients and Methods

One hundred children, aged 5-8 years, presenting for simple extraction procedures were selected to participate in the study and randomly divided into two groups (50 patients each). Exclusion criteria included children who have ASA classification III or higher, a known allergy to benzodiazepines. An upper respiratory tract infection with nasal discharge, a known liver disease or respiratory distress and known allergy to Ketamine.

Risks, possible discomforts and benefits were explained to the parents and they were required to sign an informed consent form prior to the procedure. To ensure patient safety, the clinic was well equipped with age-appropriate emergency equipment which included a

ventilation bag and mask, Oxygen and a suction device. Resuscitation equipment and medications, including reversal agents were available.

The research team included two anesthetist, four pedodontists and two nurses. The anesthetist administered the medication, two pedodontists performed the procedure, and two nurses continuously monitored the patients and documented the vital signs. Two pedodontists recorded modified Yale preoperative anxiety scale short form (mYPAS-SF) [31] modified observer pain scale (MOPS) and modified from the observer assessment of alertness and sedation scale (MOAA/S).

Control group (the C group): This included 50 patients who were treated by conventional treatment (non-pharmacological behaviour management) while sedation group (the S group) included 50 patients who were treated by intranasal sedation (3 mg/kg Ketamine and 0.5 mg/kg Midazolam).

With respect to sample size calculation, it was calculated using PS (version 3.0.43, Department of Biostatistics, Vanderbilt University, located in Nashville, United States) with the following parameters: level of anxiety used as the primary goal where power of the study was 80%, SD was ± 2, mean was 20, and α error was 0.05.

Study Design

The study was conducted in 3 stations.

Station 1 (pre-extraction)

(The S group) received 3 mg/kg Ketamine and 0.5 mg/kg Midazolam intranasally in both nostrils by the anesthetist using a mucosal atomizing device (MAD) in the waiting area as follows: After drawing the full medication dose in luer-lock syringe, using a free hand to hold the head stable the tip of the MAD gently but firmly against the nostril aiming slightly up and outward (towards the top of the ear)then the syringe plunger is rapidly compressed to deliver the medication into each nostril . Sedation and anxiety levels were assessed before administration of the study drug (baseline values) and at the time of transferring to the dental clinic. Also, the ease of child-parent separation at the time of transferring to the dental clinic was assessed. Sedation level was assessed using a 6-point sedation scale, which was modified from the observer assessment of alertness and sedation scale (MOAA/S) (Table 1) [32].

Anxiety level was assessed using the modified Yale preoperative anxiety scale- short form (mYPAS-SF) [31]. The mYPAS is an instrument developed from the modified yale preoperative anxiety scale (mYPAS) and enables the evaluation of anxiety in children preoperatively and at induction of anaesthesia. It contains 22 specific behaviors within four domains (activity, emotional expressivity, state of arousal, and vocalization,) that are reflective of an anxious state and can be performed by an observer in less than 1 min. The range is 22.92-100 with an increased score being indicative of greater anxiety [31].

Station 2 (extraction)

In the dental clinic, alphacaine topical anesthetic was applied, and a carpule 1.7 ml of Ubistesin-Forte was given to the child, and then extraction was done using extraction forceps .The level of pain was assessed using modified observer pain scale (MOPS) [33]. The score ranges from 2-10. The higher the score, it differs from objective pain score (OPS) of Broadman et al. by substituting posture assessment for blood pressure, (MOPS=sum points of 5 parameters, minimum score=0 and maximum=10) the higher the score the greater the pain experience for the child Together with (MOAA/S) and (mYPAS) for sedation and anxiety

Station 3 (post-extraction)

After extraction was completed, the level of sedation, pain and anxiety were reassessed again using the same scores, and the vital signs were also monitored until the patients met the criteria for safe discharge.

The child should be alert, with stable vital signs, and should be able to talk and sit unaided as appropriate for his age. The parents were provided with discharge instructions including information about the appropriate diet, medications, and activity level for the child.

Monitoring of vital signs including Oxygen saturation, heart rate, and blood pressure were continuously measured throughout the whole procedure also the duration of three stations was recorded and number of children failed to proceed for extraction and postponed for other session was counted for both groups.

Agitated	6
Responds readily to name spoken in normal tone (alert)	5
Lethargic response to name spoken in normal tone	4
Responds only after name is called loudly and/or repeatedly	3
Responds only after mild prodding or shaking	2
Does not respond to mild prodding or shaking	1
Does not respond to deep stimulus	0

Table 1: Modified Observer's Assessment of Alertness Sedation Scale (MOAASS).

Results

Statistical analysis was performed using computer software statistical package for the social science (SPSS, version 17.0; SPSS Inc., Chicago, Illinois, USA). Description of quantitative (numerical) variables was performed in the form of mean ± SD. Description of qualitative (categorical) data was performed in the form of number of cases and percent. Error bars represent 95% confidence interval. Analysis of unpaired numerical variable was performed using the unpaired Student t-test, whereas analysis of paired numerical variables was performed

The two groups were comparable with respect to the following variables; age, gender, weight (Table 2) also, baseline sedation and anxiety levels were comparable in both groups at time of transferal for dental clinic for extraction.

The S group achieved lower anxiety level (Table 3) and lower sedation levels (Figure 1) furthermore the S group had significantly lower level of pain during and after extraction compared to same value of control group (Figure 2). Finally the separation time (duration of station 1) and time of extraction (station 2) in S group was shorter while the time of recovery almost the same in both group (Figure 3).

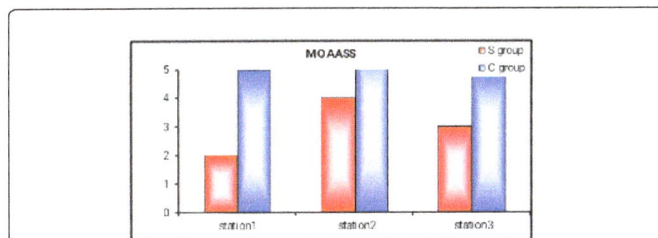

Figure 1: Modified Observer's Assessment of Alertness Sedation Scale (MOAASS).

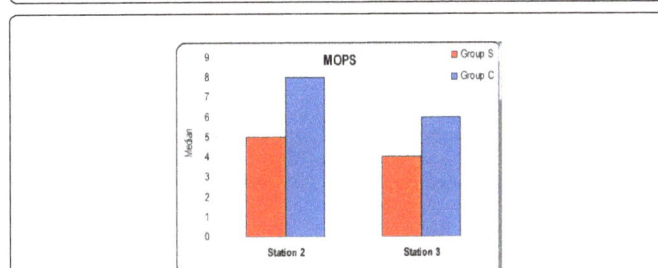

Figure 2: Modified objective pain scale (MOPS).

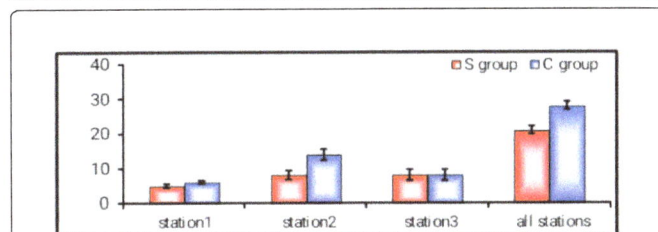

Figure 3: Total time of the whole procedural.

Demographic data

With respect to age, gender, and body weight of children, there were no statistically significant differences between both groups (p>0.05) (Table 2).

	S group	C group	Tests	
			X2/t	P-value
Sex				
Female	20 (20.0%)	17 (17.0%)	0.172	0.678
Male	30 (30.0%)	33 (33.0%)		
Age				
Range	7-Jun	8-May	1.166	0.246
Mean ± SD	7.05 ± 0.72	7.21 ± 0.65		
Weight				
Range	14-35	15-34	1.37	0.173

Mean ± SD	24.84 ± 2.3	24.15 ± 2.72		

C group: control group; S group: nasal sedation group; SD: standard deviation, %: percentage, showed no statistically significant differences between both groups (p >0.05)

Table 2: Demographic data.

Variable	Groups	S (sedation)	C (control)	Studen t t test	P value
mYPAS-SF (base line)	Mean	56.69	55.53	1.348	0.180
	± SD	3.70	4.83		
mYPAS-SF station 1	Mean	42.44	65.44	58.808	<0.001*
	± SD	1.91	2.00		
mYPAS-SF station 2	Mean	64.6	67.93	3.219	0.005*
	± SD	5.68	4.25		
mYPAS-SF station 3	Mean	46.6	48.78	2.633	0.009*
	± SD	3.25	4.87		

mYPAS: Data presented as median; mYPAS-SF: was significantly less in group S (p<0.05); C group: control group; S group: nasal sedation group; mYPAS-SF: modified Yale preoperative anxiety scale short form; station 1: pre-extraction, station 2: during extraction; station 3: post extraction; *: statically significant

Table 3: Anxiety level in the 2 groups at pre-intra and post extraction phase.

Modified observer's assessment of alertness sedation scale (MOAASS): Median MOAASS pre-extraction after sedation was 2 in group S, while it was 5 in group C while during extraction was 4 in group S and 5 in C group also, postoperatively was 4 versus 5 in group S and C respectively and this was a significant difference (p=p<0.05) show in figure 1.

Modified observer pain scale (MOPS): Median MOPS during extraction was 5 in group S and 8 in C group and, post-extraction was 4 versus 6 in group S and C respectively. This was significantly difference (p=p<0.05) shown in figure 2.

Duration of the all procedural: The S group showed decrease mean of the total time of procedural (time of separation time of operation time of discharge) 20 minute ± 3.7 versus 25 min ± 2.8 in C group and this decrease was statistically significant in comparison with the C group (p<0.05) (Figure 3).

Discussion

Anxiety and fear are the main concern of a child being introduced to dental care and procedure. Children fear the unknown and this reflects on their behaviour in the dental office. Success depends on the ability to manage this behaviour to be able to introduce treatment and minimize psychological trauma to the child.

Non pharmacological behaviour management techniques have been introduced to manage anxious children during the first and second dental visits. Although most of children can be managed with different suitable behavioural techniques pharmacological support may be the answer for resistant uncooperative children. This may include the use

of anxiolytic medications, conscious or deep sedation or general anesthesia [34].

When managing uncooperative, very young, or extremely resistant or anxious fearful children the techniques taught in most of the pediatric dental training programs include protective stabilization, sedation, and general anesthesia [34]. The merging between both stabilization and sedation is more or less controversial yet it is reported to be the alternative approach in providing a young child with a safe and comfortable treatment experience [35,36].

As far as sedation is included in dental treatment for children different drugs were used including both Midazolam and Ketamine. Midazolam is a short-acting benzodiazepine strongly recommended for pediatric dental sedation with reported success rates [37-41]. Another three studies reported that the combination between midazolam and ketamine is both safe and effective [42-44] Nitrous oxide gas was not used in the study due to manufacturing issues in Egypt.

Basic concept of the study was that the simple extraction procedure is a short technique wise procedure, doesn't consume much time yet very scary for children. The choice of general anesthesia was evaluated to be extreme with respect to the little time needed and cost benefit of the procedure. Moderate sedation was the management of choice the midazolam-ketamine combination was introduced intra nasally being more rapid in absorption compared to oral route and eliminating the need for intra venous access [16,45]. Intranasal midazolam-ketamine combination was reported as the sedation drug that makes gastric aspirates easier to perform in children. Also successful sedation with intranasal ketamine was achieved during pediatric laceration repair [46].

The midazolam-ketamine combination dose used in our study was 3 mg/kg ketamine and 0.5 mg/kg midazolam. As the use of ketamine alone might result in agitated, confuse child even in a transient manner the use of the midazolam reduces the potential of those effects and causes amnesia [47], while the ketamine eliminates the burning sensation of midazolam with its anesthetic effect [45].

During the pre-extraction phase (station 1) child separation was evaluated to be an easy process went smoothly without any tension from the child's part. Our results meet the results discussed by Weber F et al. [8] that stated that sedation with ketamine improves conditions of parent-child separation.

Children vital signs were monitored during the whole procedure through oxygen saturation and heart rate for their safety; they were recorded every 5 minutes. Children in both groups maintained normal spo2 and HR values. In our study the sedation level changes were assessed using a 6 point sedation scale, which was modified from the MOAA/S and proved to be sensitive in the assessment of sedation level changes overtime in children [32]. Anxiety level changes were assessed by means of the mYAPS-SF in order to measure child's anxiety before, during and after the extraction and whether the whole experience was satisfying or traumatic. Results of our study as regards mYPAS-SF showed (group S) 42.44+1.9, 64.6+5.68, 46.6+3.25 versus (group C) 65.44+2.00, 67.93+4.25, 48.78+4.87 in the three station respectively. Median MOAASS pre-extraction after sedation was 2 in (group S), while it was 5 in (group C) while during extraction was 4 in (group S) and 5 in (C group) also, postoperatively was 4 versus 5 in group S and C respectively and this was a -significant difference (p=p<0.05) showed in figure 1 and table 3 which in turn suggests that the sedation is of significant help in managing and reducing anxiety in children during dental procedure.

These results agree with Weber et al. [8] in the success of ketamine in reduction of anxiety in children. Also Moreira et al. [47] stated the success of the drug combination in behavioral management of the children during dental procedures describing them to be calm. They supplied exact dose of the combination yet orally.

We found that the sedated children experienced less pain during and after extraction when compared to control group (lower MOPS)

Median MOPS during extraction was 5 in groups S and 8 in C group and, post-extraction was 4 versus 6 in group S and C respectively. This was significantly difference (p=p<0.05) shown in figure 2 his may be related to ketamine persistent analgesic effects with preserving patient arousability.

Children were monitored till they fulfil age appropriate baseline criteria for a safe discharge, alertness, and stable vital signs. Most of our patients were discharged with vital signs HR 100-130 and oxygen saturation 97-100%. Our results agree with Weber et al. [8] and Audenaert et al. [23] stating that the intranasal administration of the drug combination results in no significant cardiovascular or respiratory side effects. In our study we used low ketamine dose to avoid the reported side effects including nausea, vomiting, and respiratory depression. Buonsenso et al. agrees with our results stating that the only side effect observed in the sedation group was the post-sedation agitation [46]. Other authors disagree stating that younger children required higher dosage in milligrams per kilogram of Ketamine for adequate sedation [48]. This may be explained by the faster metabolism and renal clearance leading to a shorter half-life of Ketamine in children compared to adults [28,49,50].

By the end of the process the time needed to perform a simple extraction under intranasal sedation using ketamine midazolam combination is significantly less (20.8 minutes and SD 3.68) than that of regular chair side procedure (26.8 minutes and SD 4.18), which suggests possible balanced cost benefit due to the successful elimination of child's anxiety before and during the procedure without affection of the time of recovery which later on protects the child from painful history as the combination of Midazolam-Ketamine causes amnesia on account of the Midazolam component.

Conclusion

Intranasal sedation using ketamine and midazolam was associated with lower sedation (better moderate sedation levels), lower anxiety levels, and easier child-parent separation at the time of transferring patients to the operating room than children who were not sedated. Moreover the time needed to perform a simple extraction under intranasal sedation is significantly less than that of regular chair side procedure, which suggests possible balanced cost benefit.

Clinical Implications

• Anxiety related to dental treatments in children is a problem suffered by many patients worldwide, and it remains a significant challenge in providing dental care. Midazolam-Ketamine combination has been used for different pediatric procedures for its anxiolytic and analgesic effects, in order to obtain more analgesia, less hypotension, the use of lower doses of drugs and, consequently a lower risk of respiratory depression. The effects of intranasal administered s-Ketamine and Midazolam for pediatric premedication remain unclear

• We studied intranasal sedation for pediatric dentistry versus conventional non pharmacological chair side techniques .The child's anxiety, pain, together with procedure time under intranasal sedation is significantly less than that of regular chair side. This suggests possible balanced cost benefit. The impact of intranasal sedation on the simple dental procedure done under general Anesthesia due to dental anxiety and failure of conventional chair side techniques should be further investigated.

References

1. Nigam AG, Marwah N, Goenka P, Chaudhry A (2013) Correlation of general anxiety and dental anxiety in children aged 3 to 5 years: A clinical survey. J Int Oral Health 5:18-24.

2. Gatchel RJ, Ingersoll BD, Bowman L, Robertson MC, Walker C (1983) The prevalence of dental fear and avoidance: a recent survey study. J Am Dent Assoc 107: 609-610.

3. Locker D, Liddell AM (1991) Correlates of dental anxiety among older adults. J Dent Res 70: 198-203.

4. Folayan MO1, Idehen EE, Ojo OO (2004) The modulating effect of culture on the expression of dental anxiety in children: a literature review. Int J Paediatr Dent 14: 241-245.

5. Chadwick BL, Hasey MT (2003) Child taming: How to manage children in dental practice. London: Quintessence Publishing 127.

6. Gupta A, Marya CM1, Bhatia HP, Dahiya V (2014) Behaviour management of an anxious child. Stomatologija 16: 3-6.

7. Krauss B, Krauss B, Green S (2014) Procedural sedation and analgesia in children. N Engl J Med 370: e23.

8. Weber F, Wulf H, el Saeidi G (2003) Premedication with nasal s-ketamine and midazolam provides good conditions for induction of anesthesia in preschool children. Can J Anaesth 50: 470-475.

9. Spear RM, Yaster M, Berkowitz ID, Maxwell LG, Bender KS, et al. (1991) Preinduction of anesthesia in children with rectally administered midazolam. Anesthesiology 74: 670-674.

10. Feld LH, Negus JB, White PF (1990) Oral midazolam preanesthetic medication in pediatric outpatients. Anesthesiology 73: 831-834.

11. Gutstein HB, Johnson KL, Heard MB, Gregory GA (1992) Oral ketamine preanesthetic medication in children. Anesthesiology 76: 28-33.

12. Warner DL, Cabaret J, Velling D (1995) Ketamine plus midazolam, a most effective paediatric oral premedicant. Paediatr Anaesth 5: 293-295.

13. Sekerci C, Danmez A, Ateay Y, Okten F (1996) Oral ketamine premedication in children (placebo controlled double-blind study). Eur J Anaesthesiol 13: 606-611.

14. Malinovsky JM1, Lejus C, Servin F, Lepage JY, Le Normand Y, et al. (1993) Plasma concentrations of midazolam after i.v., nasal or rectal administration in children. Br J Anaesth 70: 617-620.

15. Malinovsky JM, Servin F, Cozian A, Lepage JY, Pinaud M (1996) Ketamine and norketamine plasma concentrations after i.v., nasal and rectal administration in children. Br J Anaesth 77: 203-207.

16. Calligaris L, Davide Z, Alessandra M, De Bortoli R, Chiaretti A, et al. (2011) Concentrated midazolam for intranasal administration: a pilot study. Pediatr Emerg Care 27: 245-247.

17. Chiaretti A, Barone G, Rigante D, Ruggiero A, Pierri F, et al. (2011) Intranasal lidocaine and midazolam for procedural sedation in children. Arch Dis Child 96: 160-163.

18. Wilton NC, Leigh J, Rosen DR, Pandit UA (1988) Preanesthetic sedation of preschool children using intranasal midazolam. Anesthesiology 69: 972-975.

19. Weksler N, Ovadia L, Muati G, Stav A (1993) Nasal ketamine for paediatric premedication. Can J Anaesth 40: 119-121.

20. Diaz JH (1997) Intranasal ketamine preinduction of paediatric outpatients. Paediatr Anaesth 7: 273-278.

21. Funk W, Jakob W, Riedl T, Taeger K (2000) Oral preanaesthetic medication for children: double-blind randomized study of a combination of midazolam and ketamine vs midazolam or ketamine alone. Br J Anaesth 84: 335-340.

22. Lökken P, Bakstad OJ, Fonnelöp E, Skogedal N, Hellsten K, et al. (1994) Conscious sedation by rectal administration of midazolam or midazolam plus ketamine as alternatives to general anesthesia for dental treatment of uncooperative children. Scand J Dent Res 102: 274-280.

23. Audenaert SM, Wagner Y, Montgomery CL, Lock RL, Colclough G, et al. (1995) Cardiorespiratory effects of premedication for children. Anesth Analg 80: 506-510.

24. Hempelmann G, Kuhn DF (1997) [Clinical significance of S-(+)-ketamine]. Anaesthesist 46 Suppl 1: S3-7.

25. Adams HA, Werner C (1997) [From the racemate to the eutomer: (S)-ketamine. Renaissance of a substance?]. Anaesthesist 46: 1026-1042.

26. Doenicke A, Kugler J, Mayer M, Angster R, Hoffmann P (1992) [Ketamine racemate or S-(+)-ketamine and midazolam. The effect on vigilance, efficacy and subjective findings]. Anaesthesist 41: 610-618.

27. Kress HG (1997) [Mechanisms of action of ketamine]. Anaesthesist 46 Suppl 1: S8-19.

28. Green SM, Johnson NE (1990) Ketamine sedation for pediatric procedures: Part 2, Review and implications. Ann Emerg Med 19: 1033-1046.

29. Green SM, Krauss B (2000) The semantics of ketamine. Ann Emerg Med 36: 480-482.

30. Bahetwar SK, Pandey RK, Saksena AK, Chandra G (2011) A comparative evaluation of intranasal midazolam, ketamine and their combination for sedation of young uncooperative pediatric dental patients: a triple blind randomized crossover trial. J Clin Pediatr Dent 35:415-420.

31. Jenkins BN, Fortier MA, Kaplan SH, Mayes LC, Kain ZN (2014) Development of a short version of the modified Yale Preoperative Anxiety Scale. Anesthesia and Analgesia, September 119: 643-650.

32. Chernik DA, Gillings D, Laine H, Hendler J, Silver JM (1990) Validity and reliability of the Observer's Assessment of Alertness/Sedation Scale: study with intravenous midazolam. J Clin Psychopharmacol 10: 244-251.

33. Wilson GA, Doyle E (1996) Validation of three paediatric pain scores for use by parents. Anaesthesia 51: 1005-1007.

34. Nathan JE (1989) Management of the difficult child: a survey of pediatric dentists' use of restraints, sedation and general anesthesia. ASDC J Dent Child 56: 293-301.

35. Adair SM, Rockman RA, Schafer TE, Waller JL (2004) Survey of behavior management teaching in pediatric dentistry advanced education programs. Pediatr Dent 26: 151-158.

36. Vargas KG, Nathan JE, Qian F, Kupietzky A (2007) Use of restraint and management style as parameters for defining sedation success: a survey of pediatric dentists. Pediatr Dent 29: 220-227.

37. Kupietzky A (2004) Strap him down or knock him out: Is conscious sedation with restraint an alternative to general anaesthesia? Br Dent J 196: 133-138.

38. Lima AR, da Costa LR, da Costa PS (2003) A randomized, controlled, crossover trial of oral midazolam and hydroxyzine for pediatric dental sedation. Pesqui Odontol Bras 17: 206-211.

39. Heard C, Smith J, Creighton P, Joshi P, Feldman D, et al. (2010) A comparison of four sedation techniques for pediatric dental surgery. Paediatr Anaesth 20: 924-930.

40. Shapira J, Kupietzky A, Kadari A, Fuks AB, Holan G (2004) Comparison of oral midazolam with and without hydroxyzine in the sedation of pediatric dental patients. Pediatr Dent 26: 492-496.

41. Day PF, Power AM, Hibbert SA, Paterson SA (2006) Effectiveness of oral midazolam for paediatric dental care: a retrospective study in two specialist centres. Eur Arch Paediatr Dent 7: 228-235.

42. Wan K, Jing Q, Zhao JZ (2006) Evaluation of oral midazolam as conscious sedation for pediatric patients in oral restoration. Chin Med Sci J 21: 163-166.

43. Roelofse JA, Joubert JJ, Roelofse PG (1996) A double-blind randomized comparison of midazolam alone and midazolam combined with ketamine for sedation of pediatric dental patients. J Oral Maxillofac Surg 54: 838-844.

44. Cagiran E, Eyigor C, Sipahi A, Koca H, Balcioglu T, et al. (2010) Comparison of oral Midazolam and Midazolam-Ketamine as sedative agents in paediatric dentistry. Eur J Paediatr Dent 11: 19-22.

45. Baygin O, Bodur H, Isik B (2010) Effectiveness of premedication agents administered prior to nitrous oxide/oxygen. Eur J Anaesthesiol 27: 341-346.

46. Chiaretti A, Barone G, Rigante D, Ruggiero A, Pierri F, et al. (2011) Intranasal lidocaine and midazolam for procedural sedation in children. Arch Dis Child 96: 160-163.

47. Buonsenso D, Barone G, Valentini P, Pierri F, Riccardi R (2014) Utility of intranasal Ketamine and Midazolam to perform gastric aspirates in children: a double blind placebo controlled randomized study. BMC Pediatr 14: 67.

48. Moreira TA, Costa PS, Costa LR, Jesus-Franca CM, Antunes DE (2013) Combined oral midazolam ketamine better than midazolam alone for sedation of young children: a randomized controlled trial. Int J Paediatr Dent 23: 207-215.

49. Riavis M, Laux-End R, Carvajal-Busslinger MI, Tschäppeler H, Bianchetti MG (1998) Sedation with intravenous benzodiazepine and ketamine for renal biopsies. Pediatr Nephrol 12: 147-148.

50. Grant IS, Nimmo WS, McNicol LR, Clements JA (1983) Ketamine disposition in children and adults. Br J Anaesth 55: 1107-1111.

14

Preoperative Midodrine Use does not Predict Intraoperative Hypotension during Orthotopic Liver Transplantation

Daniel A Hansen[*], Karl A Poterack, M'hamed Temkit, Mary B Laney CRNA and Terrence L Trentman

Mayo Clinic Arizona, USA

[*]**Corresponding author:** Daniel A. Hansen, Department of Anesthesiology, Mayo Clinic Arizona, 5777 E Mayo Blvd., Phoenix AZ, USA, E-mail: Hansen.daniel1@mayo.edu

Abstract

Background: Complications of liver transplantation undermine long term benefits for patients with end-stage liver disease. Some patients awaiting liver transplantation are treated with midodrine, an oral α1 agonist. We hypothesized that preoperative use of midodrine would predict increased intraoperative hypotension with associated vasopressor and blood product administration and deleterious effects on graft survival.

Methods: We performed a retrospective, matched case control study examining patients receiving midodrine versus those not before undergoing liver transplantation. Sixty-four patients were examined and analyzed. Primary outcomes were total intraoperative vasopressor use and minutes of intraoperative hypotension.

Results: For the primary outcomes, no statistically significant difference was found between the groups. No significant differences were seen in one year patient or graft survival. Statistically significant differences were noted in American Society of Anesthesiologists (ASA) physical status, Model for End-Stage Liver Disease (MELD) scores, preoperative blood pressure metrics, use of continuous renal replacement therapy intraoperatively, cryoprecipitate, and cell saver use.

Conclusions: Preoperative use of midodrine in patients undergoing liver transplantation did not predict increased intraoperative hypotension or concomitant need for vasopressors or blood products. Midodrine use was associated with higher ASA and MELD scores, renal replacement therapy, and decreased preoperative blood pressure, but not altered graft survival.

Keywords: Midodrine; Liver transplantation; Orthotopic liver transplantation; Transplantation

Abbreviations: BMI: Body Mass Index; ASA: American Society of Anesthesiologists; MELD: Model for End-stage Liver Disease; MAP: Mean Arterial Pressure; SBP: Systolic Blood Pressure; DBP: Diastolic Blood Pressure; ERCP: Endoscopic Retrograde Cholangio Pancreatogrphy

Introduction

End stage liver disease (ESLD) and orthotopic liver transplantation (OLT) are often accompanied by severe derangements in physiologic mechanisms, and pharmacologic interventions are often required to maintain hemodynamic stability. Anesthetic management of OLT can be complicated by multiple factors, including pre-existing hypotension, chronic medications, portal hypertension, ascites, pleural effusion and pulmonary shunting, coagulopathy, renal failure and surgical manipulations.

Hypotension is a common finding in patients awaiting liver transplantation. The pathophysiology underlying hypotension in ESLD is complex, but it has been noted that excessive nitric oxide production with subsequent vasodilation and activation of the renin-angiotensin-aldosterone system plays a role [1,2]. A pharmacologic intervention employed to counter hypotension in these patients is midodrine [3].

Midodrine is a direct acting α1-adrenoceptor agonist which causes venous and arterial vasoconstriction through stimulation of α1-receptors located in the vasculature. The net result is an increase in vascular tone and systolic blood pressure. Cardiac β-receptors are unaffected and there is no significant blood brain barrier penetration. In healthy patients, an oral dose of 10 mg can increase the blood pressure 10-30 mmHg at 1 hour and remain elevated for another 3-4 hours [4]. Midodrine has been studied in patients with hepatorenal syndrome and cirrhosis, hemodialysis induced hypotension, spinal cord injury and orthostatic hypotension [5-9], but our review of the existing literature revealed scant data on midodrine use and any associated effects on liver transplantation [10].

We hypothesized that patients undergoing liver transplantation while on midodrine might have significantly more challenging intraoperative courses and adverse outcomes postoperatively; and therefore, midodrine use could serve as a marker for increased perioperative risk in liver transplantation. Clinically, we hypothesized that intraoperative hypotension would be more pronounced in patients on midodrine and they would require increased vasopressors. Additionally, they would likely require more intravenous fluids and blood products and have more tumultuous postoperative courses with potentially deleterious effects on graft outcomes.

Methods

After Institutional Review Board approval, we utilized a retrospective, matched case control design examining patients taking midodrine preoperatively versus those not taking midodrine who had undergone liver transplantation at our institution. The electronic medical record database was queried for patients who had undergone liver transplantation from 1 September 2010 through 30 June 2015, and patients were sorted into those receiving midodrine pre-transplant versus those not taking midodrine. During the study period our query extracted 324 total patients. Fifty of these were taking midodrine before receiving their transplant.

After de-identifying all patients, the midodrine cohort was demographically paired with control patients using age, gender, BMI, and donor type (live vs. deceased) to minimize confounding variables. This resulted in thirty-three demographically matched pairs. Once the two groups were finalized, the patients' medical records were reviewed by blinded reviewers and the pre-determined data points were collected (Table 1). Manual chart review was performed to verify the automatically collected data as well as to supplement any missing variables. During review of the medical records, one patient pair was removed from the study due to midodrine use only during dialysis, while all other midodrine patients were receiving midodrine daily. Dosing varied for the patients taking midodrine. The range was 2.5 mg TID to 15 mg TID. Two patients were on 2.5 mg TID, six were on 5 mg TID, nineteen were on 10 mg TID, and five were on 15 mg TID. The final analysis consisted of thirty-two matched pairs for a total sample size of sixty-four patients. After primary statistical analysis, a regression analysis was performed utilizing MELD-matched controls to re-assess outcomes when patients' MELD scores were included in the analysis.

Patient characteristics

Age

BMI

Gender

ASA physical status score

MELD score

Etiology of liver disease

Donor type

Midodrine use/dose

Perioperative data

Intraoperative continuous renal replacement therapy use

Intubation time (hours)

Length of hospital stay (days)

Preoperative blood pressure

Minutes of intraoperative hypotension

<70 mmHg

70-79 mmHg

80-90 mmHg

Surgery duration (hours)

Total intraoperative vasopressor dosing

Ephedrine (mg)

Epinephrine (mcg)

Norepinephrine (mcg)

Phenylephrine (mcg)

Vasopressin (units)

Total intravenous fluid and blood products (ml)

Cell Saver

Colloids

Cryoprecipitate

Crystalloids

Fresh frozen plasma

Packed red blood cells

Platelets

Patient/graft long term data

'Bring back' surgery (return to OR within one week of transplantation)

Death (within twelve months of transplantation)

ERCPs performed (within twelve months of surgery)

Total surgical procedures performed (within twelve months of surgery)

Table 1: Data points collected.

Statistical methods

Once all data was collected, statistical analyses were performed using the statistical software package SAS Studio 9.3 (SAS Institute, Cary, NC). Descriptive summaries such as mean, median, standard deviation, and range are provided for quantitative variables, along with frequencies and percentages for categorical data. The p-values resulting from the comparison between the two groups cases vs. controls were based on running a conditional logistic, in order to account for the clustering due to matching the cases vs. controls. The condition logistic regression model included the grouping factor (cases vs. control) and the risk factor MELD score. The significance level was at 0.05.

Results

Intraoperative vasopressor use and total minutes of intraoperative hypotension were not found to be statistically different between the two cohorts in both the primary analysis (Tables 2A and 2B) and in the regression analysis utilizing MELD scores (Table 3). Intraoperative hypotension was defined as total minutes with systolic blood pressures recordings under 90 mmHg with subset analysis of recordings under 80 and 70 mmHg respectively. Vasopressor use included comparison of ephedrine, epinephrine, norepinephrine, phenylephrine, and vasopressin.

	Control (n=32)	Midodrine (n=32)	Total (n=64)	p-value
Age	56.4	55.9	56.2	
BMI	27.4	26.8	27.1	
ASA score	3.4	3.9	3.7	0.0083
MELD score	26.4	34.9	30.6	0.0024
Crystalloids (ml)	5130.6	5339.9	5235.3	0.8306
Colloids (ml)	875.1	999.9	937.5	0.6216
Cell saver (ml)	312.2	882.9	597.6	0.0308
Packed red blood cells (ml)	1816.5	2561.9	2189.2	0.2727
Cryoprecipitate (ml)	162.6	308.7	234.5	0.0369
Platelets (ml)	274.3	384.3	328.4	0.2473
Fresh frozen plasma (ml)	1012.4	1400.7	1206.5	0.2520
Epinephrine (mcg)	631.9	722.5	677.2	0.7651
Norepinephrine (mcg)	193.8	506.3	347.6	0.2321
Phenylephrine (mcg)	5961.3	8141.0	7051.2	0.3743
Ephedrine (mg)	12.5	51.9	32.5	0.5007
Vasopressin (units)	21.0	83.7	52.4	0.4924
Preoperative MAP (mmHg)	84.2	71.2	77.7	0.0107
Preoperative SBP (mmHg)	122.2	106.3	114.3	0.0196
Preoperative DBP (mmHg)	66.5	54.8	60.6	0.0084
Intraoperative SBP <70 mmHg (mins)	9.7	8.2	8.9	0.7262
Intraoperative SBP 70-79 mmHg (mins)	17.7	18.3	18.0	0.9025
Intraoperative SBP 80-90 mmHg (mins)	42.1	59.7	50.9	0.2448
Surgical duration (mins)	268.9	258.1	263.6	0.4095
Time to extubation (hours)	27.3	30.5	28.9	0.5043
Length of hospital stay (days)	10.8	12.6	11.7	0.5318
Total surgical procedures within 12 months	2.1	1.8	2.0	0.6850
# ERCPs within 12 months	1.4	0.9	1.2	0.3104
Data summary showing mean values for control group, midodrine group, and total for selected data points.				

Table 2A: Data Analysis.

	Control (n=32)	Midodrine (n=32)	Total (n=64)	p-value
Male gender	18	18	36	
ASA emergency status	11	17	28	0.1657
Intraoperative CRRT	4	22	26	<0.0019

Bring back to OR within 1 week	5	4	9	0.7064
ERCP within 12 months	14	8	22	0.1214
Required other surgical procedures within 12 months	11	18	29	0.1000

Table 2B: Data Analysis.

	Primary analysis p-value	Regression analysis p-value
ASA Score	0.0083	0.1465
CRRT	0.0019	0.0366
Cell Saver	0.0308	0.0522
Cryoprecipitate	0.0369	0.3516
Preoperative SBP	0.0196	0.0953
Preoperative DBP	0.0084	0.0655
Preoperative MAP	0.0107	0.0711

Extracted metrics from regression analysis using MELD scores to match patients with updated p-values for selected metrics. Notice that in regression analysis only intraoperative CRRT remained statistically significant with a p-value <0.05. All omitted metrics remained statistically non-significant with p-values>0.05.

Table 3: Primary versus Regression Analysis.

In the initial demographically matched cohort analysis, statistical significant differences were noted in secondary metrics including: ASA physical status, MELD scores, all preoperative blood pressure recordings (systolic, diastolic, and mean arterial pressures), use of continuous renal replacement therapy (CRRT) intraoperatively, cryoprecipitate use, and cell saver use. Midodrine patients had mean ASA scores of 3.9 compared to 3.4 for the control group (p=0.008, SD 0.5 and 0.4 respectively). Mean MELD scores were 26.3 for the control group versus 34.9 for the midodrine group (p=0.003, SD 8.3 and 9.1 respectively). The midodrine group's preoperative blood pressure was appreciably lower, despite the effects of midodrine: mean arterial pressure was 68.8 mmHg for the midodrine group compared to 82.0 mmHg for control group (p=0.0005, SD 10.0 and 15.6 respectively). Additionally, 68.8% of the midodrine group required CRRT intraoperatively compared to 12.5% of the control group. Lastly, the midodrine group required more cryoprecipitate and cell saver products when compared to their matched pairs, but not other fluid or blood products. Midodrine patients received a mean of 883 ml of cell saver products while the control group had a mean of 312 ml. For cryoprecipitate, the midodrine group received a mean of 309 ml compared to 163 ml for the control group.

To account for MELD scores not included in the initial demographic pairing, we performed a regression analysis using MELD scores and found utilization of CRRT to remain a statistically significant difference between the cohorts with a p-value=0.036 while all other metrics failed to meet statistical significance. With the regression analysis, differences in ASA physical status, preoperative blood pressure recordings, cryoprecipitate use, and cell saver use were no longer noted.

To assess for post-operative complications we examined 'bring-back' surgery in the first week post-operatively, number of post-transplant endoscopic retrograde cholangiopancreatography procedures (ERCP), total number of surgical procedures, graft survival, and patient survival in the twelve months following transplantation. In none of these metrics did we appreciate a statistical difference. No patients were deceased within twelve months in the midodrine group and two patients were deceased in the control group. Of the deceased patients, one had a fatal intracranial bleed while the other died of complications following tacrolimus toxicity and multisystem organ failure.

Discussion

Liver transplantation is often the final treatment option for patients with acute liver failure, end-stage liver disease, and primary hepatic malignancy. The physiologic sequelae of liver disease are numerous and guide transplantation decisions as liver transplantation is not without significant risks which must be weighed against the benefits of the procedure.

Compounding the challenge of liver disease are the immediate complications associated with liver transplantation. The perioperative management of liver transplantation requires aggressive medical optimization. Anesthetic management of the intraoperative portion often necessitates significant fluid resuscitation with concomitant vasopressor and blood product utilization. However, there is considerable variation in perioperative challenges between patients and markers providing predictive value are lacking.

Midodrine has been studied in hepatorenal syndrome and cirrhosis, orthostatic hypotension, hemodialysis, and in spinal cord injuries [5-9,11-14]. As a α1 agonist available in oral formulation, midodrine is utilized as a vasopressor agent. Its current FDA indication is for the treatment of symptomatic orthostatic hypotension in doses of 5-10 mg every 3-4 hours while the patient is upright and a maximum daily dose of 30 mg [4]. Off-label uses include vasovagal syncope, hepatorenal syndrome, prevention of hypotension associated with hemodialysis, and in spinal cord dysfunction. In cirrhotic subjects midodrine has been utilized to mitigate renal function and optimize sodium excretion [15].

We hypothesized that preoperative midodrine use would predict increased intraoperative hypotension. This hypothesis was supported by the statistically significant decrease in systolic, diastolic, and mean arterial pressures preoperatively in the midodrine cohort despite midodrine use. However, we did not find a significant difference in intraoperative hemodynamics. Furthermore, we did not find a significant difference in vasopressor use, colloid or crystalloid administration, or blood product utilization with the exception of cell saver and cryoprecipitate. It is unclear why the midodrine subjects received more cell saver and cryoprecipitate while not requiring significant increases in other fluid or blood products. In regression analysis utilizing MELD scores to match the comparative groups, this difference was not noted. Comparison of the requirements for fluid resuscitation, blood products, and vasopressor therapy does suggest an overall trend towards increased fluid, blood product, and vasopressor need in the midodrine group; however this did not meet the threshold for statistical significance.

While we found midodrine use associated with higher ASA and MELD scores and the need for renal replacement therapy in demographically paired patients, it did not predict adverse intraoperative or post-operative outcomes in our patients. Indeed, our study participants were matched based on demographic data rather than ASA or MELD scores, and in spite of the elevated ASA and MELD scores for the midodrine group, they did not have increased intraoperative hypotension, increased utilization of vasopressor agents, or increased resuscitative needs. Furthermore in our study, patients did not have notably increased postoperative complications. We hypothesized that midodrine would predict more tumultuous perioperative hemodynamics and yet found minimal differences between the two groups despite the disparate ASA and MELD scores. Indeed, with regression analysis of the data using MELD scores, the outcomes remained unchanged with no significant difference between the groups in intraoperative or post-operative metrics. Due to technical and statistical limitations in the number of patients available in our database, we were unable to match patients based on MELD scores initially for this study and instead had to perform regression analysis to account for the impact of MELD scores in our comparisons.

Ultimately, the only metric found to be consistent in the initial analysis and in the regression analysis was the need for intraoperative continuous renal replacement therapy (CRRT). Likely, the association of midodrine and the need for intraoperative CRRT is driven more by the pre-existing need for renal replacement therapy than midodrine predicting the need for renal replacement therapy. There is well documented benefit from midodrine therapy while on renal replacement therapies [5,9,16]. Hemodialysis often produces hypotension as a portion of a patient's intravascular volume is removed from the effective circulation during dialysis. The addition of midodrine is one therapeutic intervention employed to elevate blood pressure so hemodialysis is hemodynamically tolerated by these patients. The finding that our midodrine group was more likely to undergo intraoperative continuous renal replacement therapy is not surprising since many of the patients were likely started on midodrine in conjunction with preoperative hemodialysis.

Medical literature database searches reveal minimal studies assessing midodrine directly in relation to OLT. Several studies have examined the outcomes of OLT when patients with hepatorenal syndrome are treated with midodrine, but to our knowledge none have directly assessed the perioperative impact of midodrine on OLT [12,17].

Limitations of our study include the relatively small size of the study population. Identifying an adequate number of patients undergoing OLT on midodrine and then pairing them with a demographically matched cohort yielded thirty-two matched pairs. Obviously, the statistical yield of our data would be improved with a larger sample population. As mentioned above, a slight trend towards increased requirements for fluid, blood, and vasopressor products might have become statistically significant with a larger study population. Midodrine dosing was varied among our patients and given the relatively small sample size; we were unable to stratify patients based on their midodrine dosing. Additionally, this was a single center study

which potentially introduces bias based on institutional practice standards. Furthermore, the study is a retrospective, matched case control study which inherently carries the risk of potential confounding factors distorting the data.

For our matching process, we focused on demographic data points to pair the midodrine patients with non-midodrine patients. Alternatively, we could have selected MELD or ASA scores to stratify our patients. Our focus on demographic data points (age, gender, donor type, and body mass index) was to account for important factors when comparing OLT patients that are not directly assessed in MELD and ASA scores. Importantly, the matching process was limited by the original population of fifty OLT patients on midodrine preoperatively and as additional variables were employed in the matching process, the total number of study patients successfully matched decreased. Ultimately, the four metrics listed above were selected as an appropriate balance between demographic matching and adequate sample size. To account for not using MELD scores to match patients, we ran a regression analysis as discussed previously.

In conclusion, preoperative use of midodrine in patients undergoing liver transplantation did not predict increased risk of intraoperative hypotension or concomitant need for vasopressors or blood products. Midodrine use was associated with higher ASA and MELD scores, renal replacement therapy, and decreased preoperative blood pressure. Regression analysis examining MELD scores was significant for increased intraoperative CRRT among the midodrine patients, but otherwise revealed no significant differences between the cohorts. No effect was detected on longer term outcomes such as one year patient and graft survival. Identifying factors predictive of perioperative and long term transplantation success are crucial as concomitant advances are made in other aspects of transplantation. Refining the precise role of midodrine in OLT will require additional prospective studies.

Funding:

Mayo Clinic Arizona

References

1. Martin PY, Ginès P, Schrier RW (1998) Nitric oxide as a mediator of hemodynamic abnormalities and sodium and water retention in cirrhosis. N Engl J Med 339: 533-541.

2. Kashani A, Landaverde C, Medici V, Rossaro L (2008) Fluid retention in cirrhosis: pathophysiology and management. QJM 101: 71-85.

3. Sourianarayanane A, Barnes DS, McCullough AJ (2011) Beneficial effect of midodrine in hypotensive cirrhotic patients with refractory ascites. Gastroenterol Hepatol (N Y) 7: 132-134.

4. Information P. Midodrine hcl oral tablets. UDL Laboratories Inc2006.

5. Hoeben H, Abu-Alfa AK, Mahnensmith R, Perazella MA (2002) Hemodynamics in patients with intradialytic hypotension treated with cool dialysate or midodrine. Am J Kidney Dis 39: 102-107.

6. Izcovich A, González Malla C, Manzotti M, Catalano HN, Guyatt G (2014) Midodrine for orthostatic hypotension and recurrent reflex syncope: A systematic review. Neurology 83: 1170-1177.

7. Jans O, Mehlsen J, Kjærsgaard-Andersen P, Husted H, Solgaard S, et al. (2015) Oral Midodrine Hydrochloride for Prevention of Orthostatic Hypotension during Early Mobilization after Hip Arthroplasty: A Randomized, Double-blind, Placebo-controlled Trial. Anesthesiology 123: 1292-1300.

8. Mukand J, Karlin L, Barrs K, Lublin P (2001) Midodrine for the management of orthostatic hypotension in patients with spinal cord injury: A case report. Arch Phys Med Rehabil 82: 694-696.

9. Prakash S, Garg AX, Heidenheim AP, House AA (2004) Midodrine appears to be safe and effective for dialysis-induced hypotension: a systematic review. Nephrol Dial Transplant 19: 2553-2558.

10. Azevedo LD, Stucchi RS, de Ataide EC, Boin IF (2015) Variables associated with the risk of early death after liver transplantation at a liver transplant unit in a university hospital. Transplant Proc 47: 1008-1011.

11. Leduc BE, Fournier C, Jacquemin G, Lepage Y, Vinet B, et al. (2015) Midodrine in patients with spinal cord injury and anejaculation: A double-blind randomized placebo-controlled pilot study. J Spinal Cord Med 38: 57-62.

12. Rice JP, Skagen C, Said A (2011) Liver transplant outcomes for patients with hepatorenal syndrome treated with pretransplant vasoconstrictors and albumin. Transplantation 91: 1141-1147.

13. Singh V, Singh A, Singh B, Vijayvergiya R, Sharma N, et al. (2013) Midodrine and clonidine in patients with cirrhosis and refractory or recurrent ascites: a randomized pilot study. Am J Gastroenterol 108: 560-567.

14. recurrent ascites: a randomized pilot study. Am J Gastroenterol 108: 560-567.

15. Wong F, Leung W, Al Beshir M, Marquez M, Renner EL (2015) Outcomes of patients with cirrhosis and hepatorenal syndrome type 1 treated with liver transplantation. Liver Transpl 21: 300-307.

16. Esrailian E, Pantangco ER, Kyulo NL, Hu KQ, Runyon BA (2007) Octreotide/Midodrine therapy significantly improves renal function and 30-day survival in patients with type 1 hepatorenal syndrome. Dig Dis Sci 52: 742-748.

17. Sourianarayanane A, Raina R, Garg G, McCullough AJ, O'Shea RS (2014) Management and outcome in hepatorenal syndrome: need for renal replacement therapy in non-transplanted patients. Int Urol Nephrol 46: 793-800.

Caraceni P, Santi L, Mirici F, Montanari G, Bevilacqua V, et al. (2011) Long-term treatment of hepatorenal syndrome as a bridge to liver transplantation. Dig Liver Dis 43: 242-245.

15

Preoperative Oral Morphine and Sub-Anesthetic Ketamine Co-Administration Reduce Acute Post-Mastectomy Pain

Montaser A Mohammad, Diab Fuad Hetta*, Rania M Abd Elemam and Shereen Mamdouh Kamal

Department of Anesthesia and Pain Management, South Egypt Cancer Institute, Assuit University, Egypt

*Corresponding author: Diab Fuad Hetta, Department of Anesthesia and Pain Management, South Egypt Cancer Institute, Assuit University, Egypt, E-mail: diabhetta25@gmail.com

Abstract

Objectives: To assess the analgesic efficacy and tolerability of co-administration of pre-emptive single oral dose of sustained release morphine and sub- anesthetic ketamine infusion for modified radical mastectomy (MRM) with axillary evacuation.

Methods: Sixty four adult female patients scheduled for MRM were divided to two groups, morphine group (n=32) received preoperative oral sustained release morphine tablet, 30 mg and placebo group (n=32) received placebo tablet. Both groups received preoperative ketamine bolus, 0.5 mg/kg followed by continuous infusion 0.1 mg/kg/h for 24 h postoperatively. VAS pain score, time to first analgesic request, 24 h analgesic consumption were reported.

Results: The mean VAS pain score during movement was significantly decreased in morphine group in comparison to placebo group from 2 h till 72 h postoperatively, 2 h (2.87 ± 1.0 *vs.* 4.53 ± 1.67) mean difference (-1.67) (95% CI)-(2.38-0.95), 72 h (1.20 ± 0.76 *vs.* 1.83 ± 0.91) mean difference (-0.63) (95% CI)-(1.07-0.20) while the mean VAS pain score during rest was significantly decreased in morphine group in comparison to placebo group from 2 h till 24 h postoperatively, 2 h (2.03 ± 0.85 *vs.* 3.47 ± 0.93) mean difference (-1.33) (95% CI)-(1.78-0.90), 24 h (1.40 ± 0.72 *vs.* 1.77 ± 0.68) mean difference (-0.37) (95% CI)-(0.73-0.01).

The median (IQ) time to first analgesic request was significantly delayed in morphine group in comparison to placebo group, 11.8 (9.7:14.2) h *vs.* 2.3 (2.1:2.5) h, (P<0.001).

The number (percentage) of patients required paracetamol in the first postoperative 24 h was significantly lower in morphine group in comparison to placebo group, 10 (33%) *vs.* 30 (100 %) (P<0.001).

Conclusion: Analgesic technique based on pre-emptive sustained release oral morphine and perioperative infusion of sub-anesthetic dose of ketamine provides satisfactory analgesia for patients undergoing MRM.

Keywords: Oral morphine; Ketamine; Mastectomy

Introduction

It is estimated that more than 50% of women will suffer moderate to severe acute pain following breast cancer surgery. It seriously affects quality of life through the combined impact of physical disability and emotional distress [1]. Surgical trauma induces hyperalgesia and allodynia. These enhanced reactions to noxious or non-noxious stimuli result from peripheral and/or central sensitization [2,3].

Pre-emptive analgesia is the administration of a drug before the onset of a painful stimulus that could reduce pain to a much greater extent than when the drug administered after the painful stimulus [4]. Opioids are considered the foundation of standard analgesic regimens for moderate-to-severe pain [5]. In addition to the broad value of morphine derivatives in clinical practice, their use as analgesic premedication before general anesthesia has aroused increasing interest [6]. Regularly dosed oral morphine has gained acceptance as the treatment of choice for patients with chronic cancer pain but is rarely used to treat acute postoperative pain. Ketamine has been used for treatment of acute pain. It is N-methyl-D-aspartate receptor

(NMDA-R) antagonist [7], exerts anti-allodynic effect through induction of synthesis and release of nitric oxide [8]. It binds to mu-receptors to increase the effectiveness of opioid-induced signalling [9]. Previous studies have found that co-administration of parenteral ketamine and morphine decrease intensity of pain as well as side effects [10,11], however, some studies revealed no benefit [12,13]. The analgesic efficacy of pre-emptive oral morphine and parenteral ketamine infusion is not studied before, so the aim of this study is to assess the analgesic efficacy and tolerability of preoperative single oral dose of sustained release morphine in patients receiving continuous infusion of sub- anesthetic dose of ketamine for patients undergoing MRM.

Methods

The study was approved by Institutional Ethics Committee of South Egypt Cancer Institute, the ethical approval number is (SECI20150196). Assuit University and a written informed consent for participation in the current clinical trial were obtained from each patient.

Inclusion and exclusion criteria

Sixty four adult women, American Society of Anesthesiologists (ASA) physical status class I and II, scheduled for modified radical mastectomy with axillary evacuation were included. The exclusion criteria were patients with known allergy or intolerance to any of the drugs used in the trial, pregnancy, history of drug abuse, preoperative opioid medication, history of postoperative nausea and vomiting (PONV), and history of ileus, liver dysfunction and patients suffering from uncontrolled hypertension or ischemic heart disease.

Randomization and blindness

Patients were randomly assigned to one of two groups: morphine group (n=32), where patients received orally 2 h before surgery sustained release morphine tablet (MST) 30 mg or placebo group (n=32), where patients received placebo tablet 2 h before surgery. The hospital pharmacists performed the randomization schedule using a computer-generated random number list. They masked the study medication by packing placebo and MST into two identical capsules in color and appearance to make the drugs unrecognizable. The study drugs were packed in opaque plastic containers labelled with the randomization numbers. The randomization code was opened at the end of the study.

Interventions

The night before surgery (in the anesthesia clinic), each patient was instructed how to evaluate their own pain intensity using the Visual Analogue Scale (VAS), scored from 0 to 10 (where 0=no pain and 10 = the worst pain imaginable).

In the preoperative area (2 hours before the operation), patients received the concerned study drug; morphine (MST) 30 mg tablet or placebo tablet according to randomization schedule.

In the operative room, monitoring probes (ECG, pulse oximeter and none invasive blood pressure) were attached and a peripheral venous line was established.

Both groups were administered intravenous ketamine bolus, 0.5 mg/kg, just before induction of anesthesia, followed by 0.1 mg/kg/h continuous intravenous infusion for 24 h postoperatively. General anesthesia was induced with propofol 2-3 mg/kg and fentanyl 2 μg/kg, followed by cisatracurium 0.15 mg/kg to facilitate endotracheal intubation. Anesthesia was maintained with sevoflurane in 40% oxygen in air and cisatracurium 0.03 mg/kg on demand. Heart rate and mean arterial blood pressure (MAP) were maintained within 20% of the preoperative baseline values by giving IV bolus doses of fentanyl 50 μg if the MAP or heart rate increased more than 20% from the baseline values. Ephedrine 10 mg was given IV as needed to keep MAP more than 65 mm Hg. Atropine 0.01 mg/kg was given IV if heart rate decreased less than 50 beat/ minute.

Before skin closure, all patients received IV paracetamol, 1 gm. The postoperative analgesia consisted of intravenous paracetamol (1 gm) infusion on demand in the first postoperative day and if the patient is still in pain, rescue analgesia with intravenous morphine, 5 mg diluted in 5 ml saline was administered by a nurse. In the subsequent postoperative days (in the home), analgesia was provided through regular paracetamol tablets, 1 gm every 8 h. Moderate to severe PONV was treated with IV ondansetron 4 mg. No other analgesics or anti-emetics were administered during the first 24 postoperative hours.

Assessments and outcomes

Time to first request for analgesic medication and the first 24 h analgesic consumption were recorded. Intensity of pain, assessed at rest and during movement, defined as (elevation of the arm from adduction to 90 degree abduction). Nausea and sedation were evaluated by the patients on a verbal rating scale scored from 0 to 3: none, light, moderate, and severe nausea or sedation. The need for anti-emetics in the first 24 hours postoperatively was recorded. Episodes of hallucinations, dizziness or nightmares were recorded by asking the patient 24 h postoperatively. Other potential side effects were recorded.

Primary outcome variable was the intensity of pain assessed with VAS pain score at rest and movement measured at the following postoperative time points (2, 6, 12, 24) h in the hospital by a nurse and at (36, 48, 72) h in home through a telephone. The secondary outcome variables were time to first analgesic request as well as 24 h analgesic consumption and morphine-ketamine related adverse events (nausea, vomiting, sedation, episodes of hallucinations and dizziness or night mares).

Statistical analysis

Statistical analysis was carried out on a personal computer using SPSS version 22 software. The primary outcome (the VAS pain score) was normally distributed using the Anderson-Darling test and comparisons between groups were done by unpaired student's t test and subsequent analysis was achieved by linear mixed effect model for repeated measures examining the following effects: group, time, and group-by-time interaction. While the secondary outcome variable, time to first analgesic request was not normally distributed and expressed as medians (IQ range) and comparison between groups was done by the Mann-Whitney U test and elucidated by Kaplan-Meier survival analysis. Qualitative data were reported as counts and percentages, and differences between groups were analyzed with the χ^2 test or Fisher exact test, as appropriate, where continuous data were described as mean ± standard division (SD) and (95% confidence interval), $P<0.05$ was considered statistically significant. Based on a preliminary pilot study of 10 patients in each group, we reported a mean ± SD of placebo group=4 ± 1.67 and a mean ± SD of morphine group=3.1 ± 1 Therefore, it was estimated that a minimum sample size of 29 patients in each study group would achieve a power of 80%, assuming a type I error of 0.05. We enrolled 64 patients to allow for dropouts.

Results

Eighty patients were assessed for eligibility and sixty patients completed the study. The flow of patients through the study was illustrated in Figure 1.

Demographic data and patient's characteristics were similar between groups (Table 1).

The mean VAS pain score during movement was significantly decreased in morphine group in comparison to placebo group at all measured time points during the first 72 h postoperatively, while the mean VAS pain score during rest was significantly decreased in morphine group in comparison to placebo group during the first postoperative 24 h only. Detailed data was shown in (Table 2).

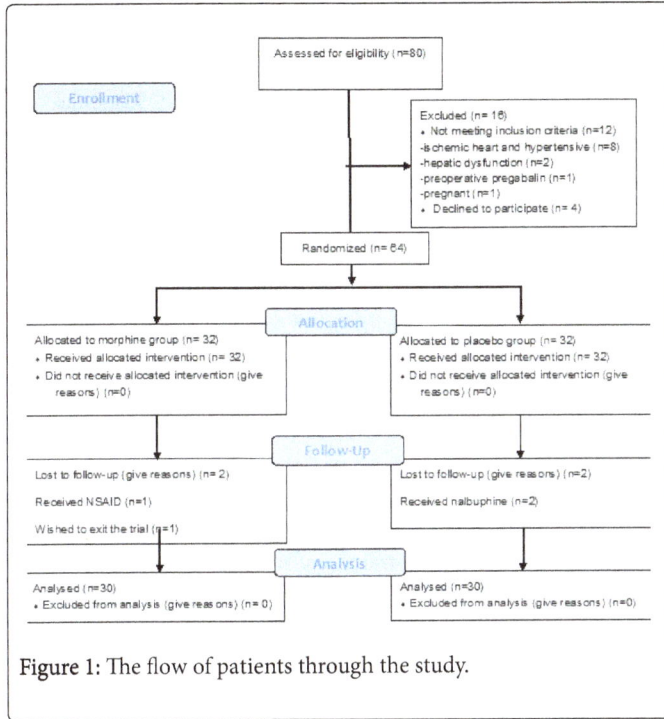

Figure 1: The flow of patients through the study.

Variable	Morphine group (n=30)	Placebo group (n=30)	P value
Age (years)	46.7 ± 7.8	43.4 ± 7.3	0.087
Weight (Kg)	79.2 ± 16.3	77.4 ± 12.4	0.120
Height (Cm)	166.9 ± 5.2	162.8 ± 5.4	0.961
ASA grade, n (%)			
I	18 (60.0%)	20 (66.7%)	0.789
II	12 (40.0%)	10 (33.3%)	
Duration of surgery (min)	140.9 ± 38.3	130.5 ± 27	0.693
Duration of anesthesia (min)	148.3 ± 38.3	142 ± 25.8	0.458

Data was presented as means ± SD or counts and percentages

Table 1: Demographic data and patient's characteristics.

Variable	Morphine N=30	Placebo N=30	Mean difference	95% CI (mean difference)
VAS at movement	Mean ± SD	Mean ± SD		
2 h	2.87 ± 1.00*	4.53 ± 1.67	-1.67	-(2.38-0.95)
6 h	2.67 ± 0.96*	4.23 ± 1.14	-1.57	-(2.11-1.02)
12 h	2.47 ± 0.81*	3.66 ± 0.88	-1.57	-(1.64-0.76)
24 h	2.10 ± 0.71*	2.93 ± 0.58	-0.83	-(1.17-0.50)
48 h	1.53 ± 0.82*	2.13 ± 0.57	-0.60	-(0.97-0.23)
36 h	1.70 ± 0.47*	2.13 ± 0.51	-0.43	-(0.69-0.18)
72 h	1.20 ± 0.76*	1.83 ± 0.91	-0.63	-(1.07-0.20)
VAS at rest	Mean ± SD	Mean ± SD		
2 h	2.03 ± 0.85*	3.47 ± 0.93	-1.33	-(1.78-0.90)
6 h	1.90 ± 0.92*	3.33 ± 0.71	-1.27	-(1.68-0.85)
12 h	1.77 ± 0.97*	2.37 ± 0.96	-0.50	-(0.98-0.02)
24 h	1.40 ± 0.72*	1.77 ± 0.68	-0.37	-(0.73-0.01)
48 h	1.10 ± 0.48	1.23 ± 0.73	-0.13	-(0.45-0.19)
36 h	1.03 ± 0.56	1.20 ± 0.66	-0.17	-(0.48-0.15)
72 h	0.60 ± 0.68	0.77 ± 0.73	-0.17	-(0.53-0.20)
Footnote: *=p value<0.05				

Table 2: postoperative VAS pain score at movement and rest.

The median (IQ) time to first analgesic request was significantly delayed in morphine group in comparison to placebo group, 11.8 (9.7:14.2) h vs. 2.3(2.1:2.5) h, (p<0.000) (Table 3).

variable	Morphine (n=30)	Placebo (n=30)	P value
Time to first analgesic request (h)	11.8(9.7:14.2)	2.3 (2.1:2.5)	0.00
Patients required analgesic in 24 h (n, %)	10 (33%)	30 (100)	0.00
paracetamol (1 gm) (n, %)	8 (26.7%)	1 (3.33%)	0.02
paracetamol (2 gm) (n, %)	2 (6.7%)	12 (40%)	0.01
paracetamol (3 gm) (n, %)	0	16 (53.3%)	0.00
Patients required morphine (5 mg) (n, %)	0	8 (26.7%)	0.00
Patients required morphine (10 mg) (n, %)	1 (3.33%)	2 (6.7%)	0.05
Footnote: Data was presented as median (1Q) range and numbers (percentages).			

Table 3: Duration of postoperative analgesia and analgesic consumption.

Regarding postoperative analgesic consumption, the number (percentage) of patients required postoperative paracetamol was significantly lower in morphine group in comparison to placebo group, 10 (33%) *vs.* 30 (100%) (p<0.001). The number (percentage) of patients required paracetamol in the first 24 h postoperatively was in morphine group *vs.* placebo group, paracetamol (1 gm) 8 (26.7%) *vs.* 1 (3.33%) (p<0.02), paracetamol (2 gm) 2 (6.7%) *vs.* 12 (40%) (p<0.01), paracetamol (3 gm) (0) *vs.* 16 (53.3%) (p<0.00) (Table 3). The number of patients required intravenous morphine was significantly lower in morphine group in comparison to placebo group 1 (3.33%) *vs.* 10 (33%) (Table 3).

The number of patients suffered from postoperative nausea and vomiting (PONV) was not statistically different between groups. The incidence of sedation was not statistically different between groups and none of the studied population suffered from excessive sedation. The number of patients complaining of dizziness was significantly increased in morphine group in comparison to placebo group (7 *vs.* 3) P<0.01). Detailed frequencies of adverse events were shown in Table 4.

Variable	Morphine (n=30)	Placebo (n=30)
Sedation (none/mild/moderate/severe, n)		
2 h	23/6/1/0	24/5/1/0
6 h	22/8/0/0	27/3/0/0
12 h	27/3/0/0	30/0/0/0
24 h	30/0/0/0	29/1/0/0
PONV (none/mild/moderate/severe, n)		
2 h	22/6/1/1	25/4/1/0
6 h	25/3/2/0	27/3/0/0
12 h	27/3/0/0	29/1/0/0
24 h	29/1/0/0	29/0/1/0
Patients required ondansetron, (n)	5	3
Dose of ondansetron (4,8,16) mg	4/1/0	2/1/0
Patients hallucinating (n)	1	2
Patients with nightmares (n)	2	1
Patients with dizziness (n)	7[*]	3
Footnote: [*]=p value<0.05		

Table 4: Postoperative adverse events in the first postoperative 24 h.

Discussion

The current study showed that preoperative medication with single dose oral morphine for patients receiving continuous infusion of sub-anesthetic dose of ketamine delayed time to first analgesic demand, reduced postoperative analgesic consumption and decreased the pain intensity during the first 72 h postoperatively without serious adverse events [14].

Opioids are still widely used prior to surgery to smooth induction of anesthesia, contribute to balanced anesthesia and provide postoperative pain relief. Morphine has been used as a premedication through different routes of administration including intra-muscular, oral sustained release and trans-buccal route [15-17].

The beneficial analgesic efficacy of combined ketamine and morphine administration was reported extensively in literature, In contrast to all previous studies that evaluated the addition of ketamine to PCA morphine for postoperative analgesia [10-12], the current study is unique in evaluation of analgesic efficacy of single oral dose of sustained release morphine for patients receiving continuous infusion of sub-anesthetic dose of ketamine. We found that two thirds of morphine group do not need any additional analgesics and expressed significantly lower VAS pain score for 72 h postoperatively.

The benefit of adding MST preoperatively is to supply the patients with a low and continuous dose of morphine in the initial postoperative phase, that should reduce overall analgesic consumption.

The rational of using continuous infusion of sub-anesthetic dosage of ketamine that started preoperatively and continued for 24 h postoperatively is firstly, acute post-mastectomy pain is essentially neuropathic due to surgical trauma of intercostal nerves, specifically intercosto-brachial nerves and ketamine is one of the effective drugs against neuropathic pain, secondly, it has been reported that perioperative ketamine may reduce the development of chronic postoperative pain *via* NMDA receptor blockade with subsequent reduction of wind-up and central sensitization [18].

The improvement in postoperative analgesia in the morphine group was consistent with previous study administered a single dose oral morphine, 10 or 20 mg for patients undergoing laparoscopic gastric bypass surgery [19].

Furthermore, it has been shown in two studies that oral and intramuscular pre-medication with morphine derivatives is able to reduce postoperative pain [20,21]. In contrast, other researchers observed no significant benefit of preoperative administration of sublingual buprenorphine or oral controlled-release morphine derivatives with regard to postoperative pain relief [22].

In the current study, we preferred to administer MST, 2 h before surgery as previous study reported that maximum plasma concentrations of morphine were recorded after 2.5 hours [23]. The smallest ketamine plasma concentration to counteract hyperalgesia while producing minimal side effects was shown to be 60 µg/ml [24]. This concentration was achieved by giving an initial bolus dose of ketamine 0.5 mg/kg, followed by a continuous infusion of 2 µg/kg/min [25], which was consistent with our study.

The improvement of analgesia produced by morphine-ketamine combination is explained by that painful stimulus activates NMDA receptors and produce hyperexcitability of dorsal root neurons. This induces central sensitization, expansion of the receptive field and wind-up phenomenon. Ketamine, a noncompetitive antagonist of NMDA receptors, can prevent the development of central sensitization caused by stimulation of peripheral nociception as well as blocking the wind-up phenomenon [26]. It has also been reported that mu-receptor activation by opioids leads to a sustained increase in glutamate synaptic effectiveness at the level of NMDA receptors. Moreover, opiates act at multiple sites in the central nervous system. Supraspinally, at locus ceruleus, nucleus raphe magnus, periaqueductal gray, medial thalamus, and limbic structures. Spinally, at the dorsal horn where the receptors are located pre- and postsynaptic [27,28]. Thus, MST when given preoperatively, it reduces pain impulses arriving to the neuroaxis and subsequently prevention of central sensitization.

Study limitation deserves mentioning is we did not follow up patients for detection of chronic post-mastectomy pain as the study was powered only for detection of changes of acute pain intensity. Future studies should concentrate on the effect of morphine-ketamine co-administration on occurrence of chronic post-mastectomy pain. This combination may be of great value for operations with severe acute postoperative pain such as thoracotomy and spine surgeries.

In conclusion, analgesic technique based on pre-emptive sustained release oral morphine and perioperative infusion of sub-anesthetic dose of ketamine provides satisfactory analgesia for patients undergoing conservative breast cancer surgery.

References

1. Katz J, Poleshuck EL, Andrus CH, Hogan LA, Jung BF, et al. (2005) "Risk factors for acute pain and its persistence following breast cancer surgery," Pain 119: 16-25.

2. Benrath J, Brechtelly C, Stark J, Sandkühler J (2005) Low dose of S (+)-ketamine prevents long-term potentiation in pain pathways under strong opioid analgesia in the rat spinal cord in vivo. Br J Anaesth 95: 518-523.

3. Sandkühler J (2000) Learning and memory in pain pathways. Pain 88: 113-118.

4. Singh H, Kundra S, Singh RM, Grewal A, Kaul TK, et al. (2013) Preemptive analgesia with Ketamine for Laparoscopic cholecystectomy. Anaesthesiol Clin Pharmacol. 29: 478-484.

5. Kelly DJ, Ahmad M, Brull SJ (2001) Preemptive analgesia I: physiological pathways and pharmacological modalities. Can J Anaesth 48: 1000-1010.

6. Rahimi M, Farsani DM, Naghibi K, Alikiaii B (2016) Preemptive morphine suppository for postoperative pain relief after laparoscopic cholecystectomy. Adv Biomed Res. 16: 5-57.

7. Mehta AK, Halder S, Khanna N, Tandon OP, Sharma KK (2012) Antagonism of stimulation-produced analgesia by naloxone and N-methyl-D-aspartate: Role of opioid and N-methyl-D-aspartate receptors. Hum Exp Toxicol 31: 51-56.

8. Romero TR, Galdino GS, Silva GC, Resende LC, Perez AC, et al. (2011) Ketamine activates the L-arginine/nitric oxide/cyclic guanosine monophosphate pathway to induce peripheral antinociception in rats. Anesth Analg 113: 1254-1259.

9. Gupta A, Devi LA, Gomes I (2011) Potentiation of mu-opioid receptor-mediated signaling by ketamine. J Neurochem 119: 294-302.

10. Adriaenssens G, Vermeyen KM, Hoffmann VL, Mertens E, Adriaensen HF (1999) Postoperative analgesia with i.v. patient controlled morphine: effect of adding ketamine. Br J Anaesth 83: 393-396.

11. Javery KB, Ussery TW, Steger HG, Colclough GW (1996) Comparison of morphine and morphine with ketamine for postoperative analgesia. Can J Anaesth 43: 212-215.

12. Reeves M, Lindholm DE, Myles PS, Fletcher H, Hunt JO (2001) Adding ketamine to morphine for patient-controlled analgesia after major abdominal surgery: a double-blinded, randomized controlled trial. Anesth Analg 93: 116-120.

13. Burstal R, Danjoux G, Hayes C, Lantry G (2001) PCA ketamine and morphine after abdominal hysterectomy. Anaesth Intensive Care 29: 246-251.

14. Aida S, Yamakura T, Baba H, Taga K, Fukuda S, et al. (2000) Preemptive analgesia by intravenous low-dose ketamine and epidural morphine in gastrectomy. Anesthesiology 92: 1624-1630.

15. Simpson KH, Tring IC, Ellis FR (1989) An investigation of premedication with morphine given by the buccal or intramuscular route. Br J Clin Pharmacol 27: 377-380.

16. Pinnock CA, Derbyshire DR, Elling AE, Smith G (1985) Comparison of slow release morphine (MST) with intramuscular morphine for premedication. Br J Anaesth 40: 1082-1085.

17. Fisher AP, Vine P, Whitelock J, Hanna M (1986) Buccal morphine premedication. Anaesthesia 41: 1104-1111.

18. Sawynok J (2014) Topical and peripheral ketamine as an analgesic. Anesth Analg 119: 170-178.

19. Hedberg J, Zacharias H, Janson L, Sundbom M (2016) Preoperative Slow-Release Morphine Reduces Need of Postoperative Analgesics and Shortens Hospital Stay in laparoscopic Gastric Bypass. Obes Surg 26: 757-761.

20. Bullingham RE, O'Sullivan G, McQuay HJ, Poppleton P, Rolfe M, et al. (1984) Mandatory sublingual buprenorphine for postoperative pain. Anaesthesia 39: 329-334.

21. Hanks GW, Rose NM, Aherne GW, Piall EM, Fairfield S (1981) Controlled-release morphine tablets. A double blind trial in dental surgery patients. Br J Anaesth 53: 1259-1264.

22. Slowey HF, Reynolds AD, Mapleson WW, Vickers MD (1985) Effect of premedication with controlled release oral morphine on postoperative pain. A comparison with intramuscular morphine. Anaesthesia 40: 438-440.

23. Hoskin PJ, Hanks GW, Aherne GW, Chapman D, Littleton P (1989) The bioavailability and pharmacokinetics of morphine after intravenous, oral and buccal administration in healthy volunteers. Br J Clin Pharmacol 27: 499-505.

24. Leung A, Wallace MS, Ridgeway B, Yaksh T (2001) Concentration effect relationship of intravenous alfentanil and ketamine on peripheral neurosensory thresholds, allodynia and hyperalgesia of neuropathic pain. Pain 91: 177-187.

25. Schmid RL, Sandler AN, Katz J (1999) Use and efficacy of low-dose ketamine in the management of acute postoperative pain: a review of current techniques and outcomes. Pain 82: 111-125.

26. Woolf CJ, Thompson SW (1991) The induction and maintenance of central sensitization is dependent on N-methyl-d-aspartate acid receptor activation: implication for the treatment of post-injury pain hypersensitivity states. Pain 44: 293-299.

27. Pert A, Yaksh T (1974) Sites of morphine induced analgesia in primate brain: Relation to pain pathways. Brain Res 80: 135-140.

28. Fields HL, Martin JB (2001) Pain: pathophysiology and management, in Braunwald E, Hauser SL, Fauci AS (eds): Harrison's Principles of Internal Medicine (ed 15). New York, NY, McGraw-Hill, pp 55-60.

16

Rapidly Metabolized Anesthetics: Novel Alternative Agents for Procedural Sedation

Joseph Colao and Daniel Rodriguez-Correa*

Department of Anesthesiology, Rutgers New Jersey Medical School, Newark, NJ, USA

***Corresponding author:** Daniel Rodriguez-Correa MD., PhD. Assistant Professor, Department of Anesthesiology, Rutgers New Jersey Medical School, Newark, NJ, USA, E-mail: dtr38@njms.rutgers.edu

Abstract

The increased demand for procedural sedation in the ambulatory setting has prompted the development of anesthetic agents that anesthesiologists and non-anesthesiologists could administer easily and safely. In this article, we discuss novel short-acting agents in development or in clinical trials that may serve as alternatives to current anesthetics for procedural sedation.

Introduction

Propofol and midazolam are the most commonly used agents for intravenous sedation and induction of anesthesia in a wide variety of surgical and nonsurgical procedures. Though both agents exert their effects by interacting with inhibitory GABA-A receptors in the central nervous system, they have different advantages and adverse effects. Midazolam is a short-acting benzodiazepine, which has sedative effects that are pharmacologically reversible by administration of flumazenil. However, midazolam has a relative long onset to produce sedation and its active metabolite, α1-hydroxymidazolam, may prolong recovery [1-3]. This can both decrease procedural efficiency and increase the risk of adverse effects, such as respiratory depression. Propofol is a sedative-hypnotic agent that is advantageous because it has a rapid onset of sedation and recovery, compared to midazolam [4-6]. It has a narrow therapeutic range and steep dose-response curve; therefore, a small increase in dose can quickly cause a large increase in depth of sedation [7]. Propofol can cause apnea and significant cardiovascular depression if too large of a dose is administered. There is no clinically available agent that can reverse its effects. Because propofol also has low solubility in aqueous solution, it is often prepared as an emulsion, which supports bacterial growth and may lead to bacteremia [8]. Propofol also produces pain on injection and it is often co-administered with lidocaine to reduce patient discomfort [9].

There has been an increase in the number of procedures requiring deep sedation, including minimally invasive surgeries and nonsurgical procedures commonly performed in outpatient settings such as upper gastrointestinal endoscopy, colonoscopy, and bronchoscopy [10]. Procedural sedation is also common in emergency departments for dislocated joint reduction, fracture care, and cardioversion, among others [11,12]. In those settings, etomidate and ketamine are agents of choice in addition to midazolam and propofol [11]. The use of propofol for sedation in these procedures is growing, and current guidelines recommend for it to be administered by anesthesiologists [13]. However, the demand for anesthesiologists' services in these procedures has exceeded anesthesiologists' availability in many clinical settings [7,10]. As a result, non-anesthesiologist administration of propofol (NAAP) by endoscopists and registered nurses is on the rise, with favorable safety data, especially for upper gastrointestinal endoscopy and colonoscopy [14-16]. Though NAAP has been supported by both American and European anesthesiology guidelines for certain procedures with low risk patients, the practice remains controversial due to concern for adverse effects occurring without a trained anesthesiologist present to manage the patient [13,17]. Ideally, anesthetic agents used for these procedures would produce rapid onset of sedation and recovery with minimal adverse effects so that anesthesiologists and non-anesthesiologists could administer them easily and safely. There is no drug approved for clinical use that possesses all of these properties. However, multiple rapidly metabolized anesthetic agents with those characteristics are currently in pre-clinical and clinical trials. This review summarizes the most recent developments in these drugs, which could shape the future of procedural sedation.

Remimazolam

Remimazolam (CNS 7056) (Figure 1) is a rapidly metabolized midazolam analogue developed by PAION for which Phase II clinical trials have recently been completed. The major shortcoming of midazolam use in sedation is that patients have prolonged recoveries due to midazolam's liver-dependent metabolism by cytochrome P450 3A4 and the accumulation of the drug's active metabolites [18]. This requires additional monitoring of patients during recovery. Remimazolam contains a carboxylic ester linkage that allows it to undergo rapid, dose-dependent hydrolysis by non-specific tissue esterases, rather than primarily by liver enzymes as with midazolam. This organ-independent metabolism allows for faster, more predictable elimination and greater procedural efficiency. Like midazolam and other benzodiazepines, remimazolam produces sedative effects by interacting with GABA-A receptors. Its carboxylic acid metabolite (CNS 7054) also has affinity for GABA-A receptors, but it is 400-fold less than remimazolam *in vitro* [19]. CNS 7054 has a terminal half-life 4 times greater than that of remimazolam but is considered inactive [20]. Phase I clinical trials demonstrated that remimazolam had a dose-dependent duration of sedation with a median time to fully alert of 10 minutes, compared to a 40 minutes for midazolam, following 1-minute IV infusions of equihypnotic doses of each drug. Remimazolam had similar adverse effects to midazolam; they were most commonly headache and somnolence. There were no significant effects on heart rate, blood pressure, respiratory rate, temperature,

ECG, or laboratory values [18]. The effects of remimazolam were easily reversed with administration of flumazenil [20]. An additional finding of note was the lack of a clear relationship between systemic clearance of remimazolam and body weight, which could suggest that dosing by body weight would not be advantageous [18].

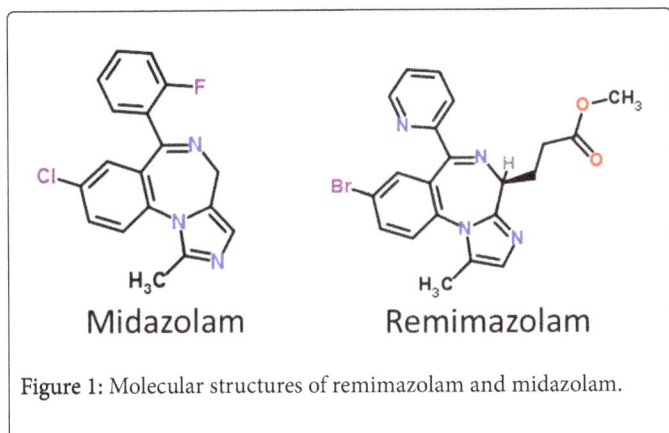

Figure 1: Molecular structures of remimazolam and midazolam.

The randomized, double-blind Phase II clinical trials, published in 2015, evaluated the safety and efficacy of remimazolam versus midazolam in upper GI endoscopy and colonoscopy to define doses for procedural sedation in future trials. In the Phase IIa trial, patients received a single dose of either remimazolam (0.10, 0.15, or 0.20 mg/kg) or midazolam (0.075 mg/kg) for an upper GI endoscopy [21]. The 0.15 and 0.20 mg/kg remimazolam study groups had greater procedure success rates (56.0% and 64.0% respectively) than the midazolam group (44.0%). The 0.10 mg/kg remimazolam group had a lower success rate of 32.0%. In all four study groups, procedure failure was solely due to the need for a rescue sedative of either propofol, midazolam, or both propofol and midazolam if sedation could not be maintained after the single dose administration. 51 of the 100 total patients in the study required rescue sedative. The percentage of patients who received rescue sedatives varied greatly from 8.3% to 78.6% among the several different clinical sites at which the procedures were performed. This likely resulted from each site waiting a different amount of time to administer the rescue sedative, which primarily determined the procedural success rates. Additionally, 25 of the recruited patients, who were evenly distributed across the four study groups, received topical anesthetic for the procedure, and only 2 (8%) of these patients required rescue sedative in comparison to the overall study rate of 51%. The authors advised for topical anesthetic administration to be standardized for all patients' in future upper GI endoscopies. All three remimazolam groups had faster onsets of sedation (1.5 to 2.5 minutes) and faster mean recoveries from of sedation (6.8 to 9.9 minutes) than the midazolam group (5 minute onset, 11.5 minute recovery). These results excluded patients who required rescue sedatives. The incidence of adverse events occurring after sedative administration was similar among all 4 study groups with the remimazolam groups (40% to 48%) having slightly less incidences than the midazolam group (52%). Both compounds had stable vital sign profiles and low risk of adverse respiratory events, suggesting that remimazolam has a typical benzodiazepine adverse effect profile, but this must be confirmed by further studies.

In contrast to the endoscopy study, the patients in the Phase IIb clinical trial received an initial body-weight-independent dose of either remimazolam (8.0, 7.0, or 5.0 mg) or midazolam (2.5 mg) for a colonoscopy [22]. The patients also received a maximum of 6 top-up

boluses of their initial drug for maintenance of sedation throughout the procedure (3.0, 2.0, or 3.0 mg for the remimazolam groups respectively or 1.0 mg for the midazolam group). Supplemental oxygen and 100 μg of fentanyl were administered to all patients prior to the procedure. Procedure success was significantly greater in the remimazolam groups (92.5% to 97.5%) than in the midazolam group (75.0%), though the greater success of the 8.0 mg remimazolam group was not statistically significant. Among the 3 remimazolam groups, the success rate increased with decreasing initial dose; the 5.0 mg group had the greatest success rate of 97.5%. All procedure failures were again due to the need for a rescue sedative if sedation could not be maintained after 2 minutes after using all 6 available top-ups. Onset of sedation was faster for the remimazolam groups (2.35 to 3.03 minutes) than for the midazolam group (4.80 minutes). Over 82.5% of the remimazolam patients were sufficiently sedated to start the procedure after the initial dose, compared to 46.3% of midazolam patients. In addition, the remimazolam groups (1.43 to 2.35) required less top-ups on average than the midazolam group (2.48). Mean recovery time was similarly short among all four study groups (11.3 to 15.2 minutes), but this is likely due to the 25% of midazolam patients who received propofol as a rescue sedative while very few remimazolam patients received rescue sedatives. The 5.0 mg remimazolam group had the best safety profile of the 4 study groups with no incidences of hypoxia, respiratory depression, or severe hypotension, which each occurred in at least 2 of the other 3 study groups. Some of these adverse events occurred shortly after fentanyl administration, so the benzodiazepines may not have been the primary cause. With the superior success rate and safety profile, a 5.0 mg initial dose of remimazolam with 3.0 mg top-ups to maintain sedation proved to be the most effective dose to pursue in future clinical trials.

Remimazolam has shown great potential among new rapidly metabolized anesthetics as a safe sedative with fast onset and short duration of action. This allows for faster procedure times and decreased risk of prolonged sedation in comparison to midazolam, the current drug of choice. The drug has made the most progress in clinical trials, and its success thus far necessitates further investigation in Phase III studies, which are ongoing.

Etomidate Analogues

Cyclopropyl-methoxycarbonyl metomidate (ABP-700)

ABP-700 (Figure 2), also known as cyclopropyl-methoxycarbonyl metomidate (CPMM), is a rapidly metabolized etomidate analogue developed by the Massachusetts General Hospital Department of Anesthesia that has recently completed Phase I clinical trials. The parent compound, etomidate, is a GABA-A receptor agonist that produces variable hypnotic recovery times after intravenous infusions and also produces adrenocortical steroid suppression that persists much longer than its hypnotic effect due to inhibition of the cytochrome P450 enzyme β-11 hydroxylase, which is necessary for cortisol, corticosterone, and aldosterone synthesis [23]. To improve recovery times and avoid adrenocortical suppression, the research team at Massachusetts General Hospital developed methoxycarbonyl etomidate (MOC-etomidate), an ester-linked etomidate analogue that is rapidly metabolized by nonspecific esterases to a significantly less potent carboxylic acid metabolite in a similar way as remimazolam [24,25]. MOC-etomidate had a significantly shorter duration of hypnotic effect and adrenocortical suppression than etomidate in animal studies, but it was determined to be too short acting for clinical use [26,27]. The research team then developed a series of MOC-etomidate analogues by incorporating various chemical groups into the compound to sterically protect the ester moiety from hydrolysis by esterases, prolonging the duration of action to a clinically useful length. CPMM (ABP-700) was the most promising of the analogues synthesized [27].

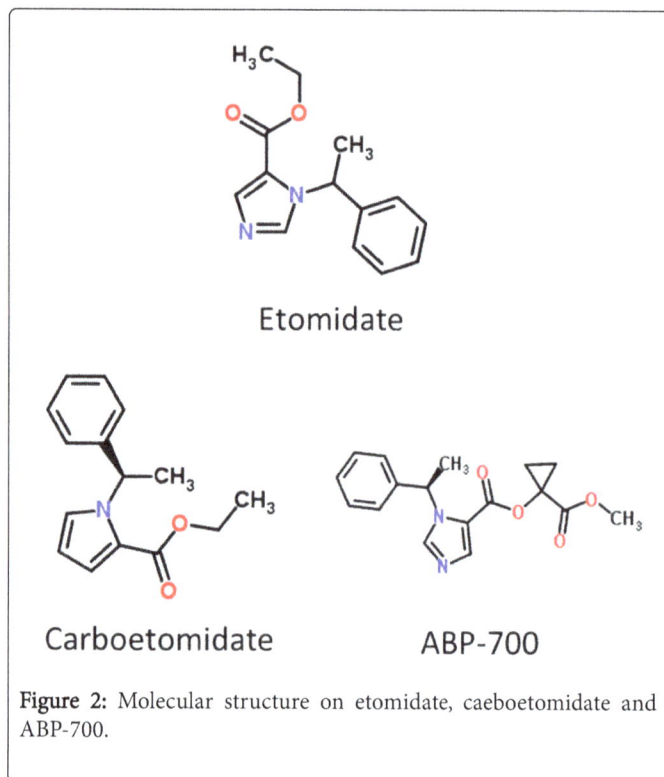

Figure 2: Molecular structure on etomidate, caeboetomidate and ABP-700.

A subsequent study comparing the effects of CPMM with those of etomidate in dogs found that single intravenous boluses of CPMM produced dose-dependent durations of sedation with significantly faster clearance than etomidate as indicated by the slopes of the dose-response curves [23]. Hypnotic recovery times after both a single bolus and a single bolus followed by a 2-hour infusion of each drug were also faster for CPMM than for etomidate. Mean recovery time did not differ significantly after single bolus administration (8 ± 3 min) than after 2-hour infusion (11 ± 3 min) demonstrating that recovery time was independent of CPMM infusion duration. In contrast, there was a greater than four-fold increase in mean hypnotic recovery time after etomidate infusion than after single bolus administration. A CPMM metabolite was also found to remain in the blood at high concentrations long after CPMM administration, but the metabolite's hypnotic potency and molecular interactions have not been determined.

Similar to etomidate, CPMM produced adrenocortical suppression during a 2-hour infusion and 30 minutes after termination of the infusion, as indicated by decreased ACTH-induced serum cortisol concentration. Adrenocortical response was normal (compared to vehicle control) 120 minutes after CPMM infusion termination, while cortisol levels remained decreased for greater than 300 minutes after etomidate infusion termination. A similar study in rats receiving infusions of either etomidate or CPMM demonstrated similarly faster adrenocortical responsiveness following CPMM infusion [24]. Adrenocortical responsiveness after a 2-hour infusion of CPMM was

also found to be similar to that of propofol within 90 minutes after infusion termination [23]. This indicated that adrenocortical suppression following CPMM administration was likely brief and clinically insignificant, further demonstrating potential for CPMM to advance to human studies. Another study found that CPMM produced reduced elevations of inflammatory cytokines in response to lipopolysaccharide challenge in rats, implicating CPMM as a safer alternative to etomidate in septic patients [28].

In October 2015, The Medicines Company issued a press release briefly summarizing the results of Phase I clinical trials for CPMM, which was renamed ABP-700 [29]. In one double-blind randomized study (ANVN-01), 60 healthy adult volunteers received either a single intravenous bolus of ABP-700 (0.03 to 1.0 mg/kg) or placebo. ABP-700 produced dose-dependent depth and duration of sedation, which was rapidly reversible at all doses. Adverse events were dose-dependent and included tachycardia, hyperventilation, apnea, muscle twitching, and myoclonus [30]. Of note, myoclonus was also observed in a significant portion of subjects in the dog study of CPMM and was reversed rapidly with midazolam administration [23]. There was no significant variance in blood pressure and low incidence of nausea and vomiting in this Phase I study.

Adrenocortical suppression was also evaluated in two separate Phase I trials mentioned in the press release. One trial was the aforementioned placebo-controlled ABP-700 bolus study, and in the other trial, subjects received placebo or 30-minute intravenous infusions of ABP-700 (0.9 to 1.97 mg/kg) or propofol (2.25 mg/kg) [29]. ACTH-induced adrenocortical responsiveness was measured one hour after bolus administration or infusion termination. In both Phase I studies, adrenocortical responsiveness after ABP-700 administration was similar to placebo and propofol, demonstrating that ABP-700 had minimal impact on adrenocortical steroid synthesis after single bolus administration or short-term infusion. These results correlated with those of the previous animal studies.

Though the complete results of these Phase I studies have not yet been published, ABP-700 has shown great potential to be used in future clinical trials due to its rapid metabolism and maintenance of etomidate's favorable hypnotic effects while producing clinically insignificant adrenocortical suppression, though this effect has not been evaluated for continuous infusions longer than 30 minutes. These characteristics of ABP-700 warrant further investigation into its potential uses in specific clinical procedures and its advantages over the sedative agents that are commonly used in those procedures.

Carboetomidate and MOC-carboetomidate

Etomidate analogs such as APB-700 and MOC-etomidate were designed to produce less adrenocortical suppression than etomidate through their rapid metabolism, resulting in a shorter duration of adrenocortical steroid production. However, these sedatives still inhibit β-11 hydroxylase by the same proposed mechanism as etomidate. The chemical structures of etomidate and its aforementioned analogs contain an imidazole ring, which has been suggested to inhibit the enzyme through the high-affinity interaction of the of its nitrogen atom with the heme iron in the enzyme's active site [31,32]. In order to create an etomidate analog that does not interact with β-11 hydroxylase, the Massachusetts General Hospital Department of Anesthesia developed carboetomidate (Figure 2), which contains a pyrrole ring rather than an imidazole ring [33]. When equihypnotic boluses of carboetomidate and etomidate were given to rats, there was significantly reduced adrenocortical suppression in those that received carboetomidate than for etomidate, indicated by a greater than two-fold less ACTH-induced serum corticosterone concentration measured 15 minutes after bolus administration. There was no statistically significant difference in adrenocortical suppression between rats that received carboetomidate and those that received placebo, suggesting that carboetomidate does not inhibit β-11 hydroxylase significantly. In a rat endotoxemia study, carboetomidate produced a smaller increase in inflammatory cytokine production and less adrenocortical suppression than etomidate, demonstrating potential usefulness in anesthetic management of septic patients [34]. However, carboetomidate had a much slower onset time than etomidate (33 ± 22 sec vs. 4.5 ± 0.6 sec), as well 1/7th the hypnotic potency [33].

Carboetomidate was modified to incorporate a metabolically labile ester group into its structure, similar to MOC-etomidate, in order to make it a more rapidly metabolized drug while maintaining its favorable adrenocortical effects. The resulting compound, MOC-carboetomidate, retained the GABA-A receptor agonist property and hemodynamic stability of carboetomidate in a rat study [35]. It had a much shorter half-life (1.3 min) than carboetomidate (>20 min) and etomidate (>20 min) but a longer half-life than MOC-etomidate (0.35 min), which was advantageous as MOC-etomidate was too short acting to be feasible for clinical use. MOC-carboetomidate also produced adrenocortical suppression that was significantly less than etomidate and similar to that of the placebo. However, MOC-carboetomidate had a similar onset time to carboetomidate, indicating that the ester linkage did not make induction of sedation faster than that of etomidate. No additional studies of MOC-carboetomidate have been published at this time. Though the reduced half-life demonstrated that MOC-carboetomidate was metabolized faster than carboetomidate and etomidate, the compound must be modified further to warrant future study as a potentially more reliable alternative to etomidate with faster onset and offset of sedation.

MR04A3

MR04A3 is a 1% aqueous solution of the compound JM-1232(-) (Figure 3) that has been evaluated for its efficacy and safety as a sedative in a human study [36]. JM-1232(-), developed by the Maruishi Pharmaceutical Company, is a water-soluble compound with a non-benzodiazepine structure that, like benzodiazepines, is a GABA-A receptor agonist. It was found to have favorable hypnotic effects in mice, and the effects were inhibited by flumazenil. Due to these results, MR04A3 (the JM-1232(-) preparation) was studied in 69 healthy male volunteers in 2010. MR04A3 produced dose-dependent durations of sedation, measured by time to eyes open on command, after both 1 minute and 10 minute infusions. Mean sedation durations ranged from 5.7 to 67.3 minutes after infusions with doses of 0.075 to 0.8 mg/kg. Ramsay sedation scores were greater with increasing doses of MR04A3. There was also a greater reduction in bispectral index and for a longer duration with larger doses. Heart rate and blood pressure were recorded for 60 minutes after the infusions, and both varied minimally throughout that time. The adverse event profile in volunteers who received MR04A3 was similar to that of those who received the placebo with a small number of volunteers developing upper airway obstruction, which was relieved by simple positional maneuvers. Overall, MR04A3 was well tolerated among the study participants. Its dose-dependent hypnotic effect and low incidence of adverse events during recovery warrant further clinical investigation. Though this study demonstrated faster onset and offset times for MR04A3 than for literature values of midazolam, future studies must compare MR04A3 directly to active control anesthetics, such as

midazolam and propofol, rather than only placebo [37]. There was also a JM-1232(-) metabolite, JM-Metabo-3, that was found in increasing arterial concentrations with greater MR04A3 infusion doses [36]. This metabolite must be investigated further to determine the risk of unexpected prolongation of sedation and other potential adverse effects.

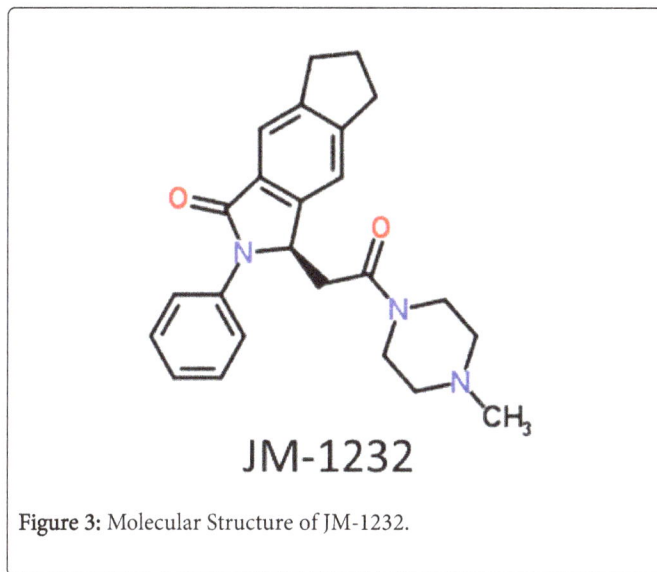

Figure 3: Molecular Structure of JM-1232.

More recently, animal studies on the cerebrovacular effects of JM-1232(-) found that intravenous administration of the compound has minimally affected vascular reactivity and further validated its safety [38,39]. However, plans for future evaluation in human studies are unclear.

Conclusion

The emerging group of rapidly metabolized anesthetics represents both pharmacokinetic and pharmacodynamic modifications to agents used clinically for intravenous induction of anesthesia, such as midazolam and etomidate. The preferred pharmacokinetic modification is an ester linkage, which is found in remimazolam, ABP-700, MOC-carboetomidate, and MOC-etomidate. The ester group allows for rapid, nonspecific metabolism by tissue esterases, leading to faster offset and less significant adverse effects due to the short duration of action. However, rapid metabolism also causes greater production of metabolites, which must be closely evaluated for the potential to prolong sedation unexpectedly and cause adverse effects. Remimazolam, MR04A3, and ABP-700, which have all at least completed Phase I clinical trials, have known metabolites under investigation, though the remimazolam metabolite is considered inactive. In contrast, carboetomidate is a pharmacodynamic modification of etomidate that significantly decreases adrenocortical suppression, which is etomidate's major adverse effect. MOC-carboetomidate is a combination of both pharmacokinetic and pharmacodynamic modifications.

Remimazolam and ABP-700 have the greatest potential to be introduced into clinical practice since they have completed Phase II and Phase I trials, respectively, with favorable results. Further trials that can continue to demonstrate these drugs' more rapid and reliable onsets and offsets of sedation may warrant their use as alternatives to midazolam, especially for short procedures. These favorable properties may also have implications for use of these drugs by non-anesthetists. While the rapidly metabolized anesthetics were compared to their parent compounds, midazolam and etomidate, an important shortcoming of the clinical trials performed thus far is the lack of direct comparison to other anesthetics commonly used outside of the operating room, such as propofol and ketamine. Inclusion of these agents for comparison in future studies would be useful in demonstrating the advantages of the novel anesthetics in procedural sedation more clearly. The last decade has yielded exciting advances in the development of rapidly metabolized anesthetics. While their exact clinical applications have yet to be defined, these drugs show great potential to produce more reliable sedation while improving procedural efficiency and patient safety.

References

1. Tuk B, van Oostenbruggen MF, Herben VM, Mandema JW, Danhof M (1999) Characterization of the pharmacodynamic interaction between parent drug and active metabolite in vivo: midazolam and alpha-OH-midazolam. J Pharmacol Exp Ther 289: 1067-1074.

2. Johnson TN, Rostami-Hodjegan A, Goddard JM, Tanner MS, Tucker GT (2012) Contribution of midazolam and its 1-hydroxy metabolite to preoperative sedation in children: a pharmacokinetic-pharmacodynamic analysis. Br J Anaesth 89: 428-437.

3. Bremer F, Reulbach U, Schwilden H, Schüttler J (2004) Midazolam therapeutic drug monitoring in intensive care sedation: a 5-year survey. Ther Drug Monit 26: 643-649.

4. Koshy G, Nair S, Norkus EP, Hertan HI, Pitchumoni CS (2000) Propofol versus midazolam and meperidine for conscious sedation in GI endoscopy. Am J Gastroenterol 95: 1476-1479.

5. Sipe BW, Rex DK, Latinovich D, Overley C, Kinser K, et al. (2002) Propofol versus midazolam/meperidine for outpatient colonoscopy: administration by nurses supervised by endoscopists. Gastrointest Endosc 55: 815-825.

6. Poulos JE, Kalogerinis PT, Caudle JN (2013) Propofol compared with combination propofol or midazolam/fentanyl for endoscopy in a community setting. AANA J 81: 31-36.

7. Tan G, Irwin MG (2010) Recent advances in using propofol by non-anesthesiologists. F1000 Med Rep 2: 79.

8. Erden IA, Gülmez D, Pamuk AG, Akincia SB, Hasçelik G, et al. (2013) The growth of bacteria in infusion drugs: propofol 2% supports growth when remifentanil and pantoprazole do not. Braz J Anesthesiol 63: 466-472.

9. Euasobhon P, Dej-Arkom S, Siriussawakul A, Muangman S, Sriraj W, et al. (2016) Lidocaine for reducing propofol-induced pain on induction of anaesthesia in adults. Cochrane Database Syst Rev 2: CD007874.

10. Burtea DE, Dimitriu A, Maloş AE, Saftoiu A (2015) Current role of non-anesthesiologist administered propofol sedation in advanced interventional endoscopy. World J Gastrointest Endosc 7: 981-986.

11. Sacchetti A, Senula G, Strickland J, Dubin R (2007) Procedural sedation in the community emergency department: initial results of the ProSCED registry. Acad Emerg Med 14: 41-46.

12. Black E, Campbell SG, Magee K, Zed PJ (2013) Propofol for procedural sedation in the emergency department: a qualitative systematic review. Ann Pharmacother 47: 856-868.

13. [Author not listed] (2016) American Society of Anesthesiology. Statement on Safe Use of Propofol.

14. Rex DK, Deenadayalu VP, Eid E, Imperiale TF, Walker JA, et al. (2009) Endoscopist-directed administration of propofol: a worldwide safety experience. Gastroenterology 137: 1229-1237.

15. Molina-Infant J, Dueñas-Sadornil C, Mateos-Rodriguez JM, Perez-Gallardo B, Vinagre-Rodríguez G, et al. (2012) Nonanesthesiologist-administered propofol versus midazolam and propofol, titrated to moderate sedation, for colonoscopy: a randomized controlled trial. Dig Dis Sci 57: 2385-2393.

16. Repici A, Pagano N, Hassan C, Carlino A, Rando G, et al. (2011) Balanced propofol sedation administered by nonanesthesiologists: The first Italian experience. World J Gastroenterol 17: 3818-3823.

17. Dumonceau JM, Riphaus A, Schreiber F, Vilmann P, Beilenhoff C, et al. (2015) Non-anesthesiologist administration of propofol for gastrointestinal endoscopy: European Society of Gastrointestinal Endoscopy, European Society of Gastroenterology and Endoscopy Nurses and Associates Guideline-Updated June 2015. Endoscopy 47: 1175-1189.

18. Antonik LJ, Goldwater DR, Kilpatrick GJ, Tilbrook GS, Borkett KM (2012) A placebo- and midazolam-controlled phase I single ascending-dose study evaluating the safety, pharmacokinetics, and pharmacodynamics of remimazolam (CNS 7056): Part I. Safety, efficacy, and basic pharmacokinetics. Anesth Analg 115: 274-283.

19. Kilpatrick GJ, McIntyre MS, Cox RF, Stafford JA, Pacofsky GJ, et al. (2007) CNS 7056: a novel ultra-short-acting Benzodiazepine. Anesthesiology 107: 60-66.

20. Worthington MT, Antonik LJ, Goldwater DR, Lees JP, Wilhelm-Ogunbiyi K, et al. (2013) A phase Ib, dose-finding study of multiple doses of remimazolam (CNS 7056) in volunteers undergoing colonoscopy. Anesth Analg 117: 1093-1100.

21. Borkett KM, Riff DS, Schwartz HI, Winkle PJ, Pambianco DJ, et al. (2015) A Phase IIa, randomized, double-blind study of remimazolam (CNS 7056) versus midazolam for sedation in upper gastrointestinal endoscopy. Anesth Analg 120: 771-780.

22. Pambianco DJ, Borkett KM, Riff DS, Winkle PJ, Schwartz HI, et al. (2016) A phase IIb study comparing the safety and efficacy of remimazolam and midazolam in patients undergoing colonoscopy. Gastrointest Endosc 83: 984-992.

23. Campagna JA, Pojasek K, Grayzel D, Randle J, Raines DE (2014) Advancing novel anesthetics: pharmacodynamic and pharmacokinetic studies of cyclopropyl-methoxycarbonyl metomidate in dogs. Anesthesiology 121: 1203-1216.

24. Ge R, Pejo E, Cotten JF, Raines DE (2013) Adrenocortical suppression and recovery after continuous hypnotic infusion: etomidate versus its soft analogue cyclopropyl-methoxycarbonyl metomidate. Crit Care 17: R20.

25. Ge RL, Pejo E, Haburcak M, Husain SS, Forman SA, et al. (2012) Pharmacological studies of methoxycarbonyl etomidate's carboxylic acid metabolite. Anesth Analg 115: 305-308.

26. Cotten JF, Husain SS, Forman SA, Miller KW, Kelly EW, et al. (2009) Methoxycarbonyl-etomidate: a novel rapidly metabolized and ultra-short-acting etomidate analogue that does not produce prolonged adrenocortical suppression. Anesthesiology 111: 240-249.

27. Husain SS, Pejo E, Ge R, Raines DE (2012) Modifying methoxycarbonyl etomidate inter-ester spacer optimizes in vitro metabolic stability and in vivo hypnotic potency and duration of action. Anesthesiology 117: 1027-1036.

28. Santer P, Pejo E, Feng Y, Chao W, Raines DE (2015) Cyclopropyl-methoxycarbonyl Metomidate: Studies in a Lipopolysaccharide Inflammatory Model of Sepsis. Anesthesiology 123: 368-376.

29. The Medicines Company (2015) Results of First-in-Man Study with Investigational Anesthetic ABP-700 Presented at ANESTHESIOLOGY® 2015 and International Society of Anesthetic Pharmacology Annual Meetings [Press Release].

30. Egan T, Raines D, Struys M, Sneyd R (2015) Update on ABP-700. Presented at American Society of Anesthesiologists 2015 Annual Meeting in San Diego, California.

31. Roumen L, Sanders MP, Pieterse K, Hilbers PA, Plate R, et al. (2007) Construction of 3D models of the CYP11B family as a tool to predict ligand binding characteristics. J Comput Aided Mol Des 21: 455-471.

32. Shanmugasundararaj S, Zhou X, Neunzig J, Bernhardt R, Cotten JF, et al. (2013) Carboetomidate: an analog of etomidate that interacts weakly with 11β-hydroxylase. Anesth Analg 116: 1249-1256.

33. Cotten JF, Forman SA, Laha JK, Cuny GD, Husain SS, et al. (2010) Carboetomidate: a pyrrole analog of etomidate designed not to suppress adrenocortical function. Anesthesiology 112: 637-644.

34. Pejo E, Feng Y, Chao W, Cotten JF, Le Ge R, et al. (2012) Differential effects of etomidate and its pyrrole analogue carboetomidate on the adrenocortical and cytokine responses to endotoxemia. Crit Care Med 40: 187-192.

35. Pejo E, Cotten JF, Kelly EW, Le Ge R, Cuny GD, et al. (2012) In vivo and in vitro pharmacological studies of methoxycarbonyl-carboetomidate. Anesth Analg 115: 297-304.

36. Sneyd JR, Rigby-Jones AE, Cross M, Tominaga H, Shimizu S, et al. (2012) First human administration of MR04A3: a novel water-soluble nonbenzodiazepine sedative. Anesthesiology 116: 385-395.

37. Sneyd JR, Rigby-Jones AE (2010) New drugs and technologies, intravenous anaesthesia is on the move (again). Br J Anaesth 105: 246-254.

38. Ikemoto K, Ishiyama T, Shintani N, Asano N, Sessler DI, et al. (2015) The effects of topical and intravenous JM-1232(-) on cerebral pial microvessels of rabbits. BMC Anesthesiol 15: 37.

39. Iwata K, Iida H, Iida M, Fukuoka N, Kito K, et al. (2015) Effects of topical and intravenous JM-1232(-) infusion on cerebrovascular reactivity in rats. J Anesth 29: 798-802.

17

Reliability and Validity of the Thai Short-Form McGill Pain Questionnaire-2 (SF-MPQ-2)

Phakapan Buppha[1], Nuj Tontisirin[1*], Pawin Numthavaj[2], Supalak Sakdanuwatwong[1], Wanida Sodsee[1] and Roderick J Finlayson[3]

[1]Department of Anesthesiology, Ramathibodi Hospital, Mahidol University, Bangkok, Thailand

[2]Department of Otorhinolaryngology, Ramathibodi Hospital, Mahidol University, Bangkok, Thailand

[3]Department of Anesthesia, Alan Edwards Pain Management Unit, McGill University, Montreal, Canada

*Corresponding author: N. Tontisirin, Department of Anesthesiology, Ramathibodi Hospital, Mahidol University, Bangkok, Thailand, E-mail: doctornuj@gmail.com; nuj.ton@mahidol.ac.th

Abstract

Background: By adding 7 neuropathic pain descriptors, the Short-form McGill Pain Questionnaire-2 (SF-MPQ-2) enables clinicians to assess not only nociceptive pain but also neuropathic pain and presents an improvement over the first version (SF-MPQ). Unfortunately, no Thai language version of this new tool was available, we therefore undertook to create and validate one.

Materials and methods: The translation included the following steps: 1) forward translation: English to Thai, 2) backward translation: Thai to English, 3) testing on patients 4) proof-reading and finalization. Adults suffering from cancer or non-cancer chronic pain completed Thai SF-MPQ and Thai SF-MPQ-2 during 2 separate visits 30 hours apart. Reliability was evaluated by assessing internal consistency and test-retest reliability. Three types of validity were investigated, including concurrent, construct and convergent validity.

Results: A total of 220 Thai patients (127F: 93 M), aged 53 ± 14 year-old, participated in this study. Cancer pain was the most common cause of pain (n=52, 24%), followed by spine related pain (n=48, 22%) and neuropathic pain (n=48, 22%). The reliability for each questionnaire item was high (Cronbach's alpha coefficient 0.771-0.993, ICC 0.985-0.996, Spearman's correlation coefficient r>0.4 p<0.001). In addition, fit indices values of each pain aspect were good. Most descriptors had an acceptable factor loading value, except gnawing and itching (factor loading value; gnawing=0.47, itching=0.49). However, all descriptor had a significant t-value and R^2 value.

Conclusion: The Thai-MPQ-2 had high reliability as well as concurrent, construct and convergent validity. It is a reliable and comprehensive tool for pain assessment in Thai patients.

Keywords: Short-form McGill pain questionnaire-2 (SF-MPQ-2); Neuropathic pain

Introduction

Pain is one of the most common complaints expressed by patients during medical visits and therefore appropriate pain assessment is critical in order to formulate a therapeutic plan [1,2]. Self-reported assessments are more reliable and accurate than observational ones, however only a limited number are available in the Thai language [3].

The McGill Pain Questionnaire (MPQ), based on a patient self-report model, was developed in 1975 and assesses the sensory, affective and evaluative aspects of pain [4]. However, the large number of items it contains makes it too time intensive for routine clinical practice. The Short-Form MPQ (SF-MPQ), developed in 1987, contains only 15 questions and is less onerous to complete [5]. Although available in a Thai version [6] and widely used, it does not adequately evaluate the sensory neuropathic aspects of pain [7]. The latter can have significant impact when selecting an optimal pharmacological regimen, as treatments for nociceptive and neuropathic pain can differ. Dworkin et al. recently developed a SF-MPQ-2 (Short-form McGill Pain Questionnaire-2), which in addition to a more accurate 10-point pain rating scale, also includes 7 questions assessing pain caused by neurological disorders [8]. In this updated version, the SF-MPQ-2 is more versatile than existing neuropathic pain questionnaires such as the DN4 [9], LANSS [10] and NPSI [11] as it is capable of evaluating nociceptive pain as well [8]. It has been shown to have a high level of reliability and validity [7,12-14] and has been translated into multiple languages [15-17]. We therefore undertook to validate a Thai version of the SF-MPQ-2.

Methods

After obtaining a translation license from Mapi Research Trust and ethics approval from the Ramathibodi Hospital Faculty of Medicine, after providing written consent, 220 patients were recruited from a university hospital based pain clinic between September 2015 and April 2016. Inclusion criteria included chronic pain from any cause with a minimum duration of 3 months, age between 18 and 70 years and good comprehension of both spoken and written Thai. Exclusion criteria included impaired cognitive function and refusal to participate in this study.

All participants were instructed on how to fill out both questionnaires and these were read to illiterate subjects if necessary.

The Thai SF-MPQ consists of a visual analogue scale (VAS), present pain intensity (PPI) measure as well as 15 pain descriptors that are each rated on a four-point scale (0-3 scale; 0=none, 1=mild, 2=moderate, 3=severe). It evaluates 3 different pain aspects, including continuous, intermittent and affective. The Thai SF-MPQ-2 contains 22 items to be rated by respondents on a 0-10 numeric scale, with "0" indicating "none" and "10" indicating "worst possible pain." It evaluates 4 different dimensions: 1) continuous pain (throbbing, cramping, gnawing, aching, heavy pain and tender), 2) intermittent pain (shooting, stabbing, sharp, splitting, electrical-shock and piercing), 3) neuropathic pain (hot-burning, cold-freezing, pain caused by light touch, itching, tingling or "pins and needles", numbness), and 4) affective aspects (tiring-exhausting, sickening, fearful, punishing-cruel). All four aspects of pain are presented as mean (± SD) and a total score obtained by adding the 22 individual scores.

Questionnaires were completed twice during visits that were separated by approximately 30 hours, an interval deemed to strike the appropriate balance between ensuring that patients did not remember their initial answers and their underlying painful condition had not changed.

A full linguistic validation process was undertaken following the methodology recommended by the Mapi Research Trust [18], which included 4 steps:

Forward translation from English to Thai by two of the clinician co-authors (PB, NT) who are fluent in both languages.

Backwards translation to English by a philologist and native Thai speaker. This version was then compared to the original English version and translated back to Thai by two clinicians.

Clinical validation of the terms used in the newly translated questionnaire by having 5 Thai-speaking patients review and complete it.

Proof reading and finalization by 5 pain physicians.

Statistical analysis

Sample size was determined according to the subjects-to-variables (STV) ratio. As there should be at least 10 cases [19,20] for each item in the instrument being studied, the total sample size was 220 patients. Data analysis was performed using SPSS for Windows version 18.5 (IBM, Armonk, New York). Demographic data was reported as mean, standard deviation (SD), frequency and percentage as appropriate. Internal consistency for each item score and total scores were analyzed using Cronbach's α coefficient and values ≥ 0.70 were deemed acceptable [21]. Test-retest reliability was assessed using intraclass correlation coefficients (ICC) and values >0.70 were considered acceptable. Concurrent validity was examined by comparing the individual items and total scores of the Thai-SF-MPQ and Thai-SF-MPQ-2 using Spearman's correlation coefficients (r). P values<0.05 and r values r>0.40 were considered significant [15].

Construct validity of the Thai-SF-MPQ-2 was analyzed using confirmatory factor analysis (CFA) and data compared to a hypothesized measurement model. Each pain aspect and overall four-factor model was analyzed. Goodness of fit indices were selected to examine the model fit including relative Chi-square ([x2/df] <3) [22,23], standardized root-mean-square residual (SRMR) (acceptable value <0.08) [24], root-mean-square error of approximation (RMSEA) (acceptable value <0.08) [25] and the comparative fit index (CFI) (value >0.95 indicating a good fit) [26]. As part of the validation

process, indices were modified to improve model fit even if the hypothesized model was found to have good construct validity and this was done by removing items, or adding an error covariance between two pain descriptors. Convergent validity was evaluated by examining the effect of loading and unloading each pain descriptor. Critical test values were t-value >1.96, R^2 (Square multiple correlation) >0.2 [27] and loading factor ≥ 0.50 [28,29].

Results

Two hundred and twenty patients were enrolled; their demographics and pain characteristics were presented in Tables 1 and 2.

Characteristics		n (%)
Gender	Male	93 (42%)
	Female	127 (58%)
Age	Mean ± SD (years)	53 ± 14
	<65 year-old	171 (78%)
	>65 year-old	49 (22%)
Duration of pain symptom	>3 months-1 year	85 (39%)
	1-5 years	75 (34%)
	6-10 years	36 (16%)
	>10 years	24 (11%)
Education level	None	5 (2%)
	Primary school	57 (26%)
	Secondary school	37 (17%)
	Diploma or Bachelor degree	91 (41%)
	Master degree or PhD	30 (14%)
Employment	Work	102 (46 %)
	Unemployed	60 (27%)
	Retired	58 (27%)
Nociceptive pain	Cancer pain	52 (24%)
	Mechanical low back pain, neck pain, spondylosis	46 (20%)
	Ischemic limb pain	4 (2%)
	Other nociceptive pain	11 (5%)
Neuropathic pain	Central neuropathic pain	8 (4%)
	Radicular pain	17 (8%)
	Post herpetic neuralgia	8 (4%)
	Painful diabetic neuropathy	4 (2%)
	Complex regional pain syndrome	22 (10%)
	Other neuropathic pain	48 (21%)

Table 1: Demographic data (n=220).

Analysis of the Thai-SF-MPQ-2 found high Cronbach's α coefficient values for total score (0.92), pain descriptors (0.96-0.98) and pain aspects (Table 3). ICC results for total score (0.996) and pain aspect (0.985-0.989) displayed similarly favorable results (Table 3). Significant correlations were found between the Thai-SF-MPQ, VAS and Thai-SF-MPQ-2, supporting concurrent validity (Table 4). In addition, confirmatory factor analysis fit indices indicated good construct validity for the four pain aspects (Table 5).

	Mean	SD	Median	Min	Max	25th percentile	75th percentile	Range (Max-Min)
MPQ-1; 15-descriptors (0-3)	17/45	11	15/45	Jan-45	41/45	Aug-45	21/45	40
VAS (0-10)	10-Jun	3	5.5/10	0	10-Oct	4.5/10	10-Aug	10
PPI (0-5)	2.7/5	1	5-Mar	0	5-May	5-Feb	3.5/5	5
SF-MPQ: McGill Short Form Questionnaire Version 1; VAS: Visual Analog Score; PPI: Present Pain Intensity								

Table 2: SF-MPQ, VAS and PPI scores for the study population.

Aspect of pain	Number of items	T1 (mean ± SD for each item)	T2 (mean ± SD for each item)	Cronbach's coefficient‡ α	Intraclass Correlation Coefficient* (ICC)	
					ICC	95% CI
1) Continuous	6	2.74 ± 2.24	2.67 ± 2.14	0.791‡	0.985†	0.990-0.994
2) Intermittent	6	2.02 ± 2.12	2.04 ± 2.08	0.800‡	0.985†	0.990-0.994
3) Affective	4	4.12 ± 3.24	4.14 ± 3.19	0.893‡	0.985†	0.972-0.984
4) Neuropathic	6	1.68 ± 1.93	1.66 ± 1.90	0.771‡	0.989†	0.993-0.996
All items	22	2.50 ± 1.96	2.49 ± 1.91	0.993‡	0.996†	0.995-0.997
T1=first data collection, T2=second data collection, ‡Acceptable Cronbach's α coefficient ≥ 0.70, †Acceptable ICC >0.70						

Table 3: Thai-SF-MPQ-2. Internal consistency and test-retest reliability.

	SF-MPQ-2 (Continuous)	SF-MPQ-2 (Intermittent)	SF-MPQ-2 (Affective)	SF-MPQ-2 (Neuropathic)	SF-MPQ-2 (Total score)
SF-MPQ-2 (Continuous)	-	-	-	-	-
SF-MPQ-2 (Intermittent)	0.529**	-	-	-	-
SF-MPQ-2 (Affective)	0.664**	0.562**	-	-	-
SF-MPQ-2 (Neuropathic)	0.456**	0.583**	0.459**	-	-
SF-MPQ-2 (Total score)	0.835**	0.782**	0.869**	0.701**	-
SF-MPQ (Sensory)	0.820**	0.756**	0.666**	0.593**	0.868**
SF-MPQ (Affective)	0.601**	0.525**	0.910**	0.429**	0.792**
SF-MPQ (Total score)	0.793**	0.718**	0.841**	0.577**	0.916**
VAS (visual analog scale)	0.521**	0.398**	0.559**	0.344**	0.574**
†Spearman's correlation; r >0.4 and **p<0.01					

Table 4: Concurrent validity (Spearman's correlation values†).

R^2 and t-values for descriptors supported convergent validity. As well, high loading factors were found for most descriptors except "gnawing and itching" (Table 6), however no significant improvement in fit indices was obtained by removing the latter. The hypothesized model was modified seven times, however new fit indices values showed a poorer model fit (Table 7).

Pain aspect	χ^2/df	SRMR	RMSEA	CFI
Continuous	1.60	0.0332*	0.0576†	0.99‡
Intermittent	2.22	0.0404*	0.0780†	0.98‡
Affective	0.53	0.0044*	0.0000†	1‡
Neuropathic	1.76	0.0376*	0.0596†	0.98‡

χ^2/df=relative Chi-Square <3, SRMR= Standardized Root Mean Square Residual; value <0.08 to show a good fit*, RMSEA=Root Mean Square Error of Approximation; value <0.08 to show adequate fit†, CFI=Comparative Fit Index; value >0.95 indicated a good fit‡

Table 5: Thai SF-MPQ-2. Fit indices values for pain aspect models.

Discussion

Our study demonstrated a high internal consistency and test-retest reliability for the Thai SF-MPQ-2, as well as good concurrent, construct and convergent validity. Internal consistency for the total score as assessed by Cronbach's α coefficient was higher (0.95) than that reported for the English version (0.92) [7] and Japanese versions (0.90) [15]. Similarly, we found a higher test-retest reliability (0.99) than the Japanese (0.83) [15] and Iranian (0.94) [17] versions. Overall four-factor model analysis (hypothesized) demonstrated good construct validity. In keeping with Melzack et al's [7] original work on the English versions and other validation studies [15], we found a good correlation between Thai-SF-MPQ and Thai-SF-MPQ-2. An exception to this was the poorer correlation found between VAS and neuropathic as well as intermittent pain.

Pain Description (item)	Standardized Factor Loadings				t-value	R^2
	Continuous	Intermittent	Affective	Neuropathic		
Throbbing pain	0.66†				10.45**	0.44
Cramping pain	0.64†				9.82**	0.4
Gnawing pain	0.47				6.82**	0.22
Aching pain	0.66†				10.42**	0.44
Heavy pain	0.67†				10.60**	0.45
Tender	0.65†				10.11**	0.42
Shooting pain		0.68†			10.87**	0.46
Stabbing pain		0.60†			9.21**	0.35
Sharp pain		0.61†			9.45**	0.37
Splitting pain		0.65†			10.28**	0.42
Electrical-shock pain		0.65†			10.33**	0.43
Piercing		0.61†			9.40**	0.37
Tiring-exhausting			0.88†		16.00**	0.77
Sickening			0.90†		16.63**	0.8
Fearful			0.71†		11.66**	0.5
Punishing-cruel			0.81†		14.31**	0.66
Hot-burning pain				0.60†	9.12**	0.36
Cold-freezing pain				0.59†	8.93**	0.37
Pain caused by light touch				0.65†	10.15**	0.43
Itching				0.49	7.18**	0.24
Tingling or 'pins and needles'				0.72†	11.52**	0.52
Numbness				0.58†	8.71**	0.33

Standardized factor loading value; acceptable at value ≥ 0.5†, t-value; significant at value ≥ 1.96 (**p<0.01), R^2= Square multiple correlation; acceptable at value >0.2

Table 6: Standardized factor loading value and t-value of the overall four-factor model.

Hypothesized model	Operating	Change of fit indices
Modified#1	Remove item Gnawing pain	less χ^2/df (less construct validity)
		less factor loading (less convergent validity)
Modified#2	Remove item itching	less χ^2/df (less construct validity)
		less factor loading (less convergent validity)
Modified#3	Add error covariance between aching pain and heavy pain	less χ^2/df (less construct validity)
Modified#4	Add error covariance between Cold-freezing pain and itching	less χ^2/df (less construct validity)
Modified#5	Add error covariance between shooting pain and sharp pain	less χ^2/df (less construct validity)
Modified#6	Add error covariance between stabbing pain and sharp pain	less χ^2/df (less construct validity)
Modified#7	Add error covariance between Tiring-exhausting and Sickening	less χ^2/df (less construct validity)

Table 7: Change of fit indices after modifying hypothesized model.

All descriptors had significant t-value and acceptable R^2 value, supporting their favorable effect on convergent validity. In addition, they also had high loading effect (value >0.5) except for itching and gnawing pain. These findings echo those of Wasuwat et al. [5], suggesting that those terms may translate poorly to Thai. A language specific effect for certain descriptors has been noted in other validation studies [15,17]. However, after modifying the model as recommended by the program, there was no significant change in fit indices and therefore the affected descriptors were not modified.

Our study presents some possible limitations. Firstly, average pain scores for individual aspects (Table 3) were lower than those reported in other languages [7,15]. This may have had an effect on the variability of patient reported scores as well as the number of descriptors that were used. However, intensity scores indicated moderate pain (Table 2: VAS 6/10, PPI 2.7/5) and findings were similar to a Thai study validating the SF-MPQ, suggesting a cultural influence. Secondly, the responsiveness to change was not evaluated. Finally, patients were recruited from a tertiary pain clinic located in a major urban center, which might limit the applicability of the results to other populations.

Conclusions

The Thai SF-MPQ-2 had high reliability as well as concurrent, construct and convergent validity. It can be used as a reliable and comprehensive tool for pain assessment in Thai patients with chronic pain including both nociceptive and neuropathic pain.

Acknowledgements

The authors would like to thank Mr. Pornchai Sakdanuwatwong PhD and Ms. Rojnarin Komonhirun for their assistance with the statistical analysis. In addition, we would also like to thank Mr.Ruangsilp Agechaosuan for his assistance with the backward translation.

- Thai Clinical Trial Registry identification number TCTR20160415001

References

1. Loeser JD, Melzack R (1999) Pain: an overview. Lancet 353: 1607-1609.

2. Breivik H, Borchgrevink PC, Allen SM, Rosseland LA, Romundstad L, et al. (2008) Assessment of pain. Br J Anaesth 101: 17-24.

3. Schug S, Palmer G, Scott D, Halliwell R, Trinca J (2015) Acute Pain Management: Scientific Evidence. (4thedn), Melbourne: Australian and New Zealand College of Anaesthetists and Faculty of Pain Medicine 45.

4. Melzack R (1975) The McGill Pain Questionnaire: major properties and scoring methods. Pain 1: 277-299.

5. Melzack R (1987) The short-form McGill Pain Questionnaire. Pain 30: 191-197.

6. Kitisomprayoonkul W, Klaphajone J, Kovindha A (2006) Thai Short-form McGill Pain Questionnaire. J Med Assoc Thai 89: 846-853.

7. Bouhassira D, Attal N (2011) Diagnosis and assessment of neuropathic pain: the saga of clinical tools. Pain 152: S74-83.

8. Dworkin RH, Turk DC, Revicki DA, Harding G, Coyne KS, et al. (2009) Development and initial validation of an expanded and revised version of the Short-form McGill Pain Questionnaire (SF-MPQ-2). Pain 144: 35-42.

9. Bouhassira D, Attal N, Alchaar H, Boureau F, Brochet B, et al. (2005) Comparison of pain syndromes associated with nervous or somatic lesions and development of a new neuropathic pain diagnostic questionnaire (DN4). Pain 114: 29-36.

10. Bennett M (2001) The LANSS Pain Scale: the Leeds assessment of neuropathic symptoms and signs. Pain 92: 147-157.

11. Bouhassira D, Attal N, Fermanian J, Alchaar H, Gautron M, et al. (2004) Development and validation of the Neuropathic Pain Symptom Inventory. Pain 108: 248-257.

12. Gauthier LR, Young A, Dworkin RH, Rodin G, Zimmermann C, et al. (2014) Validation of the short-form McGill pain questionnaire-2 in younger and older people with cancer pain. J Pain 15: 756-770.

13. Dworkin RH, Turk DC, Trudeau JJ, Benson C, Biondi DM, et al. (2015) Validation of the Short-form McGill Pain Questionnaire-2 (SF-MPQ-2) in acute low back pain. J Pain 16: 357-366.

14. Lovejoy TI, Turk DC, Morasco BJ (2012) Evaluation of the psychometric properties of the revised short-form McGill Pain Questionnaire. J Pain 13: 1250-1257.

15. Maruo T, Nakae A, Maeda L, Shi K, Takahashi K, et al. (2014) Validity, reliability, and assessment sensitivity of the Japanese version of the short-

form McGill pain questionnaire 2 in Japanese patients with neuropathic and non-neuropathic pain. Pain Med 15: 1930-1937.

16. Kachooei AR, Ebrahimzadeh MH, Erfani-Sayyar R, Salehi M, Salimi E, et al. (2015) Short Form-McGill Pain Questionnaire-2 (SF-MPQ-2): A Cross-Cultural Adaptation and Validation Study of the Persian Version in Patients with Knee Osteoarthritis. Arch Bone Jt Surg 3: 45-50.

17. Adelmanesh F, Jalali A, Attarian H, Farahani B, Ketabchi SM, et al. (2012) Reliability, validity, and sensitivity measures of expanded and revised version of the short-form McGill Pain Questionnaire (SF-MPQ-2) in Iranian patients with neuropathic and non-neuropathic pain. Pain Med 13: 1631-1636.

18. Acquadro C, Conway K, Giroudet C, Mear I (2012) Linguistic Validation Manual for Health Outcomes Assessments. (2nded), France: MAPI Institute.

19. Arrindell WA, van der Ende J (1985) An Empirical Test of the Utility of the Observations-To-Variables Ratio in Factor and Components Analysis. Appl Psychol Meas 9: 165-178.

20. Velicer WF, Fava JL (1988) Effects of Variable and Subject Sampling on Factor Pattern Recovery. Psychol Methods 3: 231-251.

21. Tavakol M, Dennick R (2011) Making sense of Cronbach's alpha. Int J Med Educ 2: 53-55.

22. Kline RB (2005) Principles and Practice of Structural Equation Modeling. (2ndedn), New York: Guilford Press.

23. Tabachnick BG, Fidell LS (2007) Using Multivariate Statistics. (5thedn), New York: Allyn and Bacon.

24. Hu LT, Bentler PM (1999) Cutoff Criteria of Fit Indexes in Covariance Structural Analysis: Conventional Criteria Versus New Alternatives. Struct Equ Modeling 6: 1-55.

25. Steiger JH (2007) Understanding the Limitations of Global Fit Assessment in Structural Equation Modeling. Pers Individ Dif 42: 893-898.

26. Bentler PM (1990) Comparative fit indexes in structural models. Psychol Bull 107: 238-246.

27. Hopper D, Coughlan J, Mullen M (2008) Structural Equation Modelling: Guidelines for Determining Model Fit. Electronic Journal of Business Research Methods 6: 53-60.

28. Parker RI, Hagan-Burke S (2007) Useful effect size interpretations for single case research. Behav Ther 38: 95-105.

29. Matsunaga M (2010) How to Factor-Analyze Your Data Right: Do's, Don'ts, and How-To's. Int J Psychol Res 3: 97-110.

18

Remifentanil can Prevent the Increase in Qt Dispersion during Modified Electroconvulsive Therapy: A Randomized Controlled Clinical Trial

Megumi Kageyama, Shinsuke Hamaguchi* and Shigeki Yamaguchi

Department of Anesthesia and Pain Medicine, Dokkyo University School of Medicine, Tochigi, Japan

***Corresponding author:** Shinsuke Hamaguchi, Professor and Chairman, Department of Anesthesia and Pain Medicine, Dokkyo University School of Medicine, 880 Kitakobayashi, Mibu, Tochigi 321-0293, Japan; E-mail: s-hama@dokkyomed.ac.jp

Abstract

Objective: To clarify the hemodynamic-stabilizing effect of remifentanil in the context of modified electroconvulsive therapy (mECT), we measured electrocardiographic alterations in the corrected QT interval (QTc) and corrected QT dispersion (QTcD), considered predictive of ventricular arrhythmia, during mECT.

Methods: Sixty patients scheduled for mECT were divided randomly into 3 groups. Patients in the low-dose remifentanil administration group (group L, N=20) were administered 0.5 µg/kg of remifentanil before mECT. Patients in the high-dose group (group H, N=20) were administered 1.0 µg/kg of remifentanil, and those in the control (group C, N=20) were administered a similar volume of normal saline solution. Modified ECT was performed in the same manner in all groups with propofol and suxamethonium. Changes in QTc and QTcD values were analyzed using a repeated measures analysis of variance, and between-group comparisons were conducted using the Bonferroni method.

Results: During mECT, an increase in the mean arterial pressure, decrease in the R wave-to-R wave interval, elongation of QTc, and increase in QTcD were observed in group C, whereas these alterations were attenuated in group L and were not observed in group H. The differences observed in group C relative to the other groups were statistically significant (P<0.05).

Conclusion: Compared with the control treatment and a 0.5 µg/kg dose, a 1.0 µg/kg dose of remifentanil had a preventive effect on ventricular arrhythmia after mECT, as well as on hemodynamic changes, according to the observed alterations in QTc and QTcD. Therefore, our results indicate that a 1.0 µg/kg dose of remifentanil could suppress hemodynamic changes, prevent myocardial ischemia or cerebral hemorrhage, and minimize the development of fatal arrhythmias such as ventricular tachycardia and/or ventricular fibrillation.

Keywords: Remifentanil; QT interval; QT dispersion; Modified electroconvulsive therapy; Ventricular arrhythmia; Hemodynamic changes; Major depression

Background

Modified electroconvulsive therapy (mECT) is used to treat patients with schizophrenia and severe depression who cannot adequately receive pharmaceutical treatment [1]. Recently, a combination of propofol and suxamethonium has been administered to induce sleep and muscle relaxation during mECT and avoid the harmful joint hyperextension and dislocation and fractures in the extremities caused by unexpected body motion. However, the extreme sympathetic instability induced by mECT can cause various arrhythmias during an electro-stimulation course. For example, bradycardia, tachycardia, and premature constriction may be observed via electrocardiograph (ECG) during mECT. In particular, ventricular premature contraction (VPC) may cause fatal arrhythmias such as ventricular tachycardia (VT) and/or ventricular fibrillation (VF). Therefore, ventricular arrhythmias must be prevented during mECT to ensure safe anesthetic management [2,3].

The QT interval (QT) is a well-known potential cause of ventricular arrhythmia. However, QT dispersion (QTD), a value obtained by subtracting the minimum QT interval from the maximum QT interval as determined using a recorded 12-lead ECG, is considered an indicator of instability during ventricle repolarization. In addition, QT and QTD appear to correlate with autonomic regulation instability [4-6] and are potential causes of ventricular arrhythmias [7] or severe cardiac adverse events [8], such as myocardial infarction or cardiac sudden death [9-13]. In addition, several reports have indicated that both values increase as a result of various perioperative surgical procedures [14,15].

Previously, we reported increased QT and QTD values during mECT in propofol and suxamethonium-treated patients with psychiatric disorders [16]. In that report, we described elongation of the QT interval and an increase in QTD, which might reflect non-uniform localized ventricle repolarization during perioperative ECG in patients taking antidepressants to treat psychiatric disorders. Our study indicated that propofol and suxamethonium could not reduce these harmful sympathetic fluctuations associated with mECT. Accordingly, we believed that a different anesthetic would better stabilize this sympathetic nerve activation. Remifentanil is a short-acting pure mu-opioid agonist with the potential to ameliorate increases in heart rate and blood pressure during the course of sympathetic nerve stimulation inhibition. However, no previous reports have discussed the effectiveness of remifentanil anesthesia for avoiding the harmful adverse events associated with mECT. Therefore, in the present study, we evaluated the QT and QTD values to determine whether remifentanil could reduce the occurrence of fatal arrhythmias caused by mECT.

Methods

Ethical considerations

This study was conducted after receiving approval from the Dokkyo Medical University Hospital Ethics Committee (registration number: 90566605, date: August 21, 2009).

Patient classification

For this randomized controlled clinical trial, we recruited 60 patients with physical status classifications of I or II from the American Society of Anesthesiologists, who were scheduled to undergo mECT for the treatment of major depression. The patients ranged in age from 20 to 65 years, and patients with a history of any heart disease or present arrhythmia were excluded. The sample size in the present study was calculated based on our previous research [16]. Accordingly, we allocated 20 patients per group to account for dropout cases.

After obtaining written, informed consent from each patient and/or their family, patients were divided into 3 groups according to a previous study by Zaballos et al. [17]: 1) control group (group C, N=20), in which all patients received a single 20-ml injection of saline solution prior to mECT; 2) low-dose remifentanil group (group L, N=20), in which all patients received a single 20-ml injection of saline solution containing 0.5 μg/kg of remifentanil prior to mECT; and 3) high-dose remifentanil group (group H, N=20), in which all patients received a single 20-ml injection of saline solution containing 1.0 μg/kg of remifentanil prior to mECT.

Monitoring and data sampling

The procedures used in this study were conducted in our operating room under various monitors. After admission to the operating room, non-invasive blood pressure (NIBP), ECG, and O₂ saturation monitors were attached to the patients. We recorded the mean arterial pressure (MAP), heart rate (HR), and 12-lead ECG, and used a multi-function electrocardiograph (FDX-4520TM, Fukuda Denshi, Tokyo, Japan) to measure QT and the corrected QT interval (QTc). These values were used to calculate the QTD and corrected QTD (QTcD) during anesthesia and mECT, as described below.

Anesthetic management

None of the patients received premedication. In all patients, we maintained an intravenous line to administer various drugs and delivered oxygen via masked inhalation at a rate of 6 L/min. Before administering 1 mg/kg of propofol to induce sleep and 1 mg/kg of suxamethonium intravenously to obtain adequate muscle relaxation, we administered 20 ml of saline solution alone (group C) or containing 0.5 μg/kg (group L) or 1.0 μg/kg of remifentanil (group H). Each solution was injected intravenously over 1 minute. After administration of the muscle relaxant, we employed manual ventilation to maintain normocapnia and normoxia.

Modified ECT

Modified ECT was performed through an electrode on the skin above both frontal lobes via a pulse-wave therapy device (ThymatronTM, Somatics LLC, Lake Bluff, IL, USA). The output current was set according to the patient's age. EEG was recorded using pulse-wave therapy equipment. Modified ECT was considered successful when the spike and wave complex wave on the EEG were observed at an interval of more than 15 seconds. All treatments were administered by psychiatrists not otherwise involved in this study.

Assessment of QTD

We measured 12-lead ECG using the previously described multi-function electrocardiograph (FDX-4520TM, Fukuda Denshi). After mECT, we calculated QTD as the difference between the minimum and maximum QT on each 12-lead ECG with QT analysis software (QTD-1TM, Fukuda Denshi) and determined the corrected QT dispersion (QTcD) for each case. A QTD that exceeded 50 msec indicated a significant increase.

Statistical analysis

Results were expressed as mean (± standard deviation) for quantitative variables. A repeated measures analysis of variance (ANOVA) was used to analyze the QT, QTC, QTD, and QTcD within groups. Between-group comparisons of data were conducted using the t post hoc test according to the Bonferroni method. All statistical analyses were conducted using SPSS (SPSS Inc., Chicago, IL, USA). A result was considered significant at a critical level of 5% ($P<0.05$).

Results

Background

No enrolled patient discontinued the study protocol. There were no significant differences in patient characteristics (e.g., age, height, weight, gender, duration of antidepressant treatment for depression) among the groups (Table 1). Additionally, no patients developed hemodynamic or neurological complications, respiratory difficulties, or other severe adverse effects.

	Group C (N=20)	Group L (N=20)	Group H (N=20)
Age (yrs)	51 ± 13	48 ± 15	47 ± 15
Height (cm)	157 ± 7	155 ± 4	159 ± 9
Weight (kg)	57 ± 18	53 ± 11	56 ± 19
Gender (male/female)	9/11	7/13	10/10
Number of treatment with psychiatric drugs			
Treatment with antidepressant	20	20	20
Treatment with major tranquilizer	6	9	8
treatment with benzodiazepine	7	8	7

Table 1: Patient characteristics. Data are shown as means ± standard deviations, with the exceptions of gender and the number of subjects

treated with various drugs. There were no significant differences in age, height, or weight between the groups.

Mean arterial pressure (MAP)

Alterations in MAP during mECT are shown in Figure 1. None of the groups exhibited a significant decrease in MAP after anesthesia induction. However, a significant increase in MAP was observed within 7 min after mECT in group C. In contrast, a significant increase in MAP was observed within 3 min in group L, whereas no significant increase in MAP was observed in group H. Groups C and L exhibited significant increases in MAP after mECT, compared with the values before mECT. Compared with group C, group L exhibited a significant decrease in MAP 2–6 min after mECT. Notably, group H exhibited a significantly lower MAP relative to group C after 10 min of mECT, and also exhibited a significantly lower MAP value after 1 min of mECT, compared with group L.

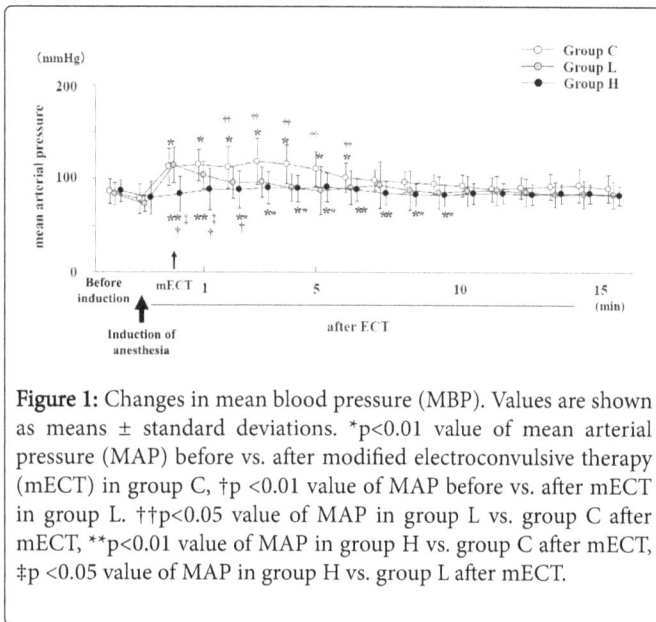

Figure 1: Changes in mean blood pressure (MBP). Values are shown as means ± standard deviations. *p<0.01 value of mean arterial pressure (MAP) before vs. after modified electroconvulsive therapy (mECT) in group C, †p <0.01 value of MAP before vs. after mECT in group L. ††p<0.05 value of MAP in group L vs. group C after mECT, **p<0.01 value of MAP in group H vs. group C after mECT, ‡p <0.05 value of MAP in group H vs. group L after mECT.

Heart rate (HR)

Variations in HR during mECT are shown in Figure 2. No significant changes in HR were observed in any group during anesthetic induction. Significant increases in the HR above the baseline were observed within 7 min in group C and 6 min in group L (P<0.05). In contrast, a significant increase in HR was observed within 3 min in group L (P<0.05). However, group H did not develop a similar significant increase in HR (P>0.05). Compared with groups C and L, group H had a significantly lower HR at 10 min after mECT (P<0.05).

QT and QTc

Previous studies have defined a normal QTc value as <450 milliseconds [16]. In the present study, no significant changes in QTc were recognized in any group, and no significant differences were observed among the groups. The variations in QTc during mECT in all groups are shown in Figure 3.

QTD and QTcD

Previous studies have defined the normal range of QTD and QTcD as 10-70 milliseconds [16]. For the present study, the variations in QTD during mECT in each group are shown in Figure 4, and the variations in QTcD during mECT are shown in Figure 5. QTD did not change significantly in any group before anesthetic induction. Significant increases in QTD were observed immediately after performing mECT in group L and within 2 min in group C (P<0.05). However, group H exhibited a significantly lower QTD compared with group C from 0 to 6 min after mECT (P<0.05).

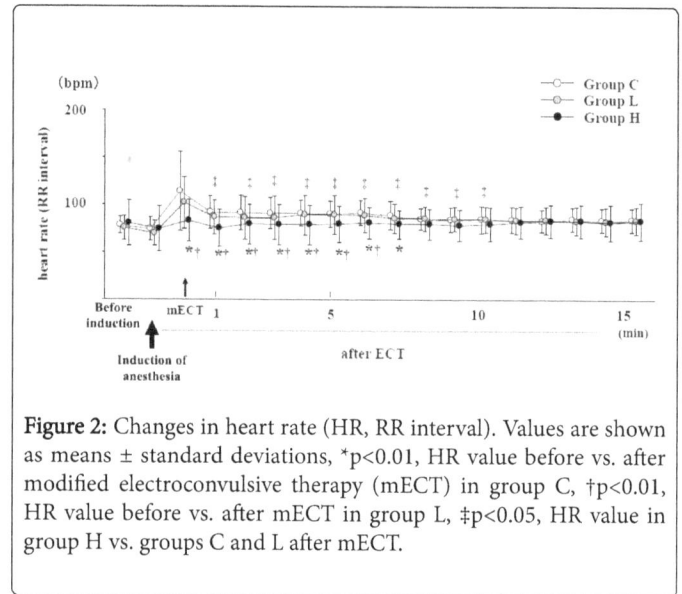

Figure 2: Changes in heart rate (HR, RR interval). Values are shown as means ± standard deviations, *p<0.01, HR value before vs. after modified electroconvulsive therapy (mECT) in group C, †p<0.01, HR value before vs. after mECT in group L, ‡p<0.05, HR value in group H vs. groups C and L after mECT.

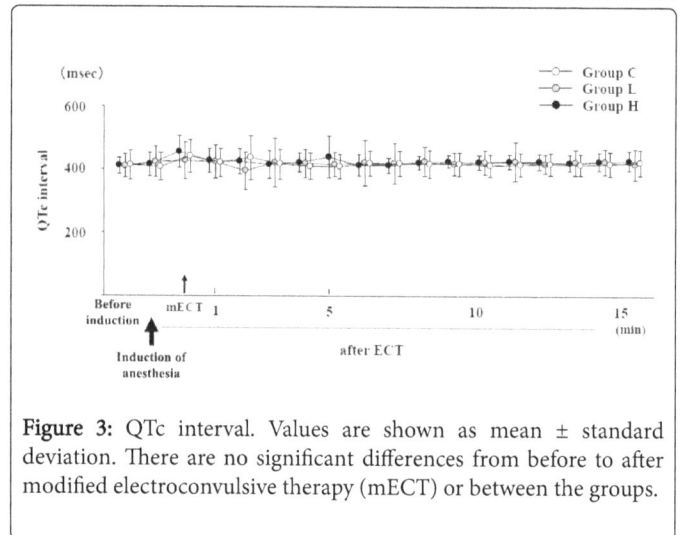

Figure 3: QTc interval. Values are shown as mean ± standard deviation. There are no significant differences from before to after modified electroconvulsive therapy (mECT) or between the groups.

The QTcD did not change significantly in any group before anesthetic induction. However, significant increases in QTcD were observed immediately after performing mECT in group L and within 3 min in group C. Notably, the QTcD of group L was significantly lower than that of group C within 2 min after mECT. However, no increases in QTD and QTcD were observed in group H over a 70 msec period (maximum mean QTcD was 69.2 msec immediately after mECT). Groups L and H exhibited significantly lower QTcD values than did group C within 2 min after mECT. Moreover, group H exhibited a significantly lower QTcD value than group L at 1 min after mECT.

Complications

No adverse events associated with remifentanil administration were observed in groups L and H. However, 3 cases of paroxysmal supraventricular tachycardia were observed in group C.

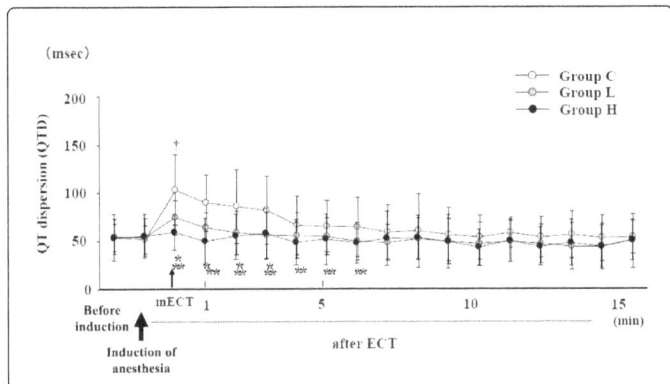

Figure 4: QT dispersion (QTD). Values are shown as mean ± standard deviation. *p<0.01 value of QTD before vs. after modified electroconvulsive therapy (mECT) in group C, †p<0.01 value of QTD before vs. after mECT in group L, **p<0.01, value of QTD in group H vs. group C after mECT

Discussion

Remifentanil, a short-acting opioid analgesic, is widely used for general anesthesia because it has a strong anti-nociceptive action [18]. Compared with other well-known opioid analgesics, remifentanil can rapidly achieve effect-site concentrations after a single injected dose. In addition, the effect-site concentration of remifentanil can decrease rapidly after the discontinuation of administration [19].

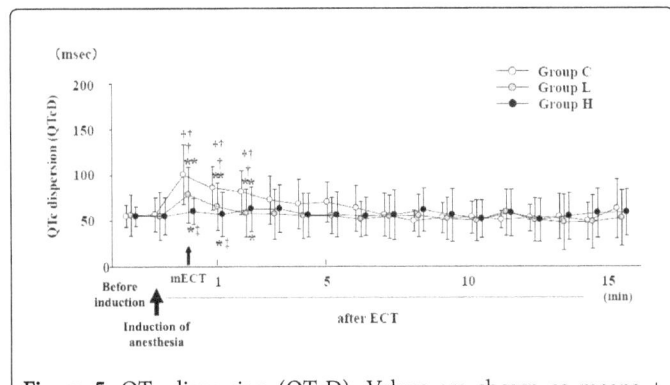

Figure 5: QTc dispersion (QTcD). Values are shown as means ± standard deviations. *p<0.01 value of QTcD before vs. after modified electroconvulsive therapy (mECT) in group C, **p<0.01 value of QTcD before vs. after mECT in group L, †p<0.05 value of QTcD in group L vs. group C after mECT, ††p<0.05, value of QTcD in group H vs. group C after mECT, ‡p<0.05, value of QTcD in group H vs. group L after mECT.

Several studies have reported the beneficial effects of remifentanil during mECT [20-22]. Anderson et al. reported the potential usefulness of remifentanil for avoiding noxious stimuli during mECT caused by a reduced anesthetic dose and for extending the significant convulsive time without delaying the resumption of spontaneous breathing [23]. However, the authors also demonstrated that remifentanil did not significantly suppress increases in MAP and HR during mECT and speculated that a too low remifentanil dose or reduction in the methohexital dose could affect hemodynamic changes. Recart et al. reported that remifentanil, when administered with methohexital, suppressed increases in the MAP [24]. Locala et al. reported that increases in HR and MAP could be suppressed by a combined single injection of methohexital and 500 μg of remifentanil [25]. A review by Chen recommended the use of remifentanil in patients with a short convulsion time, high convulsive threshold, or unstable hemodynamic condition after mECT [26].

As mentioned above, although several studies demonstrated the usefulness of remifentanil for stabilizing HR and MAP during mECT, no reports had discussed the effects of remifentanil on the prevention of fatal arrhythmias during mECT. Therefore, we used QTD and QTcD values to confirm whether administering remifentanil before mECT could prevent various arrhythmias. In previous reports, a 1.0 μg/kg dose of remifentanil stabilized the HR and MAP after mECT without serious adverse cardiac events [27]. Therefore, we selected this dose to confirm the influences of QTD and QTcD in the present study. Additionally, to confirm the beneficial effect of a low remifentanil dose, we also evaluated the preventive effect of a 0.5 μg/kg remifentanil dose against arrhythmias, using QTD and QTcD measurements.

The results of our study revealed that 1.0 μg/kg and 0.5 μg/kg doses of remifentanil could suppress increases in QTD and QTcD after mECT, when compared with the control treatment. Moreover, stronger suppression of the increases in QTD and QTcD was observed with a 1.0 μg/kg dose of remifentanil (group H) than with a 0.5 μg/kg dose (group L). In particular, increases in both QTD and QTcD during mECT were substantially suppressed by a 1.0 μg/kg dose of remifentanil. We emphasize that a 1.0 μg/kg dose of remifentanil might not only stabilize HR and MAP, but could also stabilize QTD and QTcD during mECT. Our results indicate that a 1.0 μg/kg dose of remifentanil could suppress hemodynamic changes, prevent myocardial ischemia or cerebral hemorrhage, and minimize the development of fatal arrhythmias.

Our study had some limitations. First, we stipulated a constant propofol dose, regardless of the remifentanil dose. However, several reports have indicated that a low propofol dose can help to maintain convulsion time prolongation [28]. Therefore, in future studies we must consider the appropriate dose of propofol to use with remifentanil. Such a study would be clinically essential with respect to the safety and effectiveness of mECT. Second, we did not study the usefulness of remifentanil during mECT in elderly patients. Many elderly patients may have cardiovascular complications and potential QT interval abnormalities caused by antidepressants. Moreover, increases in QTD and QTcD during elective surgery [29] and pharmacological sensitivities to remifentanil are more frequent in the elderly than in younger patients [30]. Therefore, the association between age and the effects of remifentanil should be studied in the future. Third, we have not examined the detailed mechanism by which remifentanil suppresses increase in QTD. Therefore, it is necessary to consider the effects of autonomic nervous system activity or catecholamine secretion from the adrenal medulla in response to remifentanil and mECT. Fourth, various antidepressants and antipsychotics may prolong the QT and increase the QTd prior to mECT, as shown in our previous report [15]. In fact, the prolongation in QT and QTd in patients taking these drugs prior mECT was enhanced by electrical stimulation under anesthesia in our previous report. Therefore, we should investigate the effect of these drugs in our results in future. Lastly, suxamethonium can increase QTc prolongation. However, suxamethonium was administered to all patients, including patients in our previous series study. Therefore, we reasoned that suxamethonium did not affect our results.

In conclusion, QT, QTD, and QTcD, which are potential causes of ventricular arrhythmias, increase markedly in response to mECT. Our study indicated that the administration of 1.0 μg/kg of remifentanil prior to mECT ameliorated these increases in QTc and QTcD. Therefore, we emphasize that remifentanil can prevent complications such as ventricular arrhythmias and VT or VF, which should be avoided during mECT.

Declaration of Competing Interests

The authors declare that they have no competing interests.

Authors' Contributions

Megumi Kageyama carried out general anesthesia, collected the data and wrote this manuscript. Shinsuke Hamaguchi supported this study and helped to writing this manuscript. Shigeki Yamaguchi planned this study and helped with the writing. All authors read and approved the final manuscript.

Acknowledgement

The authors wish to thank Professor William Joseph Snell, Professor at Keio University, for providing an English revision of our manuscript. We would also like to thank Editage (www.editage.jp) for English language editing.

References

1. Holmberg G, Thesleff S (1952) Succinylcholine iodide (celocurin) as a muscular relaxant in electro-shock therapy. Acta Psychiatr Neurol Scand 80: 135-138.

2. Mokriski BK, Nagle SE, Papuchis GC, Cohen SM, Waxman GJ (1992) Electroconvulsive therapy-induced cardiac arrhythmias during anesthesia with methohexital, thiamylal, or thiopental sodium. Clin Anesth 4: 208-212.

3. Kitamura T, Page AJ (1984) Electrocardiographic changes following electroconvulsive therapy. Eur Arch Psychiatry Neurol Sci 234: 147-148.

4. Molnar J, Zhang F, Weiss J, Ehlert FA, Rosenthal JE (1996) Diurnal pattern of QTc interval: how long is prolonged? Possible relation to circadian triggers of cardiovascular events. J Am Coll Cardiol 27: 76-83.

5. Ishida S, Nakagawa M, Fujino T, Yonemochi H, Saikawa T, et al. (1997) Circadian variation of QT interval dispersion: correlation with heart rate variability. Electrocardiol 30: 205-210.

6. Nakagawa M, Takahashi N, Iwao T, Yonemochi H, Ooie T, et al. (1999) Evaluation of autonomic influences on QT dispersion using the head-up tilt test in healthy subjects. Pacing Clin Electrophysiol 22: 1158-1163.

7. Lee KW, Okin PM, Kligfield P, Stein KM, Lerman BB (1997) Precordial QT dispersion and inducible ventricular tachycardia. Am Heart J 134: 1005-1013.

8. de Bruyne MC, Hoes AW, Kors JA, Hofman A, van Bemmel JH, et al. (1998) QTc dispersion predicts cardiac mortality in the elderly: the Rotterdam Study. Circulation 97: 467-472.

9. Zareba W, Moss AJ, le Cessie S (1994) Dispersion of ventricular repolarization and arrhythmic cardiac death in coronary artery disease. Am J Cardiol 74: 550-553.

10. Glancy JM, Garratt CJ, Woods KL, de Bono DP (1995) QT dispersion and mortality after myocardial infarction. Lancet 345: 945-948.

11. Zaidi M, Robert A, Fesler R, Derwael C, Brohet C (1997) Dispersion of ventricular repolarisation: a marker of ventricular arrhythmias in patients with previous myocardial infarction. Heart 78: 371-375.

12. Dabrowski A, Kramarz E, Piotrowicz R (1999) Dispersion of QT interval following ventricular premature beats and mortality after myocardial infarction. Cardiology 91: 75-80.

13. Egawa H, Minami J, Fujii K, Hamaguchi S, Okuda Y, et al. (2002) QT interval and QT dispersion increase in the elderly during laparoscopic cholecystectomy. Can J Anesth 49: 927-931.

14. Fujii K, Yamaguchi S, Egawa H, Hamaguchi S, Kitajima T, et al. (2004) Effects of head-up tilt after stellate ganglion block on QT interval and QT dispersion. Reg Anesth Pain Med 29: 317-322.

15. Tezuka, N, Egawa, H, Fukagawa D, Yamaguchi S, Hamaguchi S, et al. (2010) Assessment of QT interval and QT dispersion during electroconvulsive therapy using computerized measurements. J ECT 26: 41-46.

16. Malik M, Batchvarov VN (2000) Measurement, interpretation and clinical potential of QT dispersion. Am Coll Cardiol 36: 1749-1766.

17. Zaballos M, Jimeno C, Almendral J, Atienza F, Patiño D, et al. (2009) Cardiac electrophysiological effects of remifentanil: study in a closed-chest porcine model. Br J Anaesth 103: 191-198.

18. Glass PS, Hardman D, Kamiyama Y, Quill TJ, Marton G, et al. (1993) Preliminary pharmacokinetics and pharmacodynamics of an ultra-short-acting opioid: remifentanil (GI87084B). Anesth Analg 77: 1031-1040.

19. Kapila A, Glass PS, Jacobs JR, Muir KT, Hermann DJ, et al. (1995) Measured context-sensitive half-times of remifentanil and alfentanil. Anesthesiology 83: 968-975.

20. Staikou C, Stamelos M, Stavroulakis E (2014) Impact of anaesthetic drugs and adjuvants on ECG markers of torsadogenicity. Br J Anaesth 112: 217-230.

21. Cafiero T, Di Minno RM, Di Iorio C (2011) QT interval and QT dispersion during the induction of anesthesia and tracheal intubation: a comparison of remifentanil and fentanyl. Minerva Anestesiol 77: 160-165.

22. Kweon TD, Nam SB, Chang CH, Kim MS, Lee JS, et al. (2008) The effect of bolus administration of remifentanil on QTc interval during induction of sevoflurane anaesthesia. Anaesthesia 63: 347-351.

23. Andersen FA, Arsland D, Holst-Larsen H (2001) Effects of combined methohexitone-remifentanil anaesthesia in electroconvulsive therapy. Acta Anaesthesiol Scand 45: 830-833.

24. Recart A, Rawal S, White PF, Byerly S, Thornton L (2003) The effect of remifentanil on seizure duration and acute hemodynamic responses to electroconvulsive therapy. Anesth Analg 96: 1047-1050.

25. Locala JA, Irefin SA, Malone D, Cywinski JB, Samuel SW, et al. (2005) The comparative hemodynamic effects of methohexital and remifentanil in electroconvulsive therapy. J ECT 21: 12-15.

26. Chen ST (2011) Remifentanil: a review of its use in electroconvulsive therapy. J ECT 27: 323-327.

27. Smith DL, Angst MS, Brock-Utne JG, DeBattista C (2003) Seizure duration with remifentanil/methohexital vs. methohexital alone in middle-aged patients undergoing electroconvulsive therapy. Acta Anaesthesiol Scand 47: 1064-1066.

28. Dinwiddie SH, Glick DB, Goldman MB (2012) The effect of propofol-remifentanil anesthesia on selected seizure quality indices in electroconvulsive therapy. Brain Stimul 5: 402-407.

29. Yamaguchi S, Nagao M, Ikeda T, Fukagawa D, Kimura Y, et al. (2011) QT dispersion and rate-corrected QT dispersion during electroconvulsive therapy in elderly patients. J ECT 27: 183-188.

30. Scott JC, Stanski DR (1987) Decreased fentanyl and alfentanil dose requirements with age. A simultaneous pharmacokinetic and pharmacodynamic evaluation. Pharmacol Exp Ther 240: 159-166.

19

Serum Interleukin-6 Level after Cyclooxygenase-2 Inhibitor Treatment in Moderate Traumatic Brain Injury

Dewi Yulianti Bisri[1*], Caroline Wullur[1], Diana Ch Lalenoh[2] and Tatang Bisri[1]

[1]Department of Anesthesiology and Intensive Care, School of Medicine, Universitas Padjadjaran, Hasan Sadikin Hospital-Bandung, Indonesia

[2]Department of Anesthesiology and Intensive Care, School of Medicine, Prof. R.D. Kandou Hospital-Manado, Universitas Sam Ratulangi, Indonesia

*Corresponding author: Dewi Yulianti Bisri, Department of Anesthesiology and Intensive Care, School of Medicine, Universitas Padjadjaran, Hasan Sadikin Hospital, Indonesia, E-mail: yuliantibisri@yahoo.com

Abstract

The most clinical scoring of traumatic brain injury patient is Glasgow Coma Scale (GCS) score. Lower GCS score higher IL-6 level and higher morbidity and mortality. Neuroinflammation is one mechanism of secondary brain injury. Selective cyclooxygenase (sCOX-2) inhibitors are drugs commonly used in treatment of postoperative pain but also possess an anti-inflammatory effect. The aim of this study is to determine the role of sCOX-2 inhibitors as inhibitors of inflammatory processes in patients with head injury measured by IL-6.

This is a double blind randomized controlled study involving patients with moderate head injuries who underwent surgery in Dr. Hasan Sadikin Hospital Bandung Indonesia since December 2013 until December 2015. After obtaining approval of research ethics committees from School of Medicine Universitas Padjadjaran/Dr. Hasan Sadikin Hospital, samples were divided randomly into 5 groups: control group, COX2-group I (given sCOX-2 inhibitor ones), COX2-group II (given sCOX-2 inhibitor twice), COX2-group III (given sCOX-2 inhibitor thrice), and COX2-group IV (given sCOX-2 inhibitor four times), each group containing 6 patients. All patients received standard therapy as recommended by Traumatic Brain Foundation in 2007 as well as monitoring of GCS, blood pressure, pulse rate, respiratory rate, oxygen saturation, temperature and blood sugar in pre and postoperative stages. The data was analyzed using statistical tests Paired Samples T-test and One Way Anova, p-value <0.05 as statistical significant.

Result shows that data pretest IL-6, data posttest and IL-6 changes of both groups is not significance (p>0.05). In treatment group (Cox-2 I, Cox-2 II, Cox-2 III dan Cox-2 IV) overall are decrease of IL-6=10%, which is p 0.083<0.10, if p=0.05 that is not significance (p>0.05).

The study is concluded that sCOX-2 inhibitor has a brain protective effect by lowering IL-6 level in patients with moderate head injury.

Keywords: Moderate traumatic brain injury; Neuroinflammation; Selective COX-2 inhibitor; IL-6

Introduction

Pathophysiology of brain injury is functionally divided into 4 categories, namely: (1) primary brain injury that occurs upon impact of injury, (2) secondary injury, that involves high lactate level, free oxygen radical, interleukin, glutamate and free intracellular Ca as a response to primary injury, (3) inflammation response with further neurodenegeration involving free radicals and toxic neurochemicals, and (4) regeneration with unclear explanation [1,2].

Head injury will stimulate neural cells to synthesize and release inflammatory cytokines such as peptides from interleukin (IL) group and TNF-α. Patients with moderate head injury have increased levels of IL-1, IL-6, and TNF-α in their circulation and cerebrospinal fluid [3-6].

After head injury in mice, microglia is responsible for IL-1 and IL-6 production. Astroglial have demonstrated the relationship between upregulation with inflammatory cytokines such as IL-1α, IL-1β, and TNF-α in post-traumatic murine. In humans with head injury, as part of inflammatory response, microcelullar endothelial cells release IL-1β and TNF-α that will eventually stimulate the release of neurotoxic agents such as arachidonic acid and their metabolites [3-6].

Inflammatory response is a modulation of a direct two way relationship between brain tissue and immune system. The relationship between brain tissue and immune system is divided into 2 broad mechanisms, (1) a hormonal response, especially involving hypothalamus-pituitary-adrenal, identical to hypothalamus-pituitary-gonad (HPG); hypothalamus-pituitary-thyroid (HPT); hypothalamus-growth hormone axis, (2) autonomic nervous system, including release of noradrenaline and acetylcholine from sympathic and parasympathic nervous system, immune system also involves cytokine release [3].

Parasympathic nervous system activation results in cholinergic activation of the efferent vagus nerve fibers and release acetylcholine on the synapse. There is also inflammatory activation of vagus nerve fibers called inflammatory reflex. This is a rapid inflammatory brain response from cholinergic nerve fibers. Acetylcholine releases pro-inflammatory cytokines (TNF-α, IL-1β, IL-6 and IL-8) but not anti-inflammatory cytokine IL-10. Cytokine play an important role as a communicator and modulator between immune and neuroendocrine system. Cytokine system may modulate brain tissue though various mechanisms, including active transport in the blood brain barrier [1,3].

In head injury, inflammatory response affects injured brain tissue. Inflammatory stress response is part of the complement activation and upregulation of endothelial cells that are linked with neutrophil accumulation and cytokine production. The role of proinflammatory mediator in formation of secondary lesions has been investigated, including serial mediators such as cytokine. Among the cytokines, IL-1β, TNF-a, IL-6 and IL-8 are especially important [4,5,7].

IL-6 has both pro- and anti-inflammatory properties. High level of IL-6 in the plasma and cerebrospinal fluid are found in post-traumatic brain injury patients. IL-6 may also promote vasopression secretion and plays a role in the pathogenesis of syndrome of inappropriate antidiuretic hormone (SIADH) after traumatic brain injury [4,5,7].

COX-2 inhibitors are potent neuroprotectors both *in vitro* and *in vivo*. Inhibition of COX-2 protected neurons in mixed cultures against NMDA excitotoxicity. Significantly, COX-2 specific inhibition blocked neuronal cell death, whereas COX-1 specific inhibition did not [8].

The aim of this study is to examine whether the administration of COX-2 inhibitor will reduce IL-6 as inflammatory marker and if so, whether COX-2 inhibitor has a brain protection effect in patients with traumatic brain injury.

Subject and Method

This is an experimental double blind randomized controlled trial involving patients with moderate head injury admitted to Dr. Hasan Sadikin Hospital who will undergo neurosurgery and fulfilled inclusion and exclusion criteria.

Inclusion criteria:

- 1. Male and female between 13-60 years old.
- 2. Moderate head injury with GCS 9-12 with no other injuries.
- 3. All patients undergoing surgery (epidural hematoma, subdural hematoma, intracranial haemorrhage).
- 4. Injury <24 h.
- 5. ASA II.

Exclusion criteria:

- 1. NSAID usage within 30 days.
- 2. Unstable blood pressure (systolic blood pressure <90 mmHg).
- 3. Pregnancy and menstruation.

Drop-out criteria:

- 1. Patient died before 3 days postoperative.
- 2. Surgery >4 h.

Sample size is determined based on formula sample of five groups using Kastenbaum curve with confidence level of 95% and power test of 80% and d/s=0.5 therefore each group contains of 6 subjects. Total number of subjects is 30 patients with 10% drop out yielding 33 patients. Statistical analyses for characteristic data using One Way ANOVA, with gender variable as the exception using Chi-Square,

significant statistical difference if p<0.05 and very significant statistical difference if p<0.01.

Method

Study is conducted after obtaining ethical clearance from Ethical Commitee of Medical Faculty of Universitas Padjadjaran/Hasan Sadikin Hospital Bandung Indonesia. After obtaining informed consent, patients with moderate head injury (GCS 9-12) without other injuries were positioned 300 head up along with examination of non-invasive blood pressure, core temperature, blood glucose and SpO₂.

Sample was divided into 5 groups, treatment group COX2 and control. The treatment groups (COX2) was divided into 4 subgroups, COX2-I, COX2-II, COX2-III, and COX2-IV each consisting of 6 patients, each of whom receives 40mg of intravenous COX-2 inhibitor similar dose for analgesia in adult patient. Group COX2-I: receives 1 dose of COX-2 inhibitor; group COX2-II: receives 2 doses of COX-2 inhibitor; group COX2-III: receives 3 doses of COX-2 inhibitor; group COX2-IV: receives 4 doses of COX-2 inhibitor with 12 h interval. Control group receives 0.9% NaCl prior to anaesthetic induction.

Intravenous induction was performed using 2 mg/kgBW propofol, 0.8 mg/kgBW vecuronium bromide, 2 μgr/kgBW fentanyl, 1.5 mg/kgBW lidocaine and 1.5 MAC isoflurane with 6 L/minute oxygen. Subjects were intubated using non-kinking endotracheal tube. Maintenance of anaesthesia using 1 MAC isoflurane, 3 L/minute oxygen, 2L/minute air, continuous 0.5-1 mg/kgBW/h of propofol, and continuous 0.1 mg/kgBW/h of vecuronium. Each patient receives additional 18 G intravenous and urinary catheter placement. Ventilation was controlled throughout the surgery. Each patient receives 0.5 mg/kgBW intravenous mannitol and 500 mg metamizole as postoperative analgesia.

Depends on the subgroup, patients in COX2-II group receives another dose of COX-2 inhibitor after 12 h, 24 h for COX2-III group and 36 h for COX2-IV group after initial dose of COX-2 inhibitor prior to induction, and patients in control group receive 2cc of 0.9% NaCl. Blood samples were obtained from patients in subgroup I, II, III and IV 6 h after the last COX-2 inhibitor dose to examine the level of IL-6. In the control group, blood sampel take in the similar time with treatment group. The usual recommended dose of COX-2 inhibitor parexocib is 40 mg intravenously every 12 h (twice per day). The measuring IL-6 serum using ELISA.

Result and Discussion

General characteristics of study subjects

General characteristics including age, body weight, onset of injury, systolic blood pressure (SBP), diastolic blood pressure (DBP), blood glucose level (BGL), GCS, oxygen saturation, core temperature and duration of surgery were analyzed using One Way ANOVA, whereas gender was analyzed using Chi-Square test. Significant statistical difference if p<0.05 and very statistical significant if p<0.01.

Analysis on characteristic data shows no statistical difference with p>0.05 among the five groups therefore eligible for comparison. The result of statistical analysis of general characteristic is displayed on Table 1 below. Comparison of IL-6 in all groups can be seen in Tables 2 and 3 below.

General Characteristic	Groups					p value
	Control	COX2-I	COX2-II	COX2-III	COX2-IV	
	n=6	n=6	n=6	n=6	n=6	
Age (years)	36.17 (16.68)	31.67 (13.62)	24.67 (12.61)	28.33 (16.21)	26.83 (9.37)	0.650
Gender M	5 (83.30%)	5 (83.30%)	5 (83.30%)	6 (100%)	5 (83.30%)	0.886
F	1 (16.70%)	1 (16.70%)	1 (16.70%)	0 (0%)	1 (16.70%)	
Body weight (kg)	65.00 (10.49)	62.17 (8.50)	58.67 (7.12)	61.67 (9.31)	64.17 (11.14)	0.798
Onset of injury (h)	9.00 (2.61)	11.00 (2.53)	12.00 (5.18)	10.17 (4.71)	8.00 (3.52)	0.389
SBP (mmHg)	118.67 (12.24)	137.33 (32.63)	117.17 (30.33)	120.67 (22.99)	122.67 (16.48)	0.617
DBP (mmHg)	75.17 (6.15)	72.5 (10.62)	63.33 (20.1)	72.83 (11.43)	78.50 (5.79)	0.287
BGL (mg%)	181.33 (40.27)	142.5 (8.62)	139.67 (33.1)	138.33 (28. 9)	160.5 (26.4)	0.079
GCS	11.00 (1.26)	11.17 (1.17)	10.50 (0.84)	10.50 (1.22)	11.50 (1.38)	0.535
Core temperature (°C)	35.62 (0.84)	35.98 (1.01)	36.30 (0.53)	36.35 (0.67)	36.53 (0.79)	0.308
Oxygen saturation (%)	100 0	100 0	100 0	99.67 (082) (0.82)	99.83 (0.41)	0.537
Duration of surgery (h)	2.61 (0.45)	2.58 (0.49)	2.56 (0.35)	2.63 (0.43)	2..57 (0.34)	0.998

p-value was obtained using One Way Anova, with exception for gender variable using Chi Square test, significant statistical difference if p<0.05 and very significant statistical difference if p<0.01, COX2-I: 1 dose of COX-2 inhibitor administration; COX2-II: 2 doses of COX-2 inhibitor administration; COX2-III: 3 doses of COX-2 inhibitor administration; COX2-IV: 4 doses of COX-2 inhibitor administration; control: 0.9% NaCl administration, SBP: Systolic Blood Pressure; DBP: Diastolic Blood Pressure; BGL: Blood Glucose Level; GCS: Glasgow Coma Scale.

Table 1: General Characteristics of Study Subjects (mean-SD)).

Variable	Group						p value[a]
	COX2-I	COX2-II	COX2-III	COX2-IV	Control	All sample	
	n=6	n=6	n=6	n=6	n=6	N=30	
IL-6							
IL-6 Pre-operative	119.28 (178.16)	54.25 (79.24)	56.09 (51.92)	31.89 (26.16)	100.39 (106.51)	72.36 (100.86)	0.572
IL-6 Post-operative	48.35 (49.97)	40.21 (27.9)	19.3 (9.4)	25.63 (13.01)	36.39 (40.5)	33.97 (31.67)	0.55

	ΔIL-6 (Pre-Post)	70.93	14.03	36.8	6.26	64	38.4	0.72
		(143.64)	(81.97)	(56.53)	(27.2)	(129.21)	(94.68)	
p-value (pre-post)[b]		0.281	0.692	0.172	0.597	0.297	0.034	
p-value was obtained using: a) One Way Anova, b) paired t-test, significant statistical difference if p<0.05 and very significant statistical difference if p<0.01.								

Table 2: Comparison of IL (6 level in all groups (mean (SD)).

Variable		Group		p value[a]
		COX2 I-IV	Control	
		(n=24)	(n=6)	
IL-6				
	IL-6 Pre	65.38 (100.52)	100.39 (106.51)	0.457
	IL-6 Post	33.37 (30.10)	36.39 (40.5)	0.839
	Δ IL-6 (Pre (Post)	32.00 (86.37)	64 (129.21)	0.469
p-value (pre (post)[b]		0.083	0.279	
p-value was obtained using: a) independent (t-test, b) paired t-test, significant statistical difference if p<0.05 and very significant statistical difference if p<0.01.				

Table 3: Comparison of IL-6 between treatment (COX-2) and Control Group.

Based on the table above, there is no significant difference in either pre (operative IL-6, post (operative IL-6 or change in IL-6 between the two groups (p>0.05). In treatment group (COX2 (I, COX2 (II, COX2 (III, and COX2 (IV) there is an overall 10% reduction of IL-6 level, where p 0.083<0.10, however, using=0.05, the value is not significant (p>0.05).

Table 1 and Figure 1 show a reduction of IL-6 from preoperative to post (operative in all groups, both treatment and control. However, the reduction in IL-6 level in each group is not significant, shown by p value>0.05 using paired t-test.

Comparison of preoperative IL-6 among all groups using One Way ANOVA showed that the difference is not statistically significant with p>0.05. Similarly, comparison of postoperative IL-6 among all groups using One Way ANOVA showed no difference with p>0.05.

Table 2 and Figure 2 above show significant reduction in IL-6 (p<0.05) from 72.38 pg/mL to 33.97 pg/mL. We can conclude that there is a reduction in average level of IL-6 in all treatment group (n=30) from preoperative to postoperative, however, if assess individually for each group, where number of sample is 6, the difference is not statistically significant (p>0.05).

This may be explained by reduction of IL-6 level only occurs in a few number of samples, whereas a few other samples experience an increase in IL-6 level.

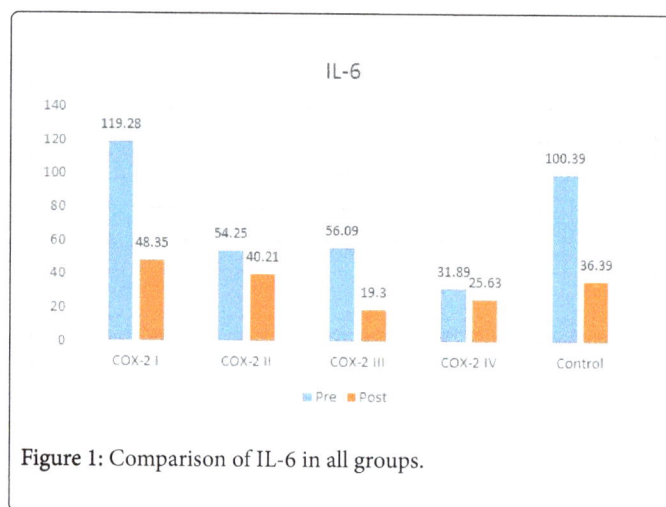

Figure 1: Comparison of IL-6 in all groups.

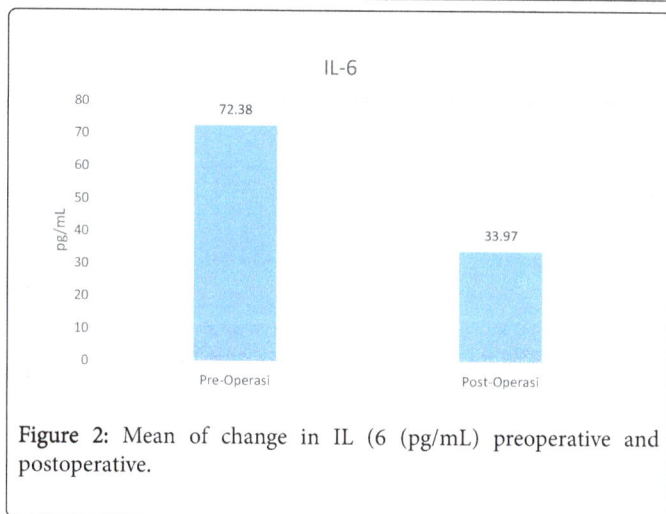

Figure 2: Mean of change in IL (6 (pg/mL) preoperative and postoperative.

Discussion

Cyclooxygenase (COX) is an enzyme that catalyzes prostaglandin synthesis from arachidonic acid. Prostaglandin mediates many processes in the body including secretion of gastric protective layer, maintenance of renal function, and platelet aggregation. Nonsteroidal anti-inflammatory drugs (NSAID) block the mechanism of COX therefore reduce the formation of prostaglandin, resulting in both positive (analgesia, anti-inflammation) and negative (gastric ulceration, reduction in renal function, bleeding) outcomes. The activity of COX is linked with 2 isoenzymes, namely COX-1 and COX-2. COX-1 is found mainly in gastric mucosa, renal parenchyme and platelet. COX-1 has minimal effect on pro (inflammatory hormonal response. This enzyme is essential in homeostasis such as platelet aggregation, maintenance of gastrointestinal mucosal integrity and renal function. On the contrary, COX-2 causes and is expressed in injured tissues (renal and brain) and mediates inflammation, fever, pain and carcinogenesis. COX-2 does not have a protective role. COX-2 expression may fascilitate a few oncogenic processes, such as tumor invasion, angiogenesis, haematemesis. Regulation of COX-2 occurs in spinal cord in response to surgical stimulation which may play an important role in central sensitization. In response to inflammation, COX-2 expression increases by 10-20 times [9-12].

Nonsteroidal antiinflamatory drugs (NSAID) suppress prostaglandin and tromboxane, which play an important role in gastric homeostasis (PGE_2 and PGI_2), renal (PGE_2) and platelets (thromboxane A_2 and PGI_2), the primary mechanism where NSAID cause some negative effects. Additionally, inhibition of prostaglandin synthesis by NSAID has been considered to contribute to bronchospasm and inhibition for new bone formation [13].

Nonsteroidal antiinflamatory drugs (NSAID) is drug with analgesia, anti (inflammatory and anti (pyretic effects. These drugs are categorized as conventionl none (specific inhibitor in two forms, COX (ibuprofen, naproxen, aspirin, acetaminofen, ketorolac) and selective COX-2 inhibitor (celecoxib, rofecoxib, valdecoxib, parecoxib). All NSAID and COX-2 inhibitors have ceiling effects and increasing their dosage will only increase the risks of toxicity. Inhibition of COX-1 is responsible for many adverse effects caused by conventional NSAID [9-13].

Non-steroidal anti-inflammatory drugs (NSAID) work peripherally (without involvement of central nervous system) and the analgesia effect is secondary to anti (inflammatory effect, caused by inhibition of prostaglandin. Inhibition of prostaglandin is also responsible for the main adverse effects namely platelet dysfunction and gastritis. NSAID are commonly used as a single agent for mild and moderate postoperative pain. NSAID have an opioid sparing effect if used in conjunction with opioid. Considering the advantages and disadvantages, they are only used to 1-2 days. NSAID are contraindicated in patients with bleeding disorder, receiving anti (coagulants, history of peptide ulcer disease and gastritis, and renal dysfunction [9-13].

Nonsteroidal anti-inflammatory drugs (NSAID) are drug with analgesia, anti (inflammatory and anti (pyretic effects. NSAID have both central and peripheral effects. Anti (pyretic is achieved centrally though hypothalamus whereas analgesia is peripherally. Latest studies showed that there is an also possible central analgesia effect through inhibition of descending pain pathway. Most dominant theory is that NSAID works peripherally through inhibition of prostaglandin synthesis therefore reducing inflammation and pain. Prostaglandin synthesis is prevented by inhibition of COX-2. Cyclooxygenase-2 (COX-2) converts arachidonic acid from cellular damage into prostaglandin D, E and F, prostacylin and thromboxane. Damaged cells and activation of phospholipase release arachidonic acid, which will be converted into prostanoid and leukotriene by COX-2 and lipooxygenase, resulting in production of reactive free radicals [13].

The role of COX (2 and its inhibition in the brain must be evaluated in a broader context than metabolism of arachidonic acid. Pertubation or brain insult will activate phospholipase, releasing arachidonic acid from membrane reserve. Cyclooxygenase-2 (COX-2) catalyses the conversion of arachidonic acid and molecular oxygen into vasoactive prostaglandin, a process which produces free radicals [9-14].

Cyclooxygenase-2 (COX-2) overexpression illustrates marker and effector from damage cells after brain injury, and in normal and pathological aging proses in the brain. Cyclooxygenase-2 (COX-2) inhibitor may have a neuroprotective effect by reducing prostanoid and free radical production, or by substituting metabolic pathway of arachidonic acid. Arachidonic shunting hypothesis states that neuroprotective effect of COX-2 inhibitor may be mediated by the increase of production of eicosinoids. Under the condition where activation of COX-2 is inhibited, accumulation of arachidonic acid or conversion into eicosanoids through lipooxygenase and cytochrome P (450-CYP) epoxygenase. A number of P450 eicosanoid have been shown to have a beneficial effect on brain tissue and/or peripherally. We suspect that shunting of arachidonic acid may play an important role in functional recovery after brain injury that alters prostanoid per se. Therefore, inhibition of COX-2 and arachidonic acid shunting has a therapeutic implication outside the suppression of prostaglandin synthesis and formation of free radicals [9-14].

The severity of neural injury appears to correlate to the degree and duration of COX-2 overexpression, mild injury yield shorter elevation ($\leq$ 24 h) of COX-2 mRNA and prostaglandin production, while moderate to severe injuries yield extended elevation ($\geq$ 3days) in brain cells. This may due to a vicious cycle, in which secondary injury cascades promulgate COX-2 expressions. Increase COX-2 expression has been observed with head trauma, cerebral ischemia, spreading depression, and seizure. Overexpression of brain COX-2 may reflect its role in chronic inflammation and neural cell death. Early on after moderate brain injury, neuron show increase COX-2 level that may persist for 1-3 days [8].

Several COX-2 specific inhibitors have been employed to treat brain injury. Their efficacy, when administered at various dose and time before or after neurological insult has not been entirely consistent, perhaps because of widely different partition coefficients across the blood-brain barrier [8]. However, the overwhelming preponderance of evidence clearly shows that protracted brain COX-2 activity mediates a toxic response that worsen functional and neuroanatomical deficits after brain and spinal cord injury. Thus, COX-2 inhibitors that benefit in the injured brain likely produce their effect primarily by reducing COX-2 activity rather than by supressing free radical-mediated brain damage or other specific mechanism [8].

In this study, administration of COX-2 inhibitor blocks the production of COX-2 which reduces overexpression of COX-2, therefore reducing neural cell damage, shown by a reduction in IL-6 level.

Conclusion

The study concludes that COX-2 inhibitor has a brain protective effect by lowering IL-6 level in patients with moderate head injury.

References

1. Ray SK, Dixon CE, Banik NL (2002) Molecular mechanisms in the pathogenesis of traumatic brain injury. Histol Histopatho 17: 1137-1152.

2. Werner C, Engelhard K (2007) Pathophysiology of traumatic brain injury. Br J Anaesth 99: 4-9.

3. Lucas SM, Rothwell NJ, Gibson RM (2006) The role inflammation in CNS injury and disease. Br J Pharmacol 147: s232-s240.

4. Veenith T, Goon SSH, Burstein RM (2009) Moleculer mechanisms of traumatic brain injury the missing link in management. World J Emerg Surg 4: 1-6.

5. Schmidt OI, Heyde CE, Ertel W, Stahel PF (2005) Closed head injury an inflammatory diseases? Brain Res Rev 48: 388-399.

6. Wen YD, Zhang HL, Qin ZH (2006) Inflammatory mechanism in ischemic neuronal injury. Neuroscience Bulletin 22: 171-182.

7. Harukuni I, Bhardwaj A (2006) Mechanisms of brain injury after global cerebral ischemia. Neurol Clin 24: 1-21.

8. Straus KI (2008) Antiinflammatory and neuroprotective actions of COX2 inhibitors in the injured brain. Brain Behav Immun 22: 285-289.

9. Minghetti L, Levi G (1998) Microglia as effector cell in brain damage and repair: focus on prostanoids and nitrit oxide. Prog Neurobiol 54: 99-125.

10. Gajraj NM (2003) Cyclooxygenase-2 inhibitor. Anesth Analg 96: 1720-1738.

11. Mirjany M, Pasinetti GM (2002) Role of Cyclooxygenase-2 in neuronal cell cycle activity and glutamate-mediated exitotoxicity. JPET 301: 494-500.

12. Huntjens DRH, Danhof M, Pasqua OED (2005) Pharmacokinetic (pharmacodynamic correlations and biomarker in development of COX-2 inhibitors. Rhematology 44: 846-859.

13. Menezes GB, Cara DC, Rezende RM (2009) Anti-inflammatory drugs: basic knowledge to safe prescripton. Odontologia. clin cientif recife 8: 7-12.

14. Allan MS, Rothwell JN (2003) Inflammation in central nervous system injury. Philos Trans R Soc Lond B Biol Sci 385: 1669-1677.

20

Severity and Risk Factors of Post-Operative Pain in University of Gondar Hospital, Northeast Ethiopa

Wosenyeleh Sahile Admassu[*], **Amare Gebregzi Hailekiros and Zewditu Denu Abdissa**

Department of Anesthesiology and Critical Care, Addis Abeba University & University of Gondar, Ethiopia

[*]**Corresponding author:** Wosenyeleh Sahile Admassu, Department of Anesthesiology and Critical Care, Addis Abeba University & University of Gondar, Atse Bekaffa ST, Gondar, Amhara, Ethiopia, E-mail: wesswub@gmail.com

Abstract

Background: Pain is a sensory and emotional experience associated with actual or potential tissue damage, or described in terms of such damage according to Association of the Study of Pain. Despite advances in medical science inadequate post-operative pain management exists in Ethiopia and worldwide. Several perioperative and pre-clinical factors are recognized in contributing to enhancement of pain severity and its adverse effect.

Objective: This study is aimed at assessing the severity and identifying the risk factors contributing to post-operative pain.

Methodology: A hospital based cross sectional study was conducted on all patients who came to Gondar university hospital, Ethiopia operating theatre from March-of April 15, 2013. Data was collected by administering questionnaires via interview and reviewing the patients chart after taking consent. Numeric rating scale was used to assess pain severity. Logistic regression was used to identify independent risk factors for post-operative pain.

Result: 150 patients are included in the prospective study. Moderate to severe pain was reported in 85(57%) of patients in the immediate post-operative period and 117(78%) in the 1st 12 hour. On multivariate analysis ASA I and II OR (4.0) P (0.013), age less than 60 OR (2.642) P (0.042), female gender with an OR (2.580) P (0.005), general anesthesia OR (5.562) P (0.000), and incision length >10cm OR (1.991) P (0.041) were identified as independent risk factors for post-operative pain severity.

Conclusion: The study confirms that post-operative pain is still severe and under managed. Identifying perioperative factors for the occurrence of moderate/severe post-operative pain may be useful for designing factor specific interventions to relieve patient suffering.

Keywords: CPSP: Chronic Post-Surgical Pain; POP: Post-Operative Pain; GUH: Gondar University Hospital; ASA: American Association of Anesthesiologists; IASP: International Association for the Study of Pain

Introduction

Pain is defined as a sensory and emotional experience associated with actual or potential tissue damage, or described in terms of such damage [1]. Although pain is a predictable part of the postoperative experience, inadequate management of pain is common and can have profound implications. Untreated post operative pain (POP) may result in clinical and psychological changes that increase morbidity and mortality also decreasing quality of life [2].

Some of the negative clinical outcomes resulting from ineffective postoperative pain management include deep vein thrombosis, pulmonary embolism, coronary ischemia, myocardial infarction, pneumonia, poor wound healing, insomnia, and demoralization, this all effects economic and medical implications, such as extended lengths of stay, readmissions, and patient dissatisfaction with medical care [3,4].

The morbidity and mortality associated with surgeries in the developing countries is high. A 5 year review of inpatient mortality in Tikur Anbessa Ethiopia, showed that there is a 7% overall and 4.5% post-operative mortality [5]. This shows us that there is still need for research on the factors that will significantly determine the perioperative morbidity and mortality.

Annually over 70 million patients in America [6] and 40 million patients in the European Union are operated [7]. Despite several advances in the understanding of pain previous researches have reported a 20-80% prevalence of moderate to severe postoperative pain [8]. Research done in Nigeria about the incidence of POP among 200 Nigerians showed that more than 68% of patients experienced moderate to severe pain while surgery conducted in the Anorectal region took 90% of the complaints [9].

Although POP is an acute response to a surgical intervention resolving spontaneously or with some analgesics sometimes it may become persistent that can lead in to chronic post-surgical pain (CPSP). In Canada surgery is a major predicting factor for chronic pain in more than 20% of persons attending pain clinic [10]. Routine procedures in GUH such as hernias and mastectomies pose greater danger [11].

Some of the risk factors are common surgical procedures that are done at the upper abdomen and thoracic region (e.g. laparatomy, Cholecystectomy, thoracotomy) [12]. Patients who have experienced acute to severe pain preoperatively are said to experience more severe pain with a tendency to develop to chronic pain [13]. Patients with ASA classification of III and above have higher tendency to develop post-operative pain [9]. Age is also another factor which has chronic relation with the development of POP. Older patients are said to experience less pain, fewer complaints and less requirements for post-operative analgesics than younger people [9]. Together with age is gender in which females and those with high pre-operative anxiety tend to develop severe post-operative pain [14]. Type of anesthesia duration and site of surgery were also other factors noted as important in increasing post-operative pain [15].

Research conducted in and out of Africa show the still uncontrolled and higher incidence of POP whilst sometimes providing the best available treatment modalities [16,17]. Currently there isn't enough evidence that shows how severe the problem is and also what the different psycho social and socio economic factors that affect POP are in developing countries.

The management of POP and prevention of all the complication that follow mainly depends on adequate knowledge on the severity of the problem. The inadequate understanding of the severity of the problem and lack of knowledge on the common risk factors POP results to poor pain management in postoperative period which has high incidence of progressing to chronic pain throughout their life. The objective of this study was to assess the severity of post-operative pain and associated risk factors.

Methodology

A hospital-based quantitative cross-sectional study was conducted from March 1- April 15, 2012 in Gondar university hospital. All patients who came to the operating theatre either for emergency or elective procedures during the study period were included except patients with the age less than 8 years, patients discharged in less than 24 h, patient with cognitive dysfunction. A pretested and structured questionnaire containing the numeric rating scale (NRS) was taken 3 times in 24 h first post operatively 2 h the return of full consciousness, second on the 12th h and third on the 24th hour. Patient's preoperative assessment, intraoperative status, medication, and post-operative events were recorded from their Medical record. Independent variables were age, sex, ASA status, premedication, type and location of surgery, type of anesthesia, previous acute or chronic painful experiences are used to predict the severity postoperative pain measured with NRS. Pain-in a NRS described as 0 -no pain, 1-3 Mild pain, 4-6 Moderate pain and 7-10 severe pain.

After obtaining ethical clearance letter from Gondar University ethical review board, Patients were interviewed at 2, 12, and 24 h after operation about the progress of pain. Two recovery room nurses were trained on numeric rating scale and patient interview by the questionnaire. Data was checked, coded and entered to SPSS version 16.0 version statistical package and analysis was made. Analytic statistics was calculated for most variables in the study. The association between the outcome and exposure variables was assessed using binary logistic regression and the chi squared test.

Results

Socio-demographic characteristics

A total of 150 patients were analyzed with patients at the age of 30-60 taking the majority (46%). The majority of the respondents were 82 (54.7%) were females, orthodox religion 144 (96%) and Amhara ethnicity 141 (94%). A total of 114 (76%) of patients were married. While the rest (23%) were unmarried that includes single, divorced and widowed (Table 1).

Variable	Frequency	Percentage
Age		
14-29	59	39
30-59	69	46
>60	22	15
Sex		
Male	68	45
Female	82	55
Religion		
Orthodox	141	94
Muslim	9	6
Marital status		
Married	114	76
Single	28	19
Divorced	5	3
Widowed	3	2
Educational status		
Illiterate	84	56
Can read and write	25	17
Primary school	17	11
Secondary school	16	11
College and above	8	5
Ethnicity		
Amhara	143	95
Tigre	7	5

Table 1: Sociodemographic of the study participants in GUH march-April 15, 2012.

Figure 1 shows the preoperative factors and the responses of patients. ASA classification showed the bulk of patients lie on ASAI and II 132(88%) while ASAIII and IV took only 18 (12%) of patients. The responsible anesthetists ordered different types of drugs for 49 (33%) of patients. While the rest of patients had none ordered, of the drugs ordered pethidine took the majority with 38 (25%) of patients and Diclofenac 7 (5%) of patients while Tramadol and paracetamol took 0.7 and 1.3% of the cases respectively, and for around 100 (62%) of patients none was ordered.

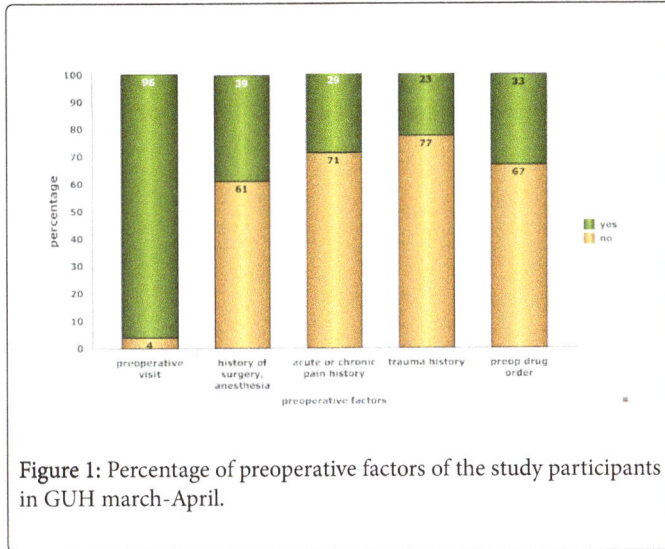

Figure 1: Percentage of preoperative factors of the study participants in GUH march-April.

Intrabdominal and Urogenital procedures took the majority of cases 100 (66%) of patients (Figure 2).

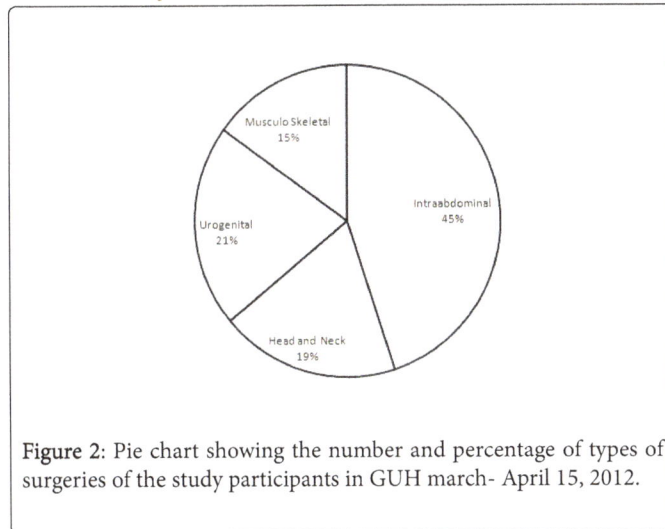

Figure 2: Pie chart showing the number and percentage of types of surgeries of the study participants in GUH march- April 15, 2012.

Intrabdominal 62% and head and neck 68 % procedures reported the most amounts of patients complaining moderate to severe pain (Figure 3).

88 (59%) patients had a greater than 10 cm surgical site incision length while the rest 41% were below 10 cm only pethidine was used as a premedication in 7 (5%) of patients. General anesthesia with inhalational maintenance was the anesthesia of choice in 56 (55%) patients.

Maintenance with Ketamine and propofol shared equal number of patients 39 (26%) each. Diclofenac 40 (27%) and pethidine 11 (7%) were the most commonly given analgesics. 18 (12%) of patients had some kind of nerve block (mostly TAP block) done for them before they went to recovery (Table 2).

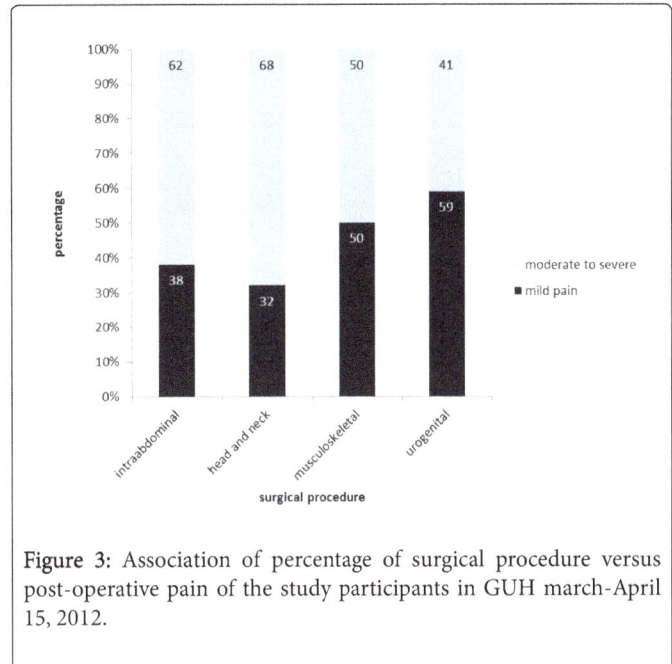

Figure 3: Association of percentage of surgical procedure versus post-operative pain of the study participants in GUH march-April 15, 2012.

Variable	Number (%)	2nd hour		12th hour	
		Mild (n)	Moderate to severe (n)	Mild (n)	Moderate to severe (n)
Type of surgery					
Intraabdominal	68 (45)	26	42	15	53
Head and neck	28 (19)	9	19	8	20
Urogenital	32 (21)	19	13	5	27
Musculoskeletal	22 (15)	11	11	5	17
Incision length					
<5 cm	27 (18)	12	15	9	18
5-10 cm	35 (23)	21	14	8	27
>10 cm	88 (59)	32	56	16	72
Premedication before induction					
Pethidine	7 (5)	1	6	1	6
None	143 (95)	64	79	32	111
Type of anesthesia					
General anesthesia	102 (68)	31	71	26	76
Spinal	46 (31)	33	13	7	39
Nerve block	2 (1)	1	1	0	2
Patient induction					
Ketamine	39 (26)	12	27	8	31
Thiopental	24 (16)	4	20	4	20

Propofol	39 (26)	15	24	14	25
Other	48 (32)	34	14	7	41
Patient maintenance					
TIVA with ketamine	15 (10)	4	11	4	11
TIVA with ketamine and propofol	8 (5)	5	3	4	4
Inhalational + Opoid	23 (15)	7	16	5	18
Inhalational	56 (37)	15	41	13	43
Other	48 (32)	34	14	7	41
Surgery time					
<1 hour	68 (45)	32	36	16	52
2-3 hour	52 (35)	26	26	13	39
>3hour	30 (20)	7	23	4	26
Anesthesia time					
<1 hour	40 (27)	17	23	7	33
2-3 hour	60 (40)	32	28	20	40
>3hour	50 (33)	16	34	6	44
Analgesic before emergence					
Diclofenac	40 (28)	18	22	8	32
Paracetamol	2 (1)	1	1	1	1
Pethidine	11 (7)	2	9	2	9
Morphine	2 (1)	1	1	1	1
Tramadol	4 (3)	2	2	1	3
None	91(61)	41	50	20	71
Nerve block before emergence					
Yes	18 (12)	10	8	6	12
No	132 (88)	55	77	27	105

Table 2: Sociodemographic of the study participants in GUH march-April 15, 2012.

The 2 hour post-operative numeric pain rating scale shows that 65 (43%) of patients experienced mild pain and 85 (57%) of patients reported that they are experiencing moderate to severe pain (Figure 4). The 12 hour pain score showed different result from that of the 2 hour in that only 33 (22%) of patients replied mild pain and the majority 117 (78%) of patients reported moderate to severe pain. At the 24th hour 71 (47%) of patients reported that they are experiencing mild pain while, 79 (53%) experience moderate to severe pain consecutively (Figure 4).

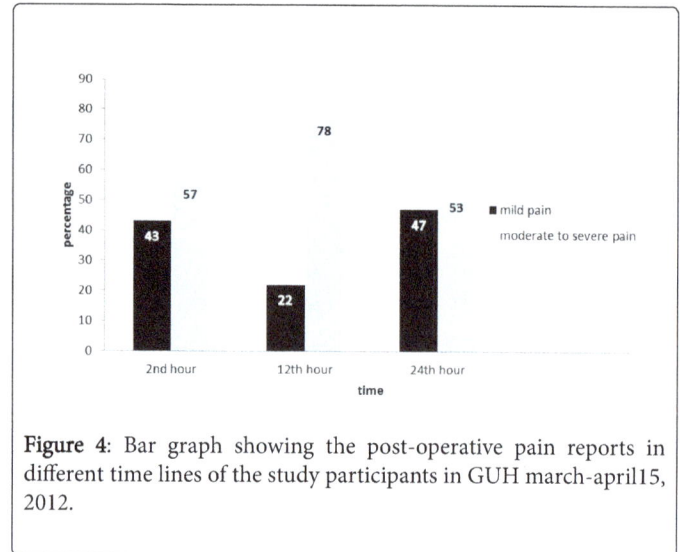

Figure 4: Bar graph showing the post-operative pain reports in different time lines of the study participants in GUH march-april15, 2012.

Univariate and multivariate analyses were carried out using the Statistical Package for the Social Sciences16 for windows. In order to control potential confounding variables, and to determine the independent association between postoperative pain and potential predictors of pain, the chi square test was employed for potential association and logistic regression was employed.

The following variables were found to have an association with moderate to severe pain post operatively.

Age OR (2.642) P (0.042) was found to show significant association with pain in the immediate post-operative period, sex with an OR (2.580) P(0.005), ASA OR (4.0) P (0.013), incision length of greater than 10 cm was another factor for causing moderate to severe post-operative pain OR (1.991) P (0.041), and type of anesthesia OR (5.562) P(0.000) (Table 3).

Variable	No or mild pain (n=150)	Moderate to severe pain (n=150)	P value	Odds ratio	95% CI
Age					
<59	51	77	0.042	2.642	(1.034-6.750)
>60	14	8			
Sex					
Male	38	30	0.005	2.58	(1.328-5.014)
Female	27	55			

ASA					
I & II	52	80	0.013	4	(1.346-11.88)
III & IV	13	15			
Incision length					
<10 cm	33	29	0.041	1.991	(1.028-3.858)
>10 cm	37	56			
Type of surgery					
Intraabdominal & Head and neck	35	61	0.025	2.179	(1.105-4.295)
Urogenital & Musculoskeletal	30	24			
Type of anesthesia					
General anesthesia	31	71	0	5.562	(2.62-11.7)
Spinal and nerve block	34	14			
Previous acute or chronic painful experiences					
Yes	23	21	0.156	1.669	(0.822-3.388)
No	42	64			
Analgesic before emergence					
Diclofenac	18	22	0.771	0.978	(0.845-1.133)
Paracetamol	1	1			
Pethidine	2	9			
Morphine	1	1			
Tramadol	2	2			
None	41	50			

Table 3: Pain severity, p value and odds ratio at the 2nd post-operative hour of the study participants in GUH march-April 15, 2012.

No significant association was found between BMI, preoperative visit, history of surgery and anesthesia, trauma history, maintenance drug surgical and anesthesia time, and whether nerve block was done or not (which were only 2 in number).

Discussion

The purpose of this study was to find out the severity of post-operative pain and to establish a relationship between the demographic, preoperative/preclinical and intraoperative factors as predictors of post-operative pain severity.

The main finding of this research is that moderate to severe pain was reported in 57% of cases 2 h after end of surgery and 78% in the first 12 hour. Despite the introduction of new standards, guidelines, and educational efforts, data from around the world suggest that postoperative pain continues to be undermanaged. Researchers agree that post-operative pain is still uncontrolled and plays a major role in the outcome of surgery. In agreement with our finding several researchers have found a 20–80% prevalence of moderate to extreme pain in post-operative patients [8]. Our observation was supported by a Meta-analysis which shows that overall, current practice standards have had minimal impact on decreasing patients' account of pain and the incidence of moderate to severe pain, and that surgical specialties such as cardiac, abdominal, and orthopaedic inpatient procedures has been reported as high as 25% to 50%, and even the incidence of moderate/severe pain after ambulatory procedures is 25% or higher [18].

In agreement with our finding a research done in Nigeria on 200 adult patients who presented for a variety of surgical procedures found out 68% of patients experienced moderate to severe post-operative pain, while the remaining 32% complained of only mild pain [9]. This is no surprise in Africa. A 5 year survey on a random sample of 250 adults who had undergone surgical procedures in the United States showed that approximately 80% of patients experienced acute pain after surgery. Of these patients, 86% had moderate, severe, or extreme pain. Experiencing postoperative pain was the most common concern in 59% of patients [19].

In Netherlands a study done to find out The prevalence of postoperative pain in 1490 surgical in patients who were receiving postoperative pain treatment according to an acute pain protocol found out that 41% of the patients on day 0 and 30% on day 1 experienced moderate to severe pain. the fact that they were in acute pain treatment and still experiencing pain shows that we need to do a lot more to avoid post-operative pain [20].

Whatever the predictors or factors involved researchers widely agree that under treatment of acute pain is an important issue in health care. Although difficult to find researches done in Africa, In the USA alone researches have estimated that only one in four surgical patients received adequate relief of acute post-operative pain [21]. One possibility to support this outcome is the wide spread patient dissatisfaction with post-operative analgesia protocols, studies show that Patients routinely receive less analgesia postoperatively than they require and nurses tend to underestimate the amount of analgesia needed [22]. Nurses usually are remiss in using pain rating scores to assess analgesia needs, a research in Sweden showed that nearly half of nurses do not use a pain rating score for assessing pain in surgical ward [23]. Our research finding shows large proportion of patients (78%) have encountered more severe pain at the 12th hour, (which is when they are usually transferred from the recovery to their respective wards) than they had in the recovery room. This implies that the pain management and follow up of patients in the wards might be poor. Some of the restricting factors might be the "absence of pain assessment and documentation practices, absence of specific written postoperative pain protocols, deficiencies in educational pain management programmes, absence of effective analgesic techniques (e.g., epidural analgesia and peripheral nerve catheters)" and if there are any; poor adherence to available guidelines [24-26].

Another finding was that "the younger the more painful", those <60 are 2 times more likely to report moderate to severe pain than the elders. Research done in Spain for predictors of post-operative pain in abdominal procedures also puts age (OR=4.72) as a major factor [8]. This might be attributed to reduction of peripheral nociceptive function which in other words means that older people experience less pain [27]. This goes in accordance with other research which also suggests that older people require less analgesia than younger for post-operative pain management [28].

The research found out that Gender was another predictive factor in the 1st 12 h postop with an OR (2.5) P (0.05). 55 (67%) of females reported moderate to severe pain compared with 30 (44%) of males. Gender-related differences in pain have been clearly shown in experimental settings. A study done in Germany on independent risk factors for postoperative pain verifies our findings: females are 1.9 times more likely to encounter severe pain post operatively than males [26], actually studies show women are more likely than men to experience a variety of recurrent pains. "Many women have moderate or severe pains from menstruation, pregnancy and childbirth. In most studies, women report more severe levels of pain, more frequent pain and pain of longer duration than do men. Women may be at greater risk for pain-related disability than men", but women also respond more aggressively to pain treatments [29]. A study has shown that females have much lower requirements for analgesia than males [30]; another study also supports this idea in that similar doses of analgesics will have the same or greater responses in females than males [31]. Gender is also a major factor in "pain perception with females typically reporting more negative responses to pain than males" [32]. One research suggests that psychosocial factors such as "sex role beliefs, pain coping strategies, mood, and pain-related expectancies may

expose females to exhibit greater sensitivity to noxious stimuli than men" [33].

Surgical incision was another major determinant of post-operative pain severity in the first 12 hours after surgery p value (0.041). In the 2nd hour of post-operative period 56 (64%) of patients with surgical incision length longer than 10 cm reported that they experienced moderate to severe pain when compared to 29 (46%) of patients with incision less than 10 cm. In accordance with our research finding a large incision together with other factors was found to be a predictive factor [34]. But one research shows that depending on surgeons experience and setup, incision length might not have any impact on post-operative outcome [35].

Our study showed that patients who had general anesthesia had a higher incidence of developing post-operative pain. Of the 102 (68%) of patients who had general anesthesia, in the second hour postoperatively, 71 (70%) of the patients (compared with 14(29%) of spinal patients) with an OR of 5.5 reported that they are experiencing moderate to severe pain. The best argument could be that spinal anesthesia has better post-operative analgesia than GA as it lasts for several hours postoperatively, but one big result is that 41 (85%) of the spinal patients reported moderate to severe pain at the 12th hour mark in relation to 76 (75%) patients in the GA group. This finding actually shows that there is an underestimation of analgesic requirement in patients who undergo surgery with neuraxial blockade in the wards. Some researchers agree that spinal anesthesia is superior in decreasing pain intensity of constant incisional pain and movement-associated incisional pain [36], but other studies results support our observation in that general anesthesia with an odds ratio of 3.96 is a significant risk factor for developing POP [16].

At the start of the study we hypothesized that those patients with a poor physical status might encounter more pain than those with a good physical status but in contrary our findings showed that those with poor physical status reported 4 times less severe pain than those with a good physical status P (0.013). This statistical result might be subject to bias in that there were 7 times more patients in the ASA I, II group than the ASA III, IV group. Researchers have a contradictory results with this aspect in that one study showed that Moderate to intense acute postoperative pain was associated with ASA III (odds ratio (OR) 1.99) [18]. While other study supports our finding in that ASA I and II patients have much more complaints of severe pain than do ASA III and IV [26].

The researcher was bound by budget and time to apply probability sampling and minimum sample size of 220, our sample size 150 from statistical point of view is few. So the research is not applicable to the larger population except for the hospital where the research is done. The data collectors were forced to collect some of the data retrospectively as it was very difficult to track down patients at the exact time of the data collection like midnight. Many of the patients included were elective schedules, which explain the lack of patients with poor physical status. The researcher believes that this might undermine or shift the severity of the outcome variable. The poor documentation system was another challenge in that it was difficult or unreliable to analyze factors such as preoperative and preinduction premedication as there was no documentation on patients chart even when the drug was given. The strengths of this study might be that this research was the first of its kind paving way for further study on the subject. And also we used the numeric rating scale which in studies proved to be the best way of documenting pain intensity.

Determining the severity and risk factors involved in postoperative pain is one way of contributing to the evaluation of health care setting in the hospital and as a Nation at large. In the present study we showed that majority of patients experienced moderate to severe pain in the first 12 h post operatively, which actually shows that the analgesic treatment and pain control are inadequate both in the recovery and the wards. We also showed that several perioperative factors have contributed to this outcome. The results from this study are even more relevant in that pain is the most important determinant factor in patient's surgical outcome.

As the research findings show that there are a large proportion of patients with acute post-operative pain. Controlling post-operative pain paves the way to avoiding complications and lessening time patients take to recover and leave from hospital, therefore decreasing any expenditure the government and the hospital has to spend. Although knowing perioperative factors for severe pain is important the researcher believes that a further study needs to focus on developing guidelines and pain services in the postoperative period.

References

1. Harvey AM (1995) Classification of Chronic Pain-Descriptions of Chronic Pain Syndromes and Definitions of Pain Terms. Clin J Pain 11: 163.

2. Carr DB, Goudas LC (1999) Acute pain. Lancet 353: 2051-2058.

3. [No authors listed] (1995) Practice guidelines for acute pain management in the perioperative setting. A report by the American Society of Anesthesiologists Task Force on Pain Management, Acute Pain Section. Anesthesiology 82: 1071-1081.

4. Twersky R, Fishman D, Homel P (1997) What happens after discharge? Return hospital visits after ambulatory surgery. Anesth Analg 84: 319-324.

5. Biluts H, Bekele A, Kottiso B, Enqueselassie F, Munie T (2009) In-patient surgical mortality in Tikur Anbessa Hospital: a five-year review. Ethiop Med J 47: 135-142.

6. [Authors not listed] (2003) Fast stats. National Center for Health Statistics Web site.

7. Fletcher D, Pogatzki-Zahn E, Zaslansky R, Meissner W (2011) Pain Out Group euCPSP: European observational study on chronic post-surgical pain. Eur J Anaesthesiol 28: 461-462.

8. Caumo W, Schmidt AP, Schneider CN, Bergmann J, Iwamoto CW, et al. (2002) Preoperative predictors of moderate to intense acute postoperative pain in patients undergoing abdominal surgery. Acta Anaesthsiol Scand 46: 1265-1271.

9. Famewo CE (1985) Study of incidence of post-operative pain among Nigerian patients. Afr J Med Med Sci 14: 175-179.

10. Liu SS, Wu CL (2007) Effect of postoperative analgesia on major postoperative complications: a systematic update of the evidence. Anesth Analg 104: 689-702.

11. Crombie IK, Davies HT, Macrae WA (1998) Cut and thrust: antecedent surgery and trauma among patients attending a chronic pain clinic. Pain 76: 167-171.

12. Perkins FM, Kehlet H (2000) Chronic pain as an outcome of surgery. A review of predictive factors. Anesthesiology 93: 1123-1133.

13. Lucille Bartholomeusz (2006) Safe anesthesia. (3rdedn). 611.

14. Kehlet H, Jensen TS, Woolf CJ (2006) Persistent postsurgical pain: risk factors and prevention. Lancet 367: 1618-1625.

15. Thomas T, Robinson C, Champion D, McKell M, Pell M (1998) Prediction and assessment of the severity of post-operative pain and of satisfaction with management. Pain 75: 177-185.

16. Aubrun F, Valade N, Coriat P, Riou B (2008) Predictive factors of severe postoperative pain in the postanesthesia care unit. Anesth Analg 106: 1535-1541.

17. [Authors not listed] (2012) The British Pain Society frequently asked questions.

18. Huang N, Cunningham F, Laurito CE, Chen C (2001) Can we do better with postoperative pain management? Am J Surg 182: 440-448.

19. McGoldrick KE (2004) Postoperative pain experience: Results from a national survey suggest postoperative pain continues to be undermanaged. Survey of Anesthesiology 48: 47-48.

20. Sommer M, de Rijke JM, van Kleef M, Kessels AG, Peters ML, et al. (2008) The prevalence of postoperative pain in a sample of 1490 surgical inpatients. Eur J Anaesthesiol 25: 267-274.

21. Wu CL, Raja SN (2011) Treatment of acute postoperative pain. Lancet 377: 2215-2225.

22. Salmon P, Manyande A (1996) Good patients cope with their pain: postoperative analgesia and nurses' perceptions of their patients' pain. Pain 68: 63-68.

23. Ene KW, Nordberg G, Bergh I, Johansson FG, Sjöström B (2008) Postoperative pain management - the influence of surgical ward nurses. J Clin Nurs 17: 2042-2050.

24. Benhamou D, Berti M, Brodner G, De Andres J, Draisci G (2008) Postoperative Analgesic THerapy Observational Survey (PATHOS): a practice pattern study in 7 central/southern European countries. Pain 136: 134-141.

25. Block BM, Liu SS, Rowlingson AJ, Cowan AR, Cowan JA Jr, et al. (2003) Efficacy of postoperative epidural analgesia: a meta-analysis. JAMA 290: 2455-2463.

26. Mei W, Seeling M, Franck M, Radtke F, Brantner B, et al. (2010) Independent risk factors for postoperative pain in need of intervention early after awakening from general anaesthesia. Eur J Pain 14: 149.

27. Perry F, Parker RK, White PF, Clifford PA (1994) Role of psychological factors in postoperative pain control and recovery with patient-controlled analgesia. Clin J Pain 10: 57-63.

28. Macintyre PE, Jarvis DA (1996) Age is the best predictor of postoperative morphine requirements. Pain 64: 357-364.

29. Unruh AM (1996) Gender variations in clinical pain experience. Pain 65: 123-167.

30. Chia YY, Chow LH, Hung CC, Liu K, Ger LP, et al. (2002) Gender and pain upon movement are associated with the requirements for postoperative patient-controllediv analgesia: a prospective survey of 2,298 Chinese patients. Can J Anesth 49: 249-255.

31. Gear RW, Miaskowski C, Gordon NC, Paul SM, Heller PH (1999) The kappa opioid nalbuphine produces gender-and dose-dependent analgesia and antianalgesia in patients with postoperative pain. Pain 83: 339-345.

32. Keogh E, Herdenfeldt M (2002) Gender, coping and the perception of pain. Pain 97: 195-201.

33. Fillingim RB (2000) Sex, gender, and pain: women and men really are different. Curr Rev Pain 4: 24-30.

34. Kalkman CJ, Visser K, Moen J, Bonsel GJ, Grobbee DE, et al. (2003) Preoperative prediction of severe postoperative pain. Pain 105: 415-423.

35. Ogonda L, Wilson R, Archbold P, Lawlor M, Humphreys P, et al. (2005) A minimal-incision technique in total hip arthroplasty does not improve early postoperative outcomes. A prospective, randomized, controlled trial. J Bone Joint Surg Am 87: 701-710.

36. Tverskoy M, Cozacov C, Ayache M, Bradley Jr EL, Kissin I et al. (1990) Postoperative pain after inguinal herniorrhaphy with different types of anesthesia. Anesth Analg 70: 29-35.

21

Specific Prevention Against Infection of Local Catheters in Postoperative Pain Management

Annekathrin Hausmann and Rupert Schupfner[*]

Surgery II, Klinikum Bayreuth, Germany

[*]**Corresponding author:** Rupert Schupfner, Surgery II, Klinikum Bayreuth, Germany, E-mail: rupert.schupfner@klinikum-bayreuth.de

Abstract

Background: The guideline for postoperative pain management therapy recommends several obligate measures and permissive provisions keeping catheters hygienic. An organized Pain Nurse is generally regarded as convenient. But some recommendations are still discussed. The guideline is based on only few large studies and the number of catheter-related infections differs from technique and risk profile. However, all recommendations for improvement have to be compared with the guideline. This prospective study was initiated to investigate the influence of catheter fixing, the frequency of changing dressings and the use of bacterium-filters on the rate of inflammation and infection.

Methods: 2545 consecutive patients, who were under treatment of the Pain Nurse, were included in the study. 1624 patients received epidural catheters, 921 patients received continuous peripheral nerve blocks. The catheters were immediately placed and fixed by stitching before performing the operation. A bacterium-filter was always interposed and after some time a second filter was added in tandem circuit. After 4 days the transparent tape was changed. The assessment of the infection severity was oriented towards the criteria of the guideline. The results of the study were statistically compared to the data of the S3-guideline.

Results: 34 (14.4%) of all catheters in the sample were colonized. Catheters placed in the groin were statistically significant more often colonized than epidural catheters (28.1% *vs.* 6.6%, p<0.01). 5 Catheters (0.2% *vs.* 4.2%, p<0.01) had signs of local inflammation. Only one fairly serious infection (placement in the groin) (0.04% *vs.* 2.4% p<0.01) and no severe infection were observed.

Conclusion: Catheter-fixing by stitching and changing catheter-dressing on the first postoperative day to avoid dampness are important measures to prevent catheter related infections. Using consequently bacterium-filters with tandem circuit is supposed to reduce the rate of catheter-related inflammations and infections.

Keywords: Hygiene catheter infection colonization bacterium-filter; Postoperative pain

Introduction

Local catheters in postoperative pain management are progressively popular in anesthesia. However, there is an incertitude concerning the implementation of hygienic measures for prevention against infection. Up till now there is no standardized hygiene policy especially for regional anesthesia catheters so far. Although hygiene deficits could lead to severe consequences for the patient, studies which consider prevention of infection in the context of local catheters in postoperative pain management are rarely.

Background

Peripheral nerve blocks are predicated as safe and highly effective in acute pain management. Specifically, in orthopedic surgeries, the patient benefits from early mobilization [1]. There are only rare severe incidents of pain catheters. But these events may have serious and in some cases life changing impacts (e. g. Mediastinitis [2], necrotizing fasciitis [3]).

Although local anesthesia catheters are frequently deployed in postoperative pain management, there is an incertitude concerning the implementation of hygienic measures for prevention against infection.

Many hygiene precepts for central venous catheters have been adapted analogously to regional anesthesia [4]. A standardized hygiene policy especially for local anesthesia catheters does not exist yet. There are many studies concerning hygienic rules for central venous catheters, but only few studies consider anesthesia catheters in postoperative pain management. It must be remembered that there could exist differences between a venous catheter and a nervous pain catheter. However, an organized pain nurse is regarded as favourable to reduce overlooked catheter infections [5].

The S3 guideline on postoperative pain management, currently being revised, recommends hygienic basic and "optional" measures regarding the management of local anesthesia catheters. Nevertheless, a significant range of variation in the recommendations for action as well as in the infection rate can be observed between the individual centers [6-9]. The scientific working group "Local Anesthesia" assumes that "prevention measures have not been used in the highest possible extent in all centers" [4].

Methods

Definitions and pathophysiology of catheter colonization

The S3 guideline on the "treatment of acute perioperative and posttraumatic pain" describes the following alternatives of catheter colonization (Figure 1).

It is important to differentiate between the terms contamination, colonization and infection (Table 1).

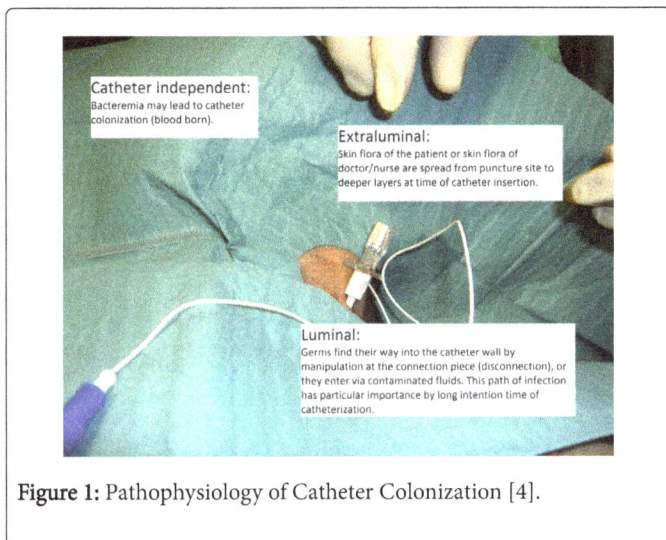

Figure 1: Pathophysiology of Catheter Colonization [4].

Open questions in hygiene management

There are only few and often several opinions concerning bandaging techniques, frequency of changing dressings, fixing catheters securely and the management of bacteria filters. Therefore, a prospective study should evaluate all these mentioned aspects in relation to occurrence, frequency and severity of infections.

Study design and test methods

The observational study lasted three years (January 1st, 2010-January 1st, 2013) and is part of the multicentric, interdisciplinary benchmark project: "Quality Control in Postoperative Pain Management" (QCPOPM).

Contamination	Colonization	Infection
Germ count <15 colony-forming units (CFU)	Germ count > 15 CFU without clinical signs of infection	Slight: flush, swelling, tenderness on palpation (two criteria at least)
		Moderately severe: purulence at puncture site, increasing inflammation parameters, temperature, required systemic antibiotic therapy (two criteria at least)
		Severe: surgical intervention required (abscess incision)

Table 1: Definitions.

An affirmative vote by the ethical review committee of Jena University Hospital is available.

The study included 2,545 consecutive patients undergoing regional anesthesia of the Klink Bayreuth. 1,624 patients had local catheters inserted close to the spinal cord, 921 patients received peripheral nerve blocks. The catheter was inserted immediately preoperative, following a standardized operating procedure (SOP) (Table 2).

The severity of infection was categorized according to the S3 guideline criteria and compared with literature incidence. There are already some well proposed studies in literature, which formed the S3 guideline.

In the following study, we eschewed attentively the control group, but matched the studies in literature of the S3 guideline (control group) against our clinical SOP group (intervention group).

The intervention is shown in Table 2. You can find three interventions regarding the bacteria filter management, dressing and fixing. These three interventions distinguish the clinical SOP group from the control group.

The study design was apart from that similar to the studies in literature (control group). The high significant lower infection rates in our study didn't allow installing a control group afterwards. It wouldn't be ethical to refuse the control group the sensationally effective hygienic procedures.

Hygiene plan
Insertion of the catheter in the preparation room.
Number of persons limited to the required minimum.
No wearing of watches or jewelry.
No routine shaving. Haired body sites are getting shaved immediately before the puncture.
No routine degreasing and cleansing of the skin; cleansing only in the case of visible contamination.
Hand disinfection according to the standards of the Robert Koch Institute.
Skin disinfection: centrifugal spray-and-wipe-and-spray disinfection with alcohol-based disinfectant and an exposure time of 1-10 minutes. Excess disinfectant absorbed by sterile compress immediately before the procedure.
Surgical mask, headgear, sterile gown.
Medical cover sheeting: large self-adhesive fenestrated drapes and spacious sterile work surfaces in order to avoid contaminations.

Medications and material: standards of the DGAI (German Society for Anesthesiology and Intensive-care Medicine) were observed.		

Bacteria filter management: By inserting the catheter, a bacteria filter is interposed. After a defined time interval an additional filter is added in tandem circuit. (epidural catheter: 48 hours, peripheral nerve blocks: 96 hours). The second filter is replaced regularly, while the first filter remains until removal of the catheter.

S3 guideline: A bacteria filter should be included, but you should abdicate a filter changing.

Dressing: Puncture site is covered with Curapor® Band-Aid, which will be exchanged with a transparent dressing after 24 hours. Renewal of the dressing after 4 days.

S3 guideline: Changing dressings only if it is unavoidable.

Fixing: After the puncture, the catheter is fixed by stitching and additionally by pasting.

S3 guideline: The catheter has to be fixed safely by pasting.

Daily supervision by the pain nurse.

Indication is verified every day.

Table 2: SOP of hygiene practices (Differences between the recommendations of the S3 guideline and the own clinical SOP is marked. 3 Interventions were different from the S3 guideline: Bacteria filter management, dressing and fixing)).

Data analysis

Incidents were indicated as numerical value with related population. In order to gain comparability, results were converted into percentage frequencies with their 95% confidence intervals. The own examination was defined as study group, the underlying works of the S3 guideline served as control group. Statistical comparisons were performed employing the Chi^2 test, using bilateral testing. Clinical significance was defined at $p<0.05$.

Results

Duration of catheterization

The mean duration of catheterization by thoracic epidural catheters lasted 5.4 days and by lumbar epidural catheters 1.8 days. The duration on the average of catheterization by femoral catheters took 5 days, while the catheters for the ischia nerve remained for 3.3 days and the catheters for the Interskalenar plexus blockade were left for 3.5 days.

Rate of colonization and infection

34 catheters (14.4%) of a random sample (236) were colonized. Femoral catheters were colonized more frequently than epidural catheters (28.1% vs. 6.6%, p<0.01). A coagulase negative staphylococcus, that means a germ of the normal skin flora, was the most frequent germ in the sample.

Slight infections (flush) occurred in 5 patients (0.2% vs. 4.2%, p<0.01), a single moderately severe infection was observed in a femoral catheter (0.04% vs. 2.4% p<0.01). No severe infections were observed.

Rate of colonization and infections in the patients were shown by following Tables 3,4,5 and 6.

	Own study (n)	Own study (%)	Morin (n)	Morin (%)	Capdevila (n)	Capdevila (%)
No colonization	202	85.6%	151	76.3%	691	71.3%
Colonization	34	14.4%	47	23.7%	278	28.7%
Divided						
One pathogen per catheter	24	70.6%	31	66.0%	242	87.1%
Two or more pathogens per catheter	10	29.4%	16	34.0%	36	12.9%
Pathogen total	45	100.0%	66	100.0%	310	100%
Normal skin microbiota						
Coagulase-neg. Staphylococcen	25	55.6%	40	60.4%	195	62.9%
Bacillus spezies	2	4.4%	9	13.6%		
Enterococcus spezies	6	13.3%	3	4.5%	21	6.8%
Facultative pathogen						
Bacillus cereus (gram positive)	4	8.9%	0	0.0%	4	1.3%

Escherichia coli	0	0.0%	5	7.8%	15	4.8%
Enterobacter spezies	1	2.0%	3	4.5%	11	3.5%
Klebsiella spezies	3	6.7%	3	4.5%	8	2.6%
Morganella morganii	1	2.0%	1	1.5%		
Nonfermenter spezies	0	0.0%	1	1.5%		
Pseudomonas aeroginosa	1	2.0%	1	1.5%	9	2.9%
Acinetobacter	0	0.0%	0	0.0%	7	2.3%
Proteus mirabilis	1	2.0%	0	0.0%	8	2.6%
Citrobacter	1	2.0%	0	0.0%	4	1.3%
Serratia	0	0.0%	0	0.0%	3	1.0%
Staphylococcus aureus	0	0.0%	0	0.0%	15	4.8%
others	0	0.0%	0	0.0%	10	3.2%
N=236						

Table 3: Comparison between the colonization rates in the own study and the control groups of the S3 guideline:

	Colonization (%)	95% VB	Chi²	Significance level	OR
Own study	14.4	[10.19-19.54]			
Morin	23.7	[17.99-30.28]	4.92	p<0.05	1.8
Capdevila	28.7	[25.86-31.65]	11.96	p<0.01	2.4

Table 4: Evaluation of the comparison between the colonization rates in the own study and the control groups of the S3 guideline.

	Colonization (%)	95% VB	Chi²	Significance level	OR
Epidural catheter	6.6	[3.07-12.19]			
Femoral catheter	28.1	[17.58-40.75]	12.18	p<0.01	5.5

Table 5: Evaluation of the comparison between the colonization rates of epidural catheters and femoral catheters in the own study.

	Slight infection (%)	95% VB	Chi²	Significance level	OR
Own study	0.2	[0.06-0.46]	95.6	p<0.01	22.1
Neuburger 2006	4.2	[3.54-4.90]			
	Moderate severe infection (%)	**95% VB**	**Chi²**	**Significance level**	**OR**
Own study	0.04	[0.01-0.22]	58,6	p<0.01	62
Neuburger 2006	2.4	[1.90-2.94]			
	Severe infection (%)	**95% VB**	**Chi²**	**Significance level**	**OR**
Own study	0				
Neuburger 2006	0.8	[0.56-1.20]			

Table 6: Evaluation and comparison between infection rate in the own study and the control group in the S3 guideline.

Discussion

As compared to literature, the present study shows a very low infection rate (Figure 2).

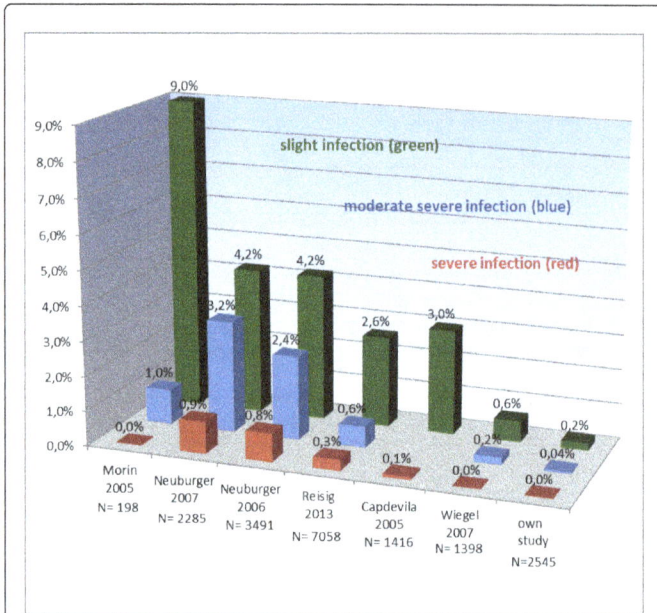

Figure 2: Frequency of infections in comparison with literature [4,6-10].

We observed a colonization rate of 14.4%. The contamination of coagulase-negative staphylococci (55.6%) was most frequent. These results confirm the observations of the control studies by Morin [11] and Capdevila [6]. Clinical signs of slight infections were observed in only 0.2% of catheterizations (Figure 3).

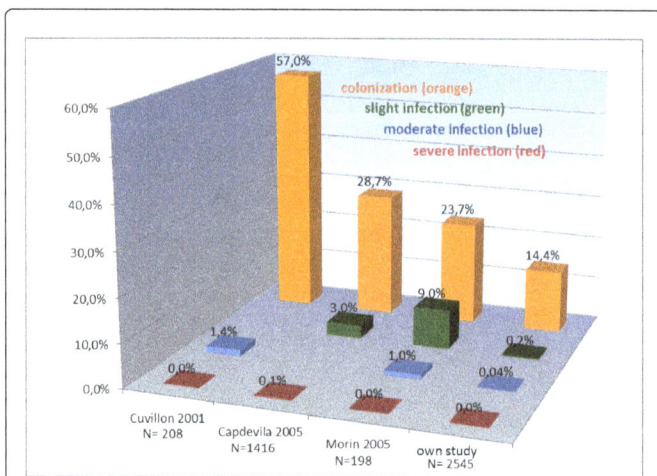

Figure 3: Colonization rate and frequency of infections in different studies [6,11,12].

Safe catheter fixing

"Catheter and connectors must be fixed safely" [4]. In the S3 guideline, it is recommended to paste the catheter with connector and plugged in filter tightly on to the skin [4]. But sole pasting with Tagaderm® can't be the best fixing of catheters, because a study, which considered the problem of well fixing catheters of pain management, showed a migration of catheters after only two days [13].

Safe catheter fixing will minimize the risk of flaw in catheters with following colonization and infection, especially if we have to change strappings frequently. Stitching the catheter for fixing is considered as satisfactory, especially if the catheter is left for less than four days [14]. An Increasing appearance of infections caused by stitching the catheter was not be observed in our own study. Conformable to the study of Bormann [15], an atraumatic insertion of the catheter and fixing the catheter by stitching is postulated to prevent infection.

Bacteria filter management

The "optional" advices of the DGAI recommend the application of a bacteria filter, "though a filter change should not be performed routinely" [4]. Studies showed that a frequent filter change increases the colonization of catheters with skin pathogens [16]. But most manufacturers claim a change of the filter after 24-72 hours. In our study, we had to face the quandary.

The DGAI recommendation does not insist of using a bacteria filter, while reducing colonization is not evidenced by documents [4]. Capdevila and associates [6] consider a bacteria filter only necessary if the catheter is left for long-term. But a Japanese study recommends already the use of microbial filters from 24 hours resting the catheter [17].

In our study, bacteria filters were always used for all the catheters in postoperative pain management. Furthermore, we educed a special bacteria filter management to guarantee the manufacturer's warranty. After a period of time (Epidural catheter: 48 hours, peripheral nerve block: 96 hours), an additional bacteria filter was added in tandem circuit. Here, we had to pay attention not to interrupt the continuity of the preoperatively added microbial filter to the catheter. A closed system was minded and the caution of De Cicco et al. was observed [16]. The second filter of the tandem circuit was changed regularly (Epidural catheter: after 48 hours, peripheral nerve block after 96 hours), while remaining the first filter in place until the catheter was removed. In case of disconnecting accidentally the first bacteria filter of the tandem circuit, the catheter was removed if possible. If it was not possible to remove the catheter, the catheter was disinfected thoroughly with an alcohol-containing antiseptic and dried according to a recommendation by Langevin [18]. Thus the proximal catheter end was cut off with a sterile instrument and then reconnected.

Dressing management

The S3 guideline [19] says: "It is assumed but not ensured that there is a positive correlation of incidence of infections with duration of catheterization, the frequency of dressing changes and catheter disconnections as well as dependence of the localization of the catheter insertion site (interskalenar, groin, caudal region)". Thus, the scientific working group "Local Anesthesia" recommends only changing strappings if it is absolutely essential. Therefore, they say: "Dressing remains as long as possible, the first dressing is the 'most abacterial'!" [4].

In Morin's study (the control group of our study) [11], three risk factors were statistically significant:

- placement in the groin,

- repetitive dressing changes and
- absence of a postoperative antibiotic prophylaxis

These risk factors, showed in our control group, were indeed associated with an increased infection rate, but they were not necessarily observed in every case of infection during Morin's study. We assume that not changing dressings by itself caused the high infection rate in the study of Morin and fellows, but the reason why. So could have leaded the reason why it was necessary to change the dressing to more bacterial growth, for example a moisture penetration of the strapping with blood or the patient's heavy perspiration. These could be the "real" risk factors [11]. To avoid a moisture penetration of the dressing we changed the strapping frequently (Table 2). It must be remembered that the most frequent germ in the colonization sample was a coagulase negative staphylococcus, a germ of the normal skin flora. We hypothesize that the significant lower infection rates in our study are due to the specific dressing management. Furthermore, we detected a higher colonization rate in femoral catheters and confirm the risk factor "location in the groin". The patient's perspiration could be the reason for this risk factor.

Conclusion for Clinical Practice

A standardized hygiene plan is necessary to minimize the risk of catheter-related infections. We conclude, that stitching the catheter for safety fixing and changing dressings on the first postoperative day in order to avoid a moisture penetration of the strapping reduce infections significantly. We recommend a strict postoperative dressing management performed by a pain nurse. Furthermore, we favor using microbial filters independent of the catheter's resting time. A special postoperative bacteria filter management (tandem circuit) with the second microbial filter being changed after a fixed period of time is profitable to reduce infections.

Adherence to Ethical Guidelines

All examinations on humans described were carried out upon approval by the responsible ethical review committee, in accordance with national legislation and according to the Declaration of Helsinki in 1975 (in the current, revised version). Informed consents of all patients involved are available.

References

1. Pogatzki-Zahn EM, Zahn PK, Brennan TJ (2007) Postoperative pain-clinical implications of basic research. Best practice & research. Clinical anaesthesiology 2: 3-13.
2. Capdevila X, Jaber S, Pesonen P, Borgeat A, Eledjam JJ (2008) Acute neck cellulitis and mediastinitis complicating a continuous interscalene block. Anesthesia and analgesia 107: 1419-1421.
3. Nseir S, Pronnier P, Soubrier S, Onimus T, Saulnier F, et al. (2004) Fatal streptococcal necrotizing fasciitis as a complication of axillary brachial plexus block. British journal of anaesthesia 92: 427-429.
4. Kerwat K, Wulf H, Morin A (2010) Hygiene standards for spinal anaesthesia. Anästhesiologie Intensivmedizin Notfallmedizin Schmerztherapie. AINS 45: 196-198.
5. Erlenwein J, Stüder D, Lange J, Bauer M, Petzke F, et al. (2012) Process optimization by central control of acute pain therapy: implementation of standardized treatment concepts and central pain management in hospitals. Anaesthesist 61: 971-983.
6. Capdevila X, Pirat P, Bringuier S, Gaertner E, Singelyn F, et al. (2005) Continuous peripheral nerve blocks in hospital wards after orthopedic surgery: a multicenter prospective analysis of the quality of postoperative analgesia and complications in 1,416 patients. Anesthesiology 103: 1035-1045.
7. Neuburger M, Breitbarth J, Reisig F, Lang D, Büttner J (2006) Complications and adverse events in continuous peripheral regional anesthesia Results of investigations on 3,491 catheters. Der Anaesthesist 55: 33-40.
8. Neuburger M, Büttner J, Blumenthal S, Breitbarth J, Borgeat A (2007) Inflammation and infection complications of 2285 perineural catheters: a prospective study. Acta anaesthesiologica Scandinavica 51: 108-114.
9. Wiegel M, Gottschaldt U, Hennebach R, Hirschberg T, Reske A (2007) Complications and adverse effects associated with continuous peripheral nerve blocks in orthopedic patients. Anesth Analg 104: 1578-1582.
10. Reisig F, Neuburger M, Zausig YA, Graf BM, Büttner J (2013) Successful infection control in regional anesthesia procedures: observational survey after introduction of the DGAI hygiene recommendations. Anaesthesist 62: 105-112.
11. Morin AM, Kerwat KM, Klotz M, Niestolik R, Ruf VE, et al. (2005) Risk factors for bacterial catheter colonization in regional anaesthesia. BMC anesthesiology 5:1.
12. Cuvillon P, Ripart J, Lalourcey L, Veyrat E, L'Hermite J, et al. (2001) The continuous femoral nerve block catheter for postoperative analgesia: bacterial colonization, infectious rate and adverse effects. Anesthesia and analgesia 93: 1045-1049.
13. Hoshi T, Tanaka M (2011) Fixation of the epidural catheter using Tegaderm. Masui. The Japanese journal of anesthesiology 60: 876-879.
14. Gastmeier P, Behnke M, Reichardt C (2004) Entwicklung einer web-basierten Datenbank für nosokomiale Ausbrüche (outbreak-Register): German Medical Science; Düsseldorf, Köln.
15. Von Bormann B, Suksompong S, Weiler J, Zander R (2014) Pure oxygen ventilation during general anaesthesia does not result in increased postoperative respiratory morbidity but decreases surgical site infection. An observational clinical study. PeerJ 2: e613.
16. De Cicco M, Matovic M, Castellani GT, Basaglia G, Santini G, et al. (1995) Time-dependent efficacy of bacterial filters and infection risk in long-term epidural catheterization. Anesthesiology 82: 765-771.
17. Haraga I, Shono S, Abe S, Higa K (2010) Aseptic precautions in epidural catheterization for surgery. Masui. The Japanese journal of anesthesiology 59: 585-588.
18. Langevin PB (2000) How should we handle epidural solutions? One view. Regional anesthesia and pain medicine 25: 343-346.
19. Laubenthal H (2008) S3-Leitlinie Behandlung akuter perioperativer und posttraumatischer Schmerzen. Köln: Dt. Ärzte-Verl,. XXXIII, 319 S. ISBN: 3-7691-0583-4.

22

SpO$_2$ and Pulse Rate Data: A Comparison of Current Technologies during Sustained Shivering in Post-Operative Patients

Kelley Dixon[*], **Austin Broussard, Mellisa Roskosky and Michael Shuler**

Athens Orthopedic Clinic, Athens, Georgia, USA

[*]**Corresponding author:** Kelley Dixon, Athens Orthopedic Clinic, 1765 Old West Broad St, Building 2, Suite 300, Athens, GA 30606, USA, E-mail: Kelley.nirs@gmail.com

Abstract

Pulse oximetry is a noninvasive method of measuring the oxygen saturation (SpO$_2$) of the arterial blood and is considered standard-of-care in post-operative settings. Patient motion or low perfusion can present challenges in obtaining accurate readings. Postoperative shivering occurs in anywhere from 5-65% of patients who have received general anesthesia and can manifest as continuous tremors and/or sporadic muscle movements.

Objective: Compare the effect of post-operative shivering on functioning capabilities of two commercially available pulse oximeters.

Methods: Two additional pulse oximeter sensors (Nonin 7500 Pulse Oximeter with 8000AA Sensor and Masimo Rad-8 with Rainbow DCI SC-200 Adult Reusable Sensor) were added to 40 shivering patients who met eligibility criteria. Shivering episodes were documented by recording the start and stop times for each episode as it occurred. Dropout rates for each device were calculated by dividing the amount of time that each instrument displayed no SpO$_2$ or pulse rate value by the total time of the test. A 2-sample T-test was performed to compare dropout times of the devices and dropout rates were compared using a z-test for 2 proportions.

Results: Drops in signal occurred in fourteen subjects. The Masimo sensor dropped 21 times, for an average of 40 seconds per drop and Nonin's dropped 16 times averaging 29 seconds per drop. Nonin's dropout rate of 0.108 was less than that of Masimo's at 0.149, however this difference was not found to be statistically significant (p=0.87).

Conclusion: The incidence of shivering was very low among patients in this particular study setting (0.1%) For 5 different subjects, both sensors experienced drops during identical time intervals indicating that motion artifact may impact readings regardless of specific technology. Clinically significant shivering varied in duration among subjects therefore individual shiver rates varied as well. This preliminary analysis shows no significant difference between Nonin and Masimo sensors.

Keywords: Pulse oximetry; Shivering; Post-operative care

Introduction

Pulse oximetry is a noninvasive method of measuring the oxygen saturation (SpO$_2$) of the arterial blood. These devices are vital and commonplace in any healthcare setting where a patient's blood oxygenation monitoring is required. Surgical procedures performed under general anesthesia rely on pulse oximetry to provide accurate readings before, during and after a patient receives anesthesia in order to ensure adequate oxygenation throughout the operation and recovery period.

The pulse oximeter device consists of a sensor, which detects the oxygen saturation and pulse rate of the patient and a monitor that displays these measurements. The sensor is designed for use on a fingertip, toe or ear lobe. Through a series of LEDs and photo-detectors, beams of light are transmitted through the tissues from one side of the probe to the other. The monitor processes and displays a value for oxygen saturation based on how much light is absorbed by the blood and tissues. The technology uses multiple wavelengths within the visible light spectrum in order to determine the percent of oxygenated hemoglobin and deoxygenated hemoglobin through the differential absorption properties of deoxy and oxy-hemoglobin using the Beer-Lambert Law [1].

Certain post-operative conditions such as patient motion, low perfusion and arrhythmias can present challenges in obtaining pulse oximetry measures [2]. In order to ensure accurate measurements, pulse oximeters must be able to function without interruption despite any potential interference. Disruptions in proper function resulting in inaccurate SpO$_2$ measures could potentially result in dangerously low levels that may not be immediately detected.

This study aimed to examine the ability of two commercially available pulse oximeters to obtain readings during a potentially challenging clinical scenario. The rate of post-operative shivering has been reported to occur in anywhere from 5-65% of patients after general anesthesia [3]. The primary outcome of the study is to determine if there is a difference in the ability to obtain readings in SpO$_2$ and pulse rate data measured by two different models of wired pulse oximeters during sustained shivering episodes in post-operative patients.

Methods

This is the first part of a two-phased, comparative, single-center, non-randomized observational study that took place at an outpatient surgery center. It was conducted under local institutional review board monitoring from May 2016-October 2016. Patients undergoing non-cardiac, outpatient surgery with general or spinal anesthesia and presented with sustained shivering post-operatively were enrolled. Sustained shivering was defined as spontaneous muscle activity or shivering-like tremors in normothermic patients immediately upon arrival to the post anesthesia care unit (PACU) [4]. For this study, the shivering episode(s) had to occur either intermittently or consistently for at least 90 seconds or longer to ensure adequate timing for test sensor placement. Patients were 18 years of age or older and were both willing and able to comply with study procedures. Exclusion criteria were less than 18 years of age; had another condition, which in the opinion of the investigator would not be suitable for participation in the study; is unwilling or unable to provide written informed consent to participate in the study or is unwilling or unable to comply with the study procedures. An a priori power analysis was performed to determine sample size. With an alpha=0.05, power=0.99 and effect size=1.28, a sample population of N=40 [5] was adequate for this simple comparison between manufacturers. Given the rarity and spontaneity of shivering occurrences, especially in the particular setting where this study was conducted, and accounting for possible missed shivering cases, a sample size of 40 shiver subjects was reasonable for the main objective of this study.

Forty healthy patients who experienced sustained shivering episodes post-operatively were enrolled and consented for participation for this study. Each subject had two additional pulse oximeter sensors placed on additional fingers. The sensors were placed on fingers that were readily available to the researcher and did not impede standard post-operative care for the patient. The two additional sensors were Nonin 7500 Pulse Oximeter with 8000AA Sensor (Minneapolis, MN, USA) and Masimo Rad-8 with Rainbow DCI SC-200 Adult Reusable Sensor (Irvine, CA, USA). After the sensors had been placed and turned on, shivering episodes were documented by recording the start and stop times of each episode as they occurred. The two additional sensors were removed when the shivering subsided. We calculated the dropout rate of each device by dividing the amount of time that each instrument displayed no SpO$_2$ or pulse rate value by the total time of the test. Since shiver documentation did not begin until both sensors were secured to the patient, the total test time for each sensor is the same. A 2-sample T-test was performed to compare the dropout times of the two devices and dropout rates were compared using a z-test for two proportions.

Results

Forty patients underwent the aforementioned protocol. Data from 36 of these subjects was used for analysis. Data was excluded from four subjects due to spontaneous, temporary lapses of function in the computer software used to mark each shivering episode. The study population consisted of 18 males and 18 females between the ages of 20 and 76. Additional demographic characteristics are reported in Table 1. The rate of shivering among subjects enrolled for this study was calculated by dividing the total amount of time that shivering occurred by the total amount of time subjects had the additional two sensors in place. The data indicate that shivering episodes accounted for 69.09% of the total time subjects were monitored.

Parameters			
Age		Mean	Min, Max
		42.5	20, 76
Sex		n	%
	Male	18	50
	Female	18	50
Race		n	%
	Black or Afrian	3	8.33
	American		
	White	33	91.67
Monitoring time		mean	SD*
Minutes		4.47	3.37
*Standard Deviation			

Table 1: Characteristics of sample population.

During the testing period, signal drops occurred in 14 subject's total. The Masimo sensor had more drops in signal than the Nonin sensor, but this difference was not found to be statistically significant. While 35.7% of subjects experienced dropouts in both Nonin and Masimo sensors, the percentage of subjects who only experienced drops in the Masimo sensor was higher than the percentage of subjects who only experienced drops in the Nonin sensor. Again, the difference in these percentages was not found to be statistically significant. Tables 2 and 3 show signal drops as they occurred between manufacturers and among test subjects, respectively.

Anesthesia/Surgical Detials		Number of Subjects
Anesthesia		
	General	17
	General with nerve block	11
	General with local anesthetic	8
Upper extremity surgeries		
	Carpal/cubital tunnel release	4
	Wrist arthroscopy with debridement	3
	Other hand/wrist operations	3
Lower extremity surgeries		
	Should arthroscopy with debridement +additional repair	5
	Knee arthroscopy with debridement+ACL/MCL/ etc. repair	12
	Other leg/Knee operations	2
	Ankle/foot/toe operations	7

Table 2: Anesthesia and operation details of sample population.

Measured values	Masimo		Nonin		t	P-value[*]
	No. of dropouts	Mean dropout time (SD)	No. of dropouts	Mean dropout time (SD)		
Overall	62	1.72 (4.62)	54	1.5 (4.55)	0.529	0.598
SpO2	30	0.84 (2.31)	27	0.75 (2.27)		
HR	32	0.89 (2.31)	27	0.75 (2.27)		
Note: Mean dropout time is displayed in minutes. [*]95% confidence interval for P-value						

Table 3: Comparison of dropout events in masimo and nonin sensors.

The dropout rate of each oximeter was calculated by dividing the total test time by the total dropout time. While the dropout rate was higher in Masimo than Nonin, the result was not statistically significant. Table 4 compares the overall dropout rate of each manufacturer as well as individual drops in SpO_2 and heart rate.

Measured values	Masimo	Nonin		
	dropout rate	dropout rate	z	P-value[*]
Total	0.385	0.335	1.96	0.67
SpO$_2$	0.186	0.168		
HR	0.199	0.168		
[*]95% confidence interval for P-value				

Table 4: Comparison of dropout rates.

The digit of sensor placement was noted for each manufacturer in every subject and dropout occurrences were recorded. The Nonin sensor had the least amount of dropouts in the middle and ring fingers while Masimo had the fewest when placed on the index finger. Table 4 shows the percentage of drops for each digit, however the differences between the Masimo and Nonin sensor were not found to be significant for any digit.

The Masimo sensor experienced the largest number of signal drops when placed on a subject's middle finger. Masimo had a greater dropout rate for every finger except for the index finger, where Nonin's dropout rate of 0.27 was just slightly greater than Masimo's of 0.25. The little finger proved to be the least reliable for maintaining signal in either sensor dropping 100% of the time in Masimo and 75% for Nonin. It is important to note however that the Masimo sensor was only placed on 1 subject's little finger compared to the Nonin sensor which was placed on 4 subjects' little fingers.

Discussion

Post-operative shivering is a fairly rare occurrence and was only observed in approximately 1% of patients throughout the duration of this study. Shivering accounted for 69% of the total time that enrolled subjects were recorded. While this study did not yield any statistically significant results, the data does provide some useful information about both sensors. Overall, more drops occurred in the Masimo sensor than in the Nonin sensor. This was also found to be true when comparing the number of subjects who experienced dropouts between the two sensors. It is important to point out that for 5 different subjects, both sensors experienced drops at the exact same time

intervals. In these cases, the ability of pulse oximetry to obtain readings regardless of specific technologies may be limited due to motion artifact.

In 4 subjects, drops in Nonin's sensor occurred when the sensor was placed on the subject's small finger. This represented 37.5% of all drops for the Nonin device. While this was only the case for 1 subject with respect to the Masimo sensor (9.5% of all losses), 80% of all readings taken from a subject's small finger were lost. Overall the small finger accounted for 19.5% of all signal losses. In the difficult patients where shivering or other factors may make obtaining readings a challenge, avoiding the small finger for monitoring may maximize overall functionality and consistency of reliable recordings.

There are some areas where limitations to this study were encountered. The sample size was 36 subjects, which may have limited the power of the study and its ability to detect a difference between technologies. Differences in fingers, difficulties in the small finger, were not known prior to the study and a standardized finger rotation or avoidance of the small finger was not utilized. Without a control device to individually compare the performance of each sensor, the two test sensors were compared with each other, which did not offer a significant indication of overall performance. Clinically significant shivering varied in length; therefore, some subjects had more time shivering compared to others.

This study is the first study to examine pulse oximetry in the setting of sustained shivering. This clinical setting proved to offer some challenges in the ability of two commercially available pulse oximetry devices. In the majority of time, the readings could be obtained. However fewer and shorter dropouts occurred in the Nonin 7500 sensor.

References

1. Chan ED, Chan MM, Chan MM (2013) Pulse oximetry: Understanding its basic principles facilitates appreciation of its limitations. Respir Med 107: 789-799.

2. World Health Organization (2011) Pulse Oximetry Training Manual; WHO Press, World Health Organization: Geneva, Switzerland.

3. Gholami A, Hadavi M (2016) Prophylactic intravenous paracetamol for prevention of shivering after general anesthesia in elective cesarean section. J Obstet Anaesth Crit Care 6: 81.

4. Horn E, Sessler DI, Standl T, Schroeder F, Bartz H, et al. (1998) Non-thermoregulatory Shivering in Patients Recovering from Isoflurane or Desflurane Anesthesia. Anesthesiology 89: 878-886.

5. Faul F, Erdfelder E, Buchner A, Lang AG (2009) Statistical power analyses using G*Power 3.1: Tests for correlation and regression analyses. Behavior Research Methods 41: 1149-1160.

23

The Anesthetic and the Akinetic Effects of 1% Ropivacaine Given in Two Different Peribulbar Blocks; Single Medial Canthus or Double Injection Technique

Mona Mohamed Mogahed* and Jehan Mohamed Ezzat Hamed

Faculty of Medicine, Tanta University, Tanta, Egypt

*Corresponding author: Mogahed MM, Anesthiology and Surgical Intensive Care, El Moatasem St, Faculty of Medicine, Tanta University, Tanta, Egypt, E-mail: monamogahedfr@hotmail.com

Abstract

Background: Owing to the advanced age of patients scheduled for cataract and IOL insertion, and the high concentrations of local anesthetic used in peribulbar blockade, the use of ropivacaine produces an effective motor blockade with minimal risks for neuro and cardiotoxicity.concerning globe injury due to multiple injection the new single injection medial canthus is theoretically preferred to decrease the frequency of globe injury.

Aim of the work: To evaluate anesthetic and akinetic Effects in single and double injection peribulbar technique to detect the better method of administration in peribulbar blockade.

Methods: This single blind randomized study was done on 60 patients ASA I-III underwent cataract and IOL insertion surgery. Patients were taken peribulbar block using 8 ml, 1% ropivacaine with 30 IU/ml hyalurinidase. Patients were classified into two equal groups; group I (n.30) is the single injection group group II (n.30) is the double injection group. Eye globe and lid akinesia and anesthesia, the need for supplementary injection and the incidence of complications like ecchemosis, high intra ocular pressure nausea, vomiting and pain were recorded.

Results: 26 patients (86.6%) of single injection group *vs.* 28 patients (93.3%) in double injection group were having complete anesthesia and akinesia after giving block; only 4 patients in group I (13.3%) needed supplementation of block *vs.* 3 patients (10%) in group II with almost no difference in absence of intra and postoperative complications.

Conclusions: Single injection peribulbar block with 1% ropivacaine is as effective as the double injection peribulbar block with 1% ropivacaine in cataract surgery providing effective block with fewer possibility for globe injury with multiple injections.

Keywords: Ropivacaine; Peribulbar block; Medial canthus; Double injection

Introduction

Ophthalmic procedures such as cataract extraction can be performed with either topical or regional anesthesia regional anesthesia are still widely used in cases of difficult and extended surgery [1]. Retrobulbar anesthesia was the standard technique for regional anesthesia in ophthalmic surgery, however peribulbar anesthesia has lesser incidence of complications [2,3].

The most common disabling injuries are related to nerve blocks, so the proposal of single rather than multiple injection technique of peribulbar anesthesia was to decrease the risks of complications [4-6]. Ropivacaine has less central nervous system and cardiac toxicity [7,8]. Several studies had demonstrated the efficacy of ropivacaine in different regional anesthetic techniques for different eye procedures including vireo retinal surgery [9,10].

The aim of this study is to evaluate the anesthetic and akinetic effects of 1% ropivacaine given in two different peribulbar blocks; single medial canthus or double injection technique.

Patients and Methods

After informed consent had taken from all patients including the surgical and the anesthetic procedures 60 adult patients ASA I-III scheduled for cataract surgery and IOL insertion with expected duration less than 70 min duration were enrolled in this prospective, single-blinded, randomized study In Tanta University Hospital between March and December 2016. Patients allergic to local anesthetic, local sepsis impairment of coagulation and orbital abnormality uncooperative patients and who refused the anesthetic technique were not included in the study. After routine preparation and evaluation, irritable patients were premedited with intra venous midazolam 1-2 mg. The patients were randomly allocated using a sealed envelope technique to 1 of 2 equal groups to receive peribulbar anesthesia with 8 ml; 1% ropivacaive and hyalurinidase 30 IU/ml using either the single injection peribulbar with a 25-gauge, 16-mm in group I (n.30) or the classic double injection pribulbar technique with a 25-gauge, 25-mm in group II (n.30). Injections were done with 25 G needle 2.5 Cm length. Non-invasive blood pressure, electrocardiogram (ECG), heart rate (HR), peripheral arterial oxygen saturation (SaO$_2$) variables were recorded every 5 min till completion of surgery. In both techniques, the patients were in supine position. In single injection peribulbar blockade patients were asked to maintain eye in the primary position, the injection site was percutaneous limited superiorly by inferior lacrimal canaliculus, medially by lateral margin of nose, laterally by imaginary line joins inferior lacrimal papilla to inferior margin of the orbit and inferiorly by inferior margin of the orbit. In double injection technique, patients were asked to maintain eye in the primary position the needle was inserted at the junction of the lateral third and the medial two thirds of the lower orbital margin injecting 4 ml, the second injection is just lateral to supratrochlear notch, injecting a volume of 3 ml then during withdrawal 1 ml was injected into orbicularis muscle. with gentle massaging for 1-2 min, Honnan balloon was inflated to 30 mmHg to promote the spread of local anesthetic solution and avoid rise of IOP (Intraocular pressure) data were collected about patients age, sex, weight, the need for supplementary injection, pain during or after injection by using NRS (numerical rating score) (0-10), complications; like ecchymosis, haematomas nausea, vomiting and retrobulbar hemorrhage. Assessment for akinesia and anesthesia was don after 10 min; eye movements in four directions superior, inferior medial and lateral was recorded using scale from (0-2) 0=no movement 1=reduced movement 2=normal movement [11]. While anesthesia score of 2=complete anesthesia 1=partial anesthesia and 0=no anesthesia. All supplementary injections were given by same kind of needle and additional assessment was performed 5 min after injection. During operation oxygen was administered under the sterile drapes postoperative analgesia was controlled by oral ketoprofen. The statistical analysis of our results was conducted using the computer program SPSS version 15.0 for Windows (SPSS, Chicago, IL). Data were expressed as mean SD or percentages. The 2-way repeated measures analysis of variance was used to compare the interval data, and Student's t-test was used as the post hoc test to determine differences between and within groups χ^2 test was used to compare nominal data or percentages. Bonferroni correction for repeated comparisons was applied if necessary. P<0.05 was considered significant.

Results

There was no statistical significant difference between the two groups in the demographic data and the duration of surgery. As regard globe anesthesia, 26 (86.6%) in single injection group comparable with 28 (93.3%) in double injection group; had complete anesthesia after the first injection.

When comparing akainesia of the globe or the lid it was more adequate in the second group resulting in 27 (90%) and 25 (83.3%) comparable with 26 (86.6%) and 23 (76.6%) in the first group, these differences were statistically insignificant. Scores for globe anesthesia, globe and lid akinesia were better in the second group than in the first but without significant differences.

Regarding the supplementary injection, there were 4 patients in group 1 comparable with 3 patients in group 2; (13.3%) vs. (10%) with no significant difference.

The incidence of postoperative nausea and vomiting was less than 5% in all cases, only 5 patients (16.6%) in group 1 and 7 patients (23.3%) in group 2 developed ecchymosis with no conjunctiva or globe hematoma the acceptance of the technique was good in all cases 27 patients in group 1 and 28 patients in group 2 would repeat the same technique in the next eye surgery (Tables 1-6).

	Group I	Group II	p. value
Male/female	14/16	18/12	0.059
Age	57 ± 14.7	59.7 ± 13.05	0.055
Weight	70 ± 11.1	68 ± 12.05	0.231
Duration of surgery (min)	47.5 ± 22	48 ± 23	0.986

Table 1: Demographic data of the patients in both groups.

	Group I	Group II	p. value
Globe anesthesia score	4.2 ± 1.1	4.3 ± 1.08*	0.236
Globe anesthesia after block	26 86.60%	28* 93.30%	0.048*

Table 2: Globe anesthesia in both groups (P=0.47*).

	Group I	Group II	p. value
Globe akinesia score	2.24 ± 1.59	1.93 ± 1.57*	0.033*
Globe akinesia after block	26 (86.6%)	27 (90%0	0.425

Table 3: Globe akinesia in both groups (P=0.47*).

	Group I	Group II	p. value
Lid akinesia score	1.17 ± 0.6	0.94 ± 0.62**	0.019*
Lid akinesia after block	23 (76.6%)	25 (83.3%)	0.058

Table 4: Lid akinesia in both groups (P=0.4**).

	Group I	Group II	p. value
Supplementary block	4 (13.3%)	3 (10%*)	0.782

Table 5: Supplementary block in both groups (p>0.05).

	Group I	Group II	p. value
Complications after block	5 (16.6%)	7 (23.3%)	0.035*

Table 6: Complications after block.

Discussion

Peribulbar anesthesia is achieved by bulk spread of local anesthetic, the choice of the technique depends on the volume of the orbit, and the preference of the anesthesiologist, however in single injection technique the site of injection is relatively a vascular, which decreases the risk of orbital hematoma [12].

In our study, we found that globe akinesia, lid akinesia, and globe anesthesia were slightly better in double injection technique than single injection but still these values were statistically insignificant.

The supplementary injection required in 13.3% of patients in group 1 and in 10% of patients in group 2 results in complete anesthesia and akinesia with pain free and both patients and surgeon's satisfaction all over the surgery.

Our results were in hands with Ballj et al. [13] who showed that adequate block can be achieved with single peribulbar injection either by inferotemporal or medial canthus injection technique, and that there was no evidence that the second primary injection decreases the rate of supplementary injection required, proposing its unnecessary with an increasing risk of globe perforation [14,15].

Also, Leonardo Rizzo et al. [12] showed that medial single injection technique is a simple and satisfactory alternative owing to its painless insertion decreased volume of anesthetic, single puncture in a relatively avascular area and needle passage with less subject to misdirection. With an ideal local anesthetic, we should have rabid onset, dense motor block, and safety.

Our results showed that with the use of 1% ropivacaine with 30 IU/ml hyalurinidase in a volume of 8 ml injection it gives initial good anesthesia and akinesia with almost fewer need for supplementary block in both groups, these results agreed with the findings of Luigi Gioia et al. [16] who studied 0.75% ropivacaine and compare it with 2% lidocaine and 0.5% bupivacaine for viteroretinal surgery and stated that the lower potential for systemic toxicity of ropivacaine enables it to be used for surgical anesthesia in concentrations up to 1%; this facilitates diffusion of local anesthetic molecules into peripheral nervous tissue and improves the onset of nerve block.

With the use of hyalurinidase 30 iu/ml this helps spread of local anesthetic and enhances its faster onset [12,17].

Pj Corke et al. [18] who compared 1% ropivacaine and a mixture of 2% lignocaine and 0.5% bupivacainefor peribulbar anesthesia in cataract surgery concluded that; 1% ropivacaine is a suitable agent for single injection peribulbar anesthesia for cataract surgery.

Short needles were associated with a lower incidence of moderate and severe pain in patients undergoing the single-injection technique [19]. So we used relatively short needles (16 or 25 mm) in single- or double injection techniques, respectively, and this was associated with a low incidence of needle-related complications (hematoma and globe perforation) in both groups. Moreover, the Ghali et al. [20] used similar needles' lengths and concluded that the single-injection technique for percutaneous peribulbar anesthesia with a short needle is a suitable alternative to the double-injection technique peribulbar anesthesia for cataract extraction.

Conclusions

1% ropivacaine is a suitable agent for single injection peribulbar anesthesia as well as double injection technique providing both good anesthesia and akinesia with few complications, however single injection peribulbar block is as effective as the double injection peribulbar block in cataract surgery providing effective block with fewer possibility for globe injury with multiple injections.

References

1. Crandall AS (2001) Anesthesia modalities for cataract surgery. Curr Opin Ophthalmol 12: 9-11.

2. Kumar CM (2006) Orbital regional anesthesia:Complications and their prevention. Indian J Ophthalmol 54: 77-84.

3. Vadivelu N, Huang Y, Kaye A, Kodumudi V, Kai A, et al. (2012) Prevention and management of comlications of regional orbital anesthesia. Middle East J Anaesthesiol 21: 775-784.

4. Ben-David B (2002) Complications of regional anesthesia an overview. Anesthesiol Clin North America 20: 665-667.

5. Ripart J, Metge L, Prat-Pradal D, Lopez FM, Eledjam JJ (1998) Medial Canthus single injection episcleral: computed tomography imaging. Anesthesia and Analgesia 87: 42-45.

6. Dareaue S, Gros T, Bassoul B (2003) Orbital hemorrhage after medial acanthus episclera anesthesia. Ann Fr Anesth Reanium 22: 474-476.

7. Jadhav V, Jadhav R, diwanmal BM (2015) Ropivacaine: A review of its use in regional anaesthesia, chronic pain management and in patients with cardiac diseases in non cardiac surgeries. IOSR-JPBS 10: 43-47.

8. McClure IH (1995) Ropivacaine. Br J Anesth 74: 458-460.

9. Govêia C, Magalhãe E (2010) Ropivacaine in peribulbar anesthesia - vasoconstrictive properties. Rev Brav Anstesiol 60: 495-512.

10. Ghali A (2012) the efficacy of 0.75% levobupivacaine versus 0.75% ropivacaine for peribulbar anesthesia on vitreoretinal surgery. Saudi J Anaesth 6: 22-26.

11. Frow MW, Miranda-Caraballo IJ, Akthar MT, Hugkulstone EC (2000) Single injection peribulbar anesthesia, total upper eye lid drop as an endpoint marker. Anesth 55: 750-756.

12. Rizzo L, Marini M, Rosati C (2005) Peribulbar anesthesia: percutaneus Single Injection. Technique With a Small Volume of Anesthesia. Anesth Analg 100: 94-96.

13. Ball JL, Woon WH, Smith S (2002) Globe perforation by the second peribulbar injection. Eye 16: 663-665.

14. Brahama AK, Pemberton CJ, Ayeko M (1994) Single medial injection peribulbar anesthesia using prilocaine. Anesth 49: 1003-1005.

15. van den, Berg AA (2005) A comparison of two double-injection techniques for peribulbar block analgesia: infero-temporal plus supero-medial vs. infero-temporal plus medial-percaruncular. Acta Anesthesiology Scand 49: 1483-1486.

16. Gioia L, Prandi E, Codenotti M, Casati A, Fanelli G, et al. (1999) Peribulbar anesthesia with either 0.75% ropivacaine or a 2% lidocaine and 0.5% bupivacaine mixture for vitreoretinal surgery: a double-blinded study. Anesth Analg 89: 739-749.

17. Allman KG, McFadyen JG, Armstrong J, Sturrock GD, Wilson IH (2001) Comparison of articaine and bupivacaine/ lidocaine for single medial canthus peribulbar anaesthesia. Br J Anaesth 87: 584-587.

18. Corke PJ, Baker J, Cammack R (1999) Comparison of 1% ropivacaine and a mixture of 2% lignocaine and 0.5% bupivacaine for peribulbar anaesthesia in cataract surgery. Anaesth Intensive Care 27: 249-252.

19. Mahfouz AK, Al Katheri HM (2007-2010) Randomized trial of superficial peribulbar compared with conventional peribulbar anesthesia for cataract extraction. Clin Ophth 1: 55-60.

20. Ghali A, Hafez A (2009) Single-Injection Percutaneous Peribulbar Anesthesia with a Short Needle as an Alternative to the Double-Injection Technique for Cataract Extraction. Anesth Analg 110: 245-247.

24

The Effect of Adding Two Different Doses of Magnesium Sulphate as Adjuvant to Ropivacaine in Peribulbar Block for Cataract Surgery

Mona Mohamed Mogahed*, **Atteia Gad Anwar and Wessam Nassar Abo-elazm**

Tanta University Faculty of Medicine, Tanta, Egypt

***Corresponding author:** Mogahed MM, Anesthiology and Surgical Intensive Care, El Moatasem St, Tanta University Faculty of Medicine, Tanta, Egypt, E-mail: monamogahedfr@hotmail.com

Abstract

Background: This study was designed to compare the effects of adding two different doses of magnesium sulphate to the local anesthesia during peribulbar block.

Patients and methods: The study comprised 105 patients undergoing cataract surgeries. The patients were divided randomly into three groups (35 patients in each group): Group I (Control group): patients received peribulbar anesthesia using a mixture of 6 ml of 0.5% ropivacaine, 1 ml (150 IU) hyaluronidase and 1 ml of normal saline, Group II (Mg 50): patients received peribulbar anesthesia using a mixture of 6 ml of 0.5% ropivacaine, 1 ml (150 IU) hyaluronidase and 50 mg of magnesium sulphate in 1 ml saline and Group III (Mg 100): patients received peribulbar anesthesia using a mixture of 6 ml of 0.5% ropivacaine, 1 ml (150 IU) hyaluronidase and 1 ml of 100 mg magnesium sulphate. Corneal sensation and motor block were evaluated, total amount of local anesthetic, duration sensory and motor block were assessed, analgesia was assessed by using visual analogue score (VAS) at the end of surgery, 1 h, 2 h, 4 h and 6 h.

Statistical analysis was done using ANOVA test, Kruskal Wallis test And Chi-square test (χ^2) to study association between qualitative variables. Whenever any of the expected cells were less than five, Fischer's Exact test with Yates correction was used. P- value of <0.05 was considered statistically significant.

Results: Patients received magnesium sulphate showed significantly rapid onset of lid and globe akinesia (P<0.0001) and significantly prolonged duration of akinesia than the control (P<0.0001). First analgesic requirement is significantly delayed in group II and group III comparison with the control group (group I) (P<0.0001). There were statistically significant differences between the three groups as regard the mean VAS in 4 and 6 hours, group II and group III have lower median pain score than group I (control group) (P<0.0001).

Conclusion: Addition of 50 mg or 100 mg of magnesium sulfate to ropivacaine in peribulbar block led to rapid onset and prolonged the duration of sensory and motor blockade without adverse effects with reduction of the postoperative analgesic requirements. The results were more significant on using 100 mg magnesium sulfate.

Keywords: Local anesthesia of the eye; Magnesium; Peribulbar block

Introduction

Topical, regional or general anesthesia can be used for ocular surgery. Among regional blocks, peribulbar block is a good choice as it provides efficient anesthesia with good lid and globe akinesia with low incidence of complications [1]. However it has a slow onset of action and frequent supplementations may be needed [2]. So many additives have been used have been used in peribulbar block to hasten the onset of akinesia and increase tissue diffusion such as hyaluronidase, [3] adrenaline, [4] clonidine, [5] corticosteroids, [6] sodium bicarbonate [7] and neuromuscular blocking agents [8]. These agents have many side-effects like allergic reaction, bradycardia, sedation, dryness of mouth, systemic neuromuscular blockade, etc.

Ropivacaine is an aminoamide local anesthetic with less central nervous system and cardiovascular toxicity but with less potent motor block as compared with bupivacaine [9].

Magnesium is the fourth most prevalent cation in the body; it has the properties of noncompetitive inhibition of NmethylDaspartate (NMDA) receptor channels and blocking of calcium influx [10]. Thus, it has been used with local anesthetics in various regional anesthesia techniques to hasten the onset time of block and to improve the quality and duration of anesthesia. [11-13].

This study was designed to examine the effect of adding two different doses of magnesium sulphate 50 mg and 100 mg to local anesthetics in peribulbar block on the onset and duration of lid and globe akinesia and postoperative analgesia to find out which dose is more efficacious in improving the quality of peribulbar block.

Patients and Methods

The study design was a prospective, double-blind, randomized, and controlled trial. Approval was obtained from the local research ethical committee. Patients were eligible for inclusion if they were ASA I–III and undergoing routine cataract extraction surgery. This study was conducted in Tanta University Hospital between June 2016 and

November 2016. The procedure of the peribulbar block and the use of visual analog scale were explained to the patients. Exclusion criteria included communication or language problems, history of allergy to amide local anesthetic agents or hyaluronidase, known anatomical abnormalities or pre-existing extra-ocular muscle palsy, severe systemic disease, active ocular infection, single eye, pregnancy, coagulopathy, taking anti-coagulants, anti-epileptic drugs, anti-psychotic medication, anti-glaucoma drugs, atrioventricular block, and obstructive apnea.

The patients were randomized through a computer-generated randomization sequence into the three groups by using 105 sealed opaque envelopes and each patient chose the envelope which determined his group. Patients were randomly allocated into one of the three following groups: Group I (Control group) (35 patients): patients received peribulbar anesthesia using a mixture of 6 ml of 0.5% ropivacaine, 1 ml (150 IU) hyaluronidase and 1 ml of normal saline. Group II (Mg 50) (35 patients): patients received peribulbar anesthesia using a mixture of 6 ml of 0.5% ropivacaine, 1 ml (150 IU) hyaluronidase (Hyalase 1500 IU, Wockhardt, UK) and 50 mg of magnesium sulphate in 1 ml saline. And Group III (Mg100) (35 patients): patients received peribulbar anesthesia using a mixture of 6 ml of 0.5% ropivacaine, 1 ml (150 IU) hyaluronidase and 1 ml of 100 mg magnesium sulphate.

On arrival at the operating room, an IV line was placed. Routine monitoring including the electrocardiogram, pulse oximetry and noninvasive blood pressure were applied in all patients. A nasal cannula was applied and supplemental oxygen was given throughout the procedure at 2-3 L/min. The eye was prepared with a 5% povidone iodine solution.

The study solutions were prepared by anesthesiologists not participating in the study. According to the randomizing table, the drug to be injected in the peribulbar block was prepared in 10 ml syringes to equal volume of 8 ml in all three groups and labeled indicating only the serial number of the patient. The peribulbar anesthesia was performed by a senior anesthesiologist. Both the anesthesiologist performing the anesthesia and the patient were masked the composition of the anesthetic mixture.

Peribulbar anesthesia was done through single transcutaneous inferolateral injection technique using a 25-gauge, 25 mm bevel disposable needle. Patients were asked to maintain the eye in the primary position. The injection site was identified at the junction of the lateral one-third and medial two-third of the inferior orbital rim in the inferotemporal quadrant. The needle was advanced in an antero-posterior, slightly medial, and cephalad direction. After aspiration, the anesthetic solution was injected in approximately 30 seconds; the local anesthetic was injected until the presence of a complete drop and fullness of the upper eyelid. Slight external manual pressure with of 4-5 layers of gauze piece was applied over the eye immediately after injection for 5 minutes to promote the spread of local anesthetics and softening of the globe. IOP was measured using indentation tonometry at 5 min before injection and 1, 5 and 10 minutes after injection. Corneal sensation was evaluated using cotton wick at 1, 2, 3, 5 and 10 minutes till the onset of anesthesia, it was assessed on 0-2 scale where 0=no anesthesia, 1=partial but acceptable anesthesia, 2=complete anesthesia. Ocular movement were evaluated before blocking, then 3, 5, and 10 minutes after the block in all four directions using 3-point scale (0-complete akinesia, 1-limited movement, 2- normal movement) for each direction. Optimal time to start the surgery was defined as presence of corneal anesthesia together with the total ocular movement score $\leq$ 1 and eyelid squeezing score of 0. If one or more of the components of ocular movement showed inadequate motor blockade (akinesia score >3) 10 min after block, supplementary anesthesia (2-3 mL) was injected into the involved quadrant using the same length needle as for the primary block. After that, an additional assessment was performed 5 min later. Any complications were recorded. The total volume of LA solution injected (mL) was calculated. Duration of operation, duration sensory and motor block were assessed by onset of pain and recovery of eyeball movement respectively. Degree of pain was assessed at the end of surgery, 1 h, 2 h, 4 h and 6 h postoperatively by using VAS (0-10 cm; zero cm representing no pain and 10 cm representing the most severe pain). A tablet of paracetamol 500 mg was given if VAS >4. Total analgesic requirement in 6 hours were recorded.

Statistical analysis of the collected data: Results were collected, tabulated and statistically analyzed by an IBM compatible personal computer with SPSS statistical package version 20 (SPSS Inc. Realesed 2011. IBM SPSS statistics for windows, version 20.0, Armnok, NY: IBM Corp.). Two types of statistical analysis were done: a) Descriptive statistics e.g. was expressed in: Number (No), percentage (%) mean ($\bar{x}$) and standard deviation (SD). b) Analytic statistics e.g. ANOVA test was used for comparison of quantitative variables between more than two groups of normally distributed data with LSD test as post Hoc test while; Kruskal Wallis test was used for comparison of quantitative variables between more than two groups of not normal distributed data with Tamhane's test as post hoc test. And Chi-square test ($\chi 2$) was used to study association between qualitative variables. Whenever any of the expected cells were less than five, Fischer's Exact test with Yates correction was used. P- value of <0.05 was considered statistically significant.

Results

	Group I (n=45) Mean ± SD	Group II (n=45) Mean ± SD	Group III (n=45) Mean ± SD	ANOVA	P value
Age	58.93 ± 5.65	59.13 ± 4.59	58.91 ± 5.15	0.02	0.97
Weight	74.53 ± 4.94	74.88 ± 5.55	74.56 ± 5.53	0.15	0.85

Table 1: Mean age and weight distribution among the studied group.

Table 1 Shows mean age and weight showed no significant difference between the 3 groups.

	Group I (n=45)		Group II (n=45)		Group III (n=45)		χ^2	P value
	No.	%	No	%	No.	%		
Gender								
Male	24	53.3	25	55.6	24	53.3		
Female	21	46.7	20	44.4	21	46.7	0.06	0.97

Table 2: Percentage distribution of gender among the studied groups.

Table 2 shows there was no significant difference between male and female distribution between the three groups.

	Group I (n=45) Mean ± SD	Group II (n=45) Mean ± SD	Group III (n=45) Mean ± SD	Kruskal Wallis test	P value
Axial length	24.86 ± 0.90	24.72 ± 0.99	24.79 ± 0.92	F=0.25	0.77
ASA	1.82 ± 0.61	1.73 ± 0.61	1.57 ± 0.62	3.82	0.14
(median)	-2	-2	-3		

Table 3: Mean axial length and ASA among the studied group.

Table 3 shows the axial length and ASA showed no significant difference between the 3 groups.

	Group I (n=45) Mean ± SD	Group II (n=45) Mean ± SD	Group III (n=45) Mean ± SD	Kruskal wallis test	P value	Post Hoc
Motor akinesia score of the 4 intraocular muscles at 3 min	6.31 ± 2.26 (8.00)	3.13 ± 0.78 (3.00)	2.44 ± 0.96 (3.00)	70.26	<0.0001	P1<0.0001 P2<0.0001 P3 0.001
Motor akinesia score of the 4 intraocular muscles at 5 min	1.06 ± 1.73 (0.00)	0.00 ± 0.00 (0.00)	0.00 ± 0.00 (0.00)	28.48	<0.0001	P1<0.0001 P2<0.0001
Motor akinesia score of the 4 intraocular muscles at 10 min	0.44 ± 1.03 (0.00)	0.00 ± 0.00 (0.00)	0.00 ± 0.00 (0.00)	19.11	<0.0001	P1 0.01 P2 0.01
Lid squeeze at 3 min	1.80 ± 0.40 (2.00)	0.84 ± 0.36 (1.00)	0.86 ± 0.34 (1.00)	98.18	<0.0001	P1<0.0001 P2<0.0001 P3 0.98
Lid squeeze at 5 min	2.8 ± 0.50 (0.00)	0.00 ± 0.00 (0.00)	0.00 ± 0.00 (0.00)	26.34	<0.0001	P1 0.001 P2 0.001
Lid squeezing score at 10 min	0.24 ± 0.52 (0.00)	0.00 ± 0.00 (0.00)	0.00 ± 0.00 (0.00)	19.28	<0.0001	P1 0.01 P2 0.01

Table 4: Mean motor akinesia score at different time measures among the three groups.

Table 4 shows P1 for comparison between group I and group II, P2 for comparison between group I and group III, p3 for comparison between group II and group III

This table shows regarding the motor akinesia score at 3 min; group I was significantly higher than both group II and group III, also group II was significantly higher than group III, however, at 5 and 10 min, group I was significantly higher than both group II and group III. And regarding lid squeezing score, group I was significantly higher than both group II and group III at 3, 5 and 10 min.

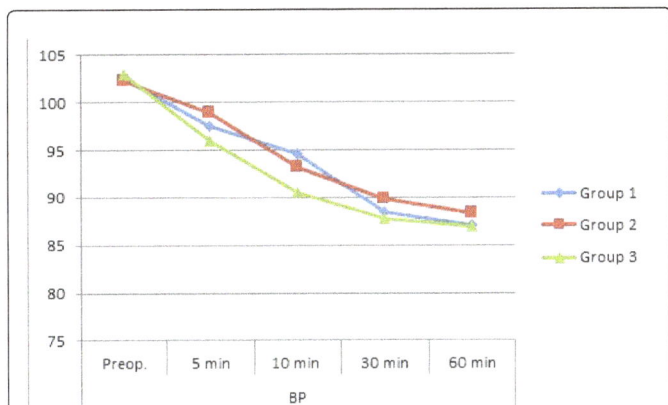

Figure 1: Blood pressure at different time measures in the 3 groups.

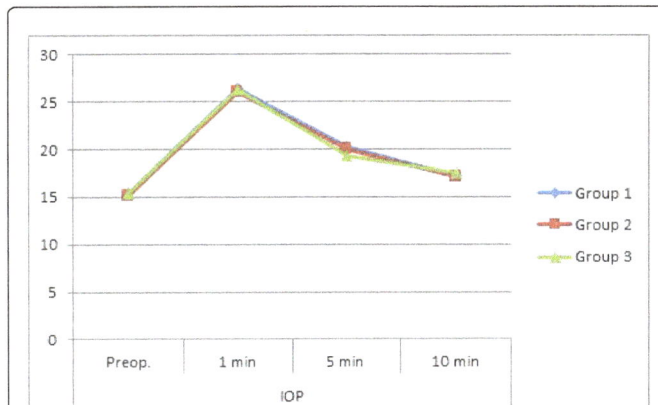

Figure 2: Heart rate at different time measures in the 3 groups.

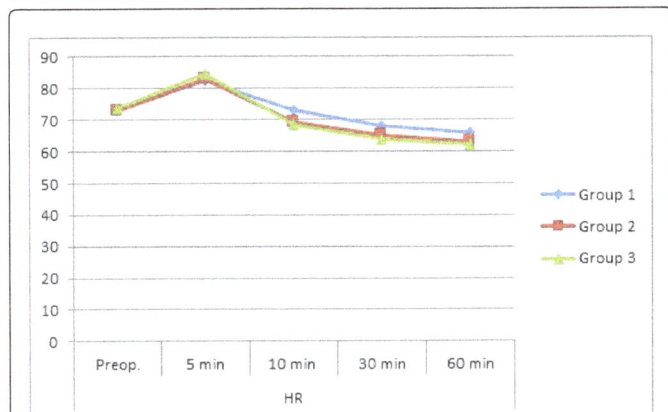

Figure 3: IOP at different time measures in the 3 groups.

Table 5 shows that the mean of corneal sensation at 1 min was significantly lower in group I than group III, at 2 min was significantly lower in group I than both group II and III, also group II was significantly lower than group III. And at 3 and 5 min was significantly lower in group I than both group II and III. Blood pressure, heart rate and IOP at different time measures in the 3 groups are shown in Figures 1-3, respectively.

Table 6 shows that there was no significant difference between the 3 groups regarding post-operative pain score at the end of surgery, post-operative pain score at 1h, post-operative pain score at 2h and duration of operation, regarding volume of anesthetic, optimal time to start surgery, postoperative pain score at 4 h and total amount of paracetamol; group I was significantly higher than both groups II and III. While regarding postoperative pain score at 6 h, group I was significantly higher than both group I and II and also group II was higher than group III, and regarding duration of sensory block and motor block, group I was significantly lower than both group I and II. Also, group II was lower than group III.

	Group I (n=45) Mean ± SD	Group II (n=45) Mean ± SD	Group III (n=45) Mean ± SD	Kruskal wallis test	P value	Post Hoc
Corneal sensation at 1 min	0.95 ± 0.36	1.08 ± 0.51	1.22 ± 0.42	7.93	0.01	P1 0.40 P2 0.006 P3 0.45
Corneal sensation s at 2 min	1.42 ± 0.58	1.77 ± 0.42	2.00 ± 0.00	34.35	<0.0001	P1 0.004 P2 <0.001 P3 003
Corneal sensation s at 3 min	1.66 ± 0.52	2.00 ± 0.00	2.00 ± 0.00	30.98	<0.0001	P1 <0.001 P2 <0.001 P3 1.00
Corneal sensation s at 5 min	1.75 ± 0.52	2.00 ± 0.00	2.00 ± 0.000	19.12	<0.0001	P1 0.01 P2 0.01 P3 1.00
Corneal sensation s 10	1.86 ± 0.45	2.00 ± 0.00	2.00 ± 0.00	8.18	0.01	P1 0.04 P2 0.04

						P3 1.00

Table 5: Mean corneal sensation at different time measures.

	Group I (n=45) Mean ± SD	Group II (n=45) Mean ± SD	Group III (n=45) Mean ± SD	Kruskal wallis test	P value	Post hoc
Total volume of anesthetic mixture	8.33 ± 0.95	8.00 ± 0.00	8.00 ± 0.00	F=5.50	0.005	P1 0.005 P2 0.005 P3 1.00
Optimal time to start surgery	6.51 ± 2.75	3.93 ± 0.25	3.77 ± 0.42	112.37	<0.0001	P1<0.001 P2<0.001 P3 0.10
Post-operative pain score at the end of surgery:	0.00 ± 0.00	0.00 ± 0.00	0.00 ± 0.00	-------	-------	-------
Post-operative pain score at 1 h	0.00 ± 0.00	0.00 ± 0.00	0.00 ± 0.00	-------	-------	-------
Post-operative pain score at 2 h	0.00 ± 0.00	0.00 ± 0.00	0.00 ± 0.00	-------	-------	-------
Post-operative pain score at 4 h	3.35 ± 0.90	0.00 ± 0.00	0.00 ± 0.00	124.5	<0.0001	P1<0.001 P2<0.001 P 3 -
Post-operative pain score at 6 h	4.20 ± 0.89	1.75 ± 0.98	0.44 ± 0.58	104.66	<0.0001	P1<0.001 P2<0.001 P3<0.001
Total amount of Paracetamol:	322.22 ± 414.99	22.22 ± 104.20	0.00 ± 0.00	37.19	<0.0001	P1<0.001 P2<0.001 P3 0.40
Duration of sensory block	232.37 ± 8.78	315.31 ± 11.86	360.55 ± 12.80	F=1493.2	<0.0001	P1<0.001 P2<0.001 P3<0.001
Duration of motor block	209.28 ± 8.45	283.33 ± 15.46	330.11 ± 11.71	F=1118.5	<0.0001	P1<0.001 P2<0.001 P3<0.001
Duration of operation	54.24 ± 6.92	52.02 ± 8.59	51.40 ± 7.34	F=1.71	0.18	-------

Table 6: Mean Post-operative pain score at different time measures.

Discussion

The goal of this study was to compare the effect of two different doses of magnesium sulphate as an adjuvant to ropivacaine in the peribulbar block in cataract surgery. Few studies used magnesium as an additive in the peribulbar block [14-16]; however, to our knowledge no one compared between the effects of adding different concentration of magnesium sulphate to the local anesthetic in the peribulbar block.

Magnesium is an additive drug with analgesic and antinociceptive characters. It is used with local anesthetic to prolong the analgesia by blocking NmethylDaspartate (NMDA) channels in voltage dependent fashion and prevent the induction of central sensitization by peripheral nociceptive stimulation [17]. These properties have prompted using magnesium as an adjuvant for local anesthetics in different techniques as magnesium improves the effect of local anesthetics on peripheral nerve [18,19].

Our study showed significant enhancement of the motor and sensory blocks between the three groups; mean score of motor movement of the four ocular muscles was 6.31 ± 2.26 in the group I, 3.13 ± 0.78 in group II and 2.44 ± 0.96 in group III, but after 5 min it was 1.06 ± in the first group while the second and third groups showed complete motor block. Mean score of lid squeezing of the 1.80 ± 0.40 in the group I, 0.84 ± 0.36 in group II and 0.86 ± 0.34 in group III, but after 5 min it was 2.8 ± 0.50 in the first group while the second and third groups showed complete motor block.

At 2 min, complete block of the corneal sensation occurred in group III, and at 3 min in group II. So, the optimal time to start surgery was shorter in group III (3.77 ± 0.42 min), and group II (3.93 ± 0.25 min) in comparison with group I (6.51 ± 2.75 min).

These results were in agreement with Sinha R et al. [16] who found that adding magnesium sulfate as an adjuvant in peribulbar block results in the earlier onset of akinesia and establishment of suitable conditions to start the ophthalmic surgeries. On the other hand, Tamer Y et al. [14] showed that adding rocuronium to the local anesthetic mixture provides a better akinesia score and faster establishment of suitable conditions to start ophthalmic surgery compared with those in the magnesium and placebo groups. El-Hamid AM et al. [15] found that co-administration of peribulbar magnesium local anesthetic provides predictable rapid onset of anesthesia without any side-effects.

Dogru et al. who added magnesium to levobupivacaine for axillary brachial plexus block in chronic renal failure patients scheduled for arteriovenous fistula surgery and found statistically shorter motor and sensory block onset times [20].

Ekmekci P found that magnesium can reduce the use of non-steroidal anti-inflammatory drugs that causes side effects in postoperative pain management [21].

This was in consistence with our results in which total paracetamol rescue analgesia in the first 6 hours postoperatively was much higher in group I (322.22 ± 414.99), than what was needed in group II (22.22 ± 104.20) while no analgesia was needed in group III.

Our results showed longer durations of sensory and motor blocks in group III (360.55 ± 12.80) and (330.11 ± 11.71), they were (315.31 ± 11.86) and (283.33 ± 15.46) in group II and (232.37 ± 8.78) and (209.28 ± 8.45) respectively.

This was in consistence with many studies that have shown that magnesium associated with decreasing the total analgesic requirements and reducing pain postoperatively by different routes [22-24]. When magnesium sulphate was added as an adjuvant to bupivacaine in ultrasoundguided transversus abdominis plane block in patients underwent total abdominal hysterectomy by subarachnoid block there was a decrease in VAS score postoperatively, and a prolongation in the duration of analgesia and decrease the total amount of rescue analgesia [25]. Also, magnesium sulphate was added to local anesthetic for femoral nerve block and better postoperative pain control was obtained; as it prolongs the sensory and motor block duration without increasing side effects, enhances the quality of postoperative analgesia and increases the time of motor block and decreases the requirements of the rescue analgesic [21], Malleeswaran et al. [26] found that the addition of magnesium to spinal local anesthesia increased the duration of spinal anesthesia by 42 min, Turan et al. [27] made a study on patients who were scheduled for elective hand surgery, they added 10 ml of 15% magnesium to lidocaine in intravenous regional anesthesia (IVRA) and found that the addition of magnesium to lidocaine in IVRA decreased sensory and motor block onset, prolonged the duration of the block and the time to first analgesic requirement but decreased postoperative pain and total amount of rescue analgesic consumption, Hossam A et al. found that adding magnesium sulfate to bupivacaine during femoral nerve block provided a marked prolongation of the duration of both sensory and motor block, and a significant decrease in postoperative pain scores and total dose of analgesic requirements in the first postoperative day. [28] Aytac et al. [29] concluded that the use of magnesium with prilocaine during the block causes pronounced prolongation of

sensory and motor block without side effects, they are suggesting the magnesium as a useful adjuvant to local anesthetics.

Bondok et al. [30] showed that Intra-articular magnesium is effective for postoperative analgesia in arthroscopic knee surgery; as it provided a significant decrease in the postoperative VAS in the first 24 h and a significant decrease in the dose of postoperative rescue analgesia concluding that intra-articular magnesium can be a good alternative for postoperative analgesia. Furthermore, Kashefi et al. [31] Added magnesium sulphate to lidocaine for intravenous regional anesthesia and showed that magnesium sulfate improves the quality of anesthesia and analgesia during regional intravenous anesthesia without causing side effects. Also, it was proved that adding the dose of 100 mg, magnesium in comparison with fentanyl showed better hemodynamic stability with fewer side effects [32].

Many studies compared different doses of magnesium sulphate as an adjuvant to local anesthetics in different surgeries rather than ocular surgery. Nety LK et al. compared three different doses 50, 75, or 100 mg of magnesium sulphate as adjuvant to bupivacaine in spinal anesthesia and noticed prolongation of the duration of sensory and motor blockade without major side effects [33], Also Jabalameli M et al. [34] added three different doses of magnesium i.e. 50, 75 and 100 mg to 0.5% bupivacaine in caesarean section and found that the100 mg group provided maximum duration of sensory and motor block, Sayed JA et al. [35] compared two different doses of intrathecal magnesium sulphate to bupivacain fentanyl spinal anesthesia in mild preeclamptic patients undergoing caesarean section. And found the prolongation of onset as well as time to regression of sensory block was more with 100 mg of magnesium as compared to 50 mg.

Jabalameli M et al. added different doses 50, 75, or 100 mg of intrathecal magnesium sulfate to hyperbaric bupivacaine for spinal anesthesia in the cesarean section in a prospective double blind randomized trial and found significant delay in the onset of both sensory and motor block, and prolonged the duration of sensory and motor blockade without increasing side effects [36].

Conclusion

Co-administration of 50 mg or 100 mg of magnesium sulfate to ropivacaine in peribulbar block enhances the onset and prolong the duration of sensory and motor blockade without adverse effects with reduction of the postoperative analgesic requirements. The results were more significant on using 100 mg magnesium sulfate.

References

1. Dempsey GA, Barrett PJ, Kirby IJ (1997) Hyaluronidase and peribulbar block. Br J Anaesth 78: 671–674.

2. Wong DH (1993) Regional anesthesia for intraocular surgery. Can J Anaesth 40: 635-657.

3. Zahl K, Jordan A, McGroarty J, Gotta AW (1990) pH-adjusted bupivacaine and hyaluronidase for peribulbar block. Anesthesiology 72: 230-232.

4. Sarvela J, Nikki P, Paloheimo M (1993) Orbicular muscle akinesia in regional ophthalmic anesthesia with pH-adjusted bupivacaine: Effects of hyaluronidase Can J Anaesth 40: 1028-1033.

5. Bharti N, Madan R, Kaul HL, Khokhar SK, Mishra S (2002) Effect of addition of clonidine to local anaesthetic mixture for peribulbar block. Anaesth Intensive Care 30: 438-441.

6. Weijtens O, Schoemaker RC, Lentjes EG, Romijn FP, Cohen AF, et al. (2000) Dexamethasone concentration in the subretinal fluid after a

subconjunctival injection, a peribulbar injection, or an oral dose. Ophthalmology 107: 1932-1938.

7.   Roberts JE, MacLeod BA, Hollands RH (1993) Improved peribulbar anesthesia with alkalinization and hyaluronidase. Can J Anaesth 40: 835-838.

8.   Aissaoui Y, Belyamani L, Kamili ND (2010) Effect of the addition of rocuronium to local anesthetics for peribulbar block. Acta Anaesthesiol Belg 61: 51-54.

9.   Knudsen R, Suurkula MD, Blomberg S, Sjovali J, Edvardsson N (1997) Central nervous and cardiovascular effects of i.v. infusions of ropivacaine, bupivacaine and placebo in volunteers. Br J Anaesth 1997: 78: 507-514.

10. Nath MP, Garg R, Talukdar T, Choudhary D, Chakrabarty A (2012) To evaluate the efficacy of intrathecal magnesium sulphate for hysterectomy under subarachnoid block with bupivacaine and fentanyl: A prospective randomized double blind clinical trial. Saudi J Anaesth 6: 254-258.

11. Malleeswaran S, Panda N, Mathew P, Bagga R (2010) A randomised study of magnesium sulphate as an adjuvant to intrathecal bupivacaine in patients with mild preeclampsia undergoing caesarean section. Int J Obstet Anesth 19: 161-166.

12. Yousef AA, Amr YM (2010) The effect of adding magnesium sulphate to epidural bupivacaine and fentanyl in elective caesarean section using combined spinal-epidural anesthesia: A prospective double blind randomised study. Int J Obstet Anesth 19: 401-404.

13. Ghatak T, Chandra G, Malik A, Singh D, Bhatia VK (2010) Evaluation of the effect of magnesium sulphate vs. clonidine as adjunct to epidural bupivacaine. Indian J Anaesth 54: 308-313

14. Hamawy TY, Bestarous JN (2013) Rocuronium versus magnesium as an adjuvant to local anesthetics in peribulbar block Bestarous Ain-Shams. J Anesthesiol 6: 317-321.

15. El-Hamid AM (2011) Evaluation of the effect of magnesium sulphate vs. clonidine as adjuvant to local anesthetic during peribulbar block. Ain Shams J Anesthesiol 4: 21-26.

16. Sinha R, Sharma A, Ray BR, Chandiran R, Chandralekha C, et al. (2016) Effect of addition of magnesium to local anesthetics for peribulbar block: A prospective randomized double-blind study.Saudi Journal of Anesthesia 10: 64-67.

17. Soave PM, Conti G, Costa R, Arcangeli A (2009) Magnesium and anaesthesia. Curr Drug Targets 10: 734-743.

18. Kara H, Sahin N, Ulusan V, Aydogdu T (2002) Magnesium infusion reduces postoperative pain. Eur J Anesthesiol 19:52-56

19. Ko SH, Lim HR, Kim DC, Han YJ, Choe H, et al. (2001) Magnesium sulfate does not reduce postoperative analgesic requirements. Anesthesiology 95: 640-646.

20. Dogru K, Yildirim D, Ulgey A, Aksu R, Bicer C, et al. (2012) Adding magnesium to levobupivacaine for axillary brachial plexus block in arteriovenous fistule surgery. Bratisl Lek Listy 113: 607-609.

21. Ekmekci P, Bengisun Z, AkanB, Kazbek B, Ozkan K, et al. (2013) The effect of magnesium added to levobupivacaine for femoral nerve block on postoperative analgesia in patients undergoing ACL reconstruction. Knee Surg Sports Traumatol Arthrosc 21: 1119-1124.

22. Bilir A, Gulec S, Erkan A, Ozcelik A (2007) Epidural magnesium reduces postoperative analgesic requirement. Br J Anaesth 98: 519-523.

23. Arcioni R, Palmisani S, Tigano S, Santorsola C, Sauli V, et al. (2007) Combined intrathecal and epidural magnesium sulfate supplementation of spinal anesthesia to reduce post-operative analgesic requirements: a prospective, randomized, double-blind, controlled trial in patients undergoing major orthopedic surgery. Acta Anaesthesiol Scand 51: 482-489.

24. Hwang JY, Na HS, Jeon YT, Ro YJ, Kim CS, et al. (2010) I.V. infusion of magnesium sulphate during spinal anaesthesia improves postoperative analgesia. Br J Anaesth 104: 89-93.

25. Rana S, Verma R, Singh J, Chaudhary S, Chandel A (2016) Magnesium sulphate as an adjuvant to bupivacaine in ultrasoundguided transversus abdominis plane block in patients scheduled for total abdominal hysterectomy under subarachnoid block. Indian J Anaesth 60: 174-179.

26. Malleeswaran S, Panda N, Mathew P, Bagga R (2010) A randomised study of magnesium sulphate as an adjuvant to intrathecal bupivacaine in patients with mild preeclampsia undergoing caesarean section. Int J Obstet Anesth 19: 161-166.

27. Turan A, Memis D, Karamanlioglu B, Guler T, Pamukcu Z (2005) Intravenous regional anesthesia using lidocaine and magnesium. Anesth Analg 100: 1189-1192.

28. ELShamaa HA, Ibrahim M, Eldesuky EL (2014) Magnesium sulfate in femoral nerve block, does postoperative analgesia differ? A comparative study. Eg J Anaesth 30: 169-173.

29. Aytac G, Ayten B, Sacit G (2006) Magnesium added to Prilocaine prolongs the duration of Axillary Plexus block. Reg Anesth Pain Med 31: 233-236.

30. Bondok RS, Abd El-Hady AM (2006) Intra-articular magnesium is effective for postoperative analgesia in arthroscopic knee surgery. Br J Anesth 97: 389-392.

31. Kashefi P, Montazeri K, Honarmand A, Masoomi G (2008) Adding magnesium sulphate to lidocaine for intravenous regional anesthesia. Reg Anesth Pain Med 33: 97.

32. Katiyar S, Dwivedi C, Tipu S, Jain R (2015) Comparison of different doses of magnesium sulphate and fentanyl as adjuvants to bupivacaine for infraumbilical surgeries under subarachnoid block. Indian J Anaesth 59: 471-475.

33. Nety LK, ChandarD, Rathore S, Maravi G (2016) Comparsion of Three Different Doses of Magnisium Sulphate As Adjuvant To Bupivacaine in Spinal Anaesthesia For Abdominal Hystrectomies GJRA 5: 274-276.

34. Jabalameli M, Pakzadmoghadam SH (2012) Adding different doses of intrathecal magnesium sulfate for spinal anesthesia in the cesarean section: A prospective double blind randomized trial. Adv Biomed Res 1: 7.

35. Sayed JA, Fathy MA (2012) Maternal and Neonatal Effects of Adding Two Different Doses of Intrathecal Magnesium Sulphate to Bupivacain Fentanyl Spinal Anesthesia in Mild Preeclamptic Patients Undergoing Caesarean Section. J Am Sci 8.

36. Jabalameli M, Pakzadmoghadam (2012) Adding different doses of intrathecal magnesium sulfate for spinal anesthesia in the cesarean section: A prospective double blind randomized trial. Adv Biomed Res 1: 11.

25

The Effect of a Preoperative Single Dose of Magnesium Sulfate *versus* Preoperative Ultrasound Guided Bilateral Transversus Abdominis Plane Block on Hemodynamics and Postoperative Analgesic Requirements in Patients Undergoing Colorectal Surgery

Sabry Mohamed Amin[*] and Rabab Mohamed Mohamed

Departments of Anesthesiology and Surgical Intensive Care, Faculty of Medicine, Tanta University, Egypt

[*]**Corresponding author:** Sabry Mohamed Amin, Departments of Anesthesiology and Surgical Intensive Care, Faculty of Medicine, Tanta University, Egypt, E-mail: sabry_amin@yahoo.com

Abstract

Background: The transversus abdominis plane (TAP) block is a peripheral nerve block, utilized to anesthetize the sensory nerves by local anesthetic injection in the neurovascular plane. Magnesium sulfate can prevent the induction of central sensitization from peripheral nociceptive stimuli at the spinal action site by blocking N-methyl-D-aspartate (NMDA) receptors. The aim of our study is to compare the effect of preoperative single-dose of Magnesium sulfate versus preoperative ultrasound guided bilateral transversus abdominis plane block on hemodynamics, and postoperative analgesia in patients undergoing colorectal surgical operations.

Patients and methods: This study was conducted on 40 adult patients ASA I and II scheduled for colorectal surgical operations under general anesthesia. The patients were randomly divided into two equal groups as follow:

Group I: Patients received magnesium sulfate 50 mg/kg IV as single-dose before induction of anesthesia.

Group II: Bilaterally TAP block was performed before induction of anesthesia under ultrasound guidance.

In both groups, general anesthesia was used. Measurements: HR and MABP, Intraoperative fentanyl, atracurium, and isoflurane consumption, operative time, postoperative analgesia, duration of anesthesia, and side-effects such as nausea, vomiting, and shivering.

Results: There were no significant differences between the 2 groups as regards to age, weight, duration of surgery, and the duration of anesthesia. There were no significant differences in the time of the first analgesic request in both groups. Pain score was statistically insignificant between both groups. The incidences of postoperative nausea, vomiting and shivering were more in group II than group I.

Conclusion: Preoperative administration of a single dose of magnesium sulfate (50 mg/kg) versus preoperative ultrasound guided bilateral transversus abdominis plane block in patients undergoing colorectal surgery was associated in both groups with reduction in the analgesic requirements postoperatively, with less postoperative nausea, vomiting and shivering in the magnesium sulfate group.

Keywords: Preventive analgesia; TAP block; Perioperative magnesium

Introduction

Postoperative pain after colorectal surgeries results from surgical incision in addition to intense inflammatory response as a result of surgical trauma [1-3]. Postoperative pain can be associated with physiological and psychological derangements which may adversely affect perioperative outcome and sometimes may even cause mortality. Acute perioperative pain results in poor patient satisfaction, delays mobilization and if left untreated can lead to chronic pain [4,5].

Postoperative pain after colorectal surgeries may be visceral, or somatic which become worst with movement, visceral pain takes upper hand in the first 48 h postoperatively [6].

Proper and effective plane was needed for the treatment of postoperative pain to prevent its adverse effects. Prevention of this pain has been dubbed as the "holy grail of anesthesiology" [7].

The transversus abdominis plane (TAP) block is a peripheral nerve block, utilized to anesthetize the sensory nerves supplying the anterior abdominal wall by injection of local anesthetic in the neurovascular plane between internal oblique and transversus abdominis muscle layers [8-9]. The triangle of Petit is a single entry point for performing transversus abdominis plane (TAP) block *via* description of the landmark technique to access a number of abdominal wall nerves and providing more widespread analgesia [10]. Ultrasound guided TAP block has been described, it helps us to locate the neurovascular plane between internal oblique and transversus abdominis muscle layers easily and local anesthetic was deposited with accuracy [11].

Magnesium sulfate has been used as an anticonvulsant or antiarrhythmic drug. The interference with calcium channels and N-methyl-D-aspartate (NMDA) receptors may be the mechanism of the its analgesic effect. Magnesium sulfate can prevent the induction of central sensitization from peripheral nociceptive stimuli at the spinal action site by blocking NMDA receptors in a voltage-dependent manner. Reduction of catecholamine release with decrease in sympathetic stimulation may be another mechanism which lead to decrease the stress response to the surgery. NMDA receptor antagonists like magnesium sulfate with low doses have an effect on pain threshold and could prevent pain perception [12-16]. Magnesium sulfate was used as an adjuvant agent to increase the analgesic effect of the other analgesic drugs. Magnesium sulfate was found to be effective in reducing the perioperative pain and analgesic consumption through block the somatic, autonomic and endocrinal response to painful stimulus [17,18].

The Hypothesis of this Study

- Preoperative administration of single dose magnesium sulfate will be effective as preincistional TAP block in reducing anesthetic requirements.
- Preoperative administration of single dose magnesium sulfate will be effective as preincistional TAP block in reducing postoperative pain score, reduce the postoperative opioid consumption and prolong the time of first analgesic request.
- Preoperative administration of single dose magnesium sulfate will be associated with less postoperative nausea, vomiting, and shivering.

The aim of our study is to compare the effect of preoperative single-dose of magnesium sulfate versus preincisional ultrasound guided bilateral transversus abdominis plane block on hemodynamics, anesthetic requirements and postoperative analgesia in patients undergoing colorectal surgical operations. Primary outcomes of our study were reduction in opioid consumption in the first 24 h postoperatively and postoperative pain scores, while the secondary outcomes were the time to fist analgesic administration; and adverse events including, nausea, vomiting, and shivering.

Patients and Methods

This randomized double blinded study was carried out in Tanta University Hospital at the surgical Department on the time period from 3/2016 to 11/2016, after approval of the hospital ethical committee and obtaining verbal and written informed consent from each patient. All patients' data were confidential with secret codes and were used for the current study only. Any unexpected risk appears during the course of the study was cleared to the patient and the ethical committee on time and the proper measures were taken to overcome these risks.

The approval code of ethical committee was 30822/3/16.

Exclusion criteria

Patients refusal to share in the study, liver disease, coagulopathy, patients on anticoagulant or thrombolytic therapy, Patients who had prior abdominal surgeries, allergy to Magnesium sulfate or local anesthetic drugs. Figure 1 shows the patients flow diagram.

Randomization

The randomization was performed using sealed numbered envelopes indicating the group of each patient. A nurse blinded to study who did not participate in patients follow up, read the number and made group assignments. All operating room personals were blind to study.

The process of inclusion in the study went on until the required number of patients was reached. Infusion pumps and syringes which used for drugs administration were identical, covered, encoded Group I, and Group II by anesthesiologist and nurse blinded to study and did not participate in the study or data collection.

Preoperative preparation

All patients underwent preoperative assessment by history taking, physical examination and laboratory investigations which include complete blood count, liver function test, renal function test, prothrombin time, INR, ECG, blood group and chest X-ray.

Premedication

All patients received 150 mg ranitidine and 10 mg of metoclopramide one hour before anesthesia.

Intraoperative management

On arrival to operating room an intravenous line was inserted. All patients preloaded with 10 ml/kg ringers solution and were attached to monitor displaying the following: ECG, HR, NIBP, $ETCO_2$ and O_2 saturation.

The patients were randomly divided into two equal groups as follows:

Group I: Patients received magnesium sulfate 50 mg/kg in 250 ml of isotonic sodium chloride solution intravenously (IV) as single-dose before induction of anesthesia and placebo TAP block was considered where the needle was inserted and 20 ml of normal saline was injected bilaterally into the transversus abdominis neuro-facial plane.

Group II: Bilaterally TAP block was performed before induction of anesthesia under ultrasound guidance with the patient in the supine position, the ultrasound probe is placed in a transverse plane in a sterile manner between the lower costal margin and the iliac crest in the midaxillary line. Once the external oblique abdominis muscle, the internal oblique abdominis muscle, and the transversus abdominis muscles were visualized at the level of the anterior axillary line between the 12th rib and the iliac crest, the block was performed with a 20-G, 100 mm Facetted tip needle, the needle is advanced between the aponeurosis of the internal oblique abdominis muscle and the transversus abdominis muscle. Once the needle was placed in the space between the internal oblique abdominis muscle and transversus abdominis muscle, intermittent aspiration is done to exclude intravascular injection, 20 ml 0.25% levobupivacaine was deposited bilateral into the transversus abdominis neuro-facial plane after negative aspiration. The drug was seen spreading in the TAP as a dark oval shape.

Also patients in group II received placebo 250 ml of normal saline intravenously before induction of anesthesia.

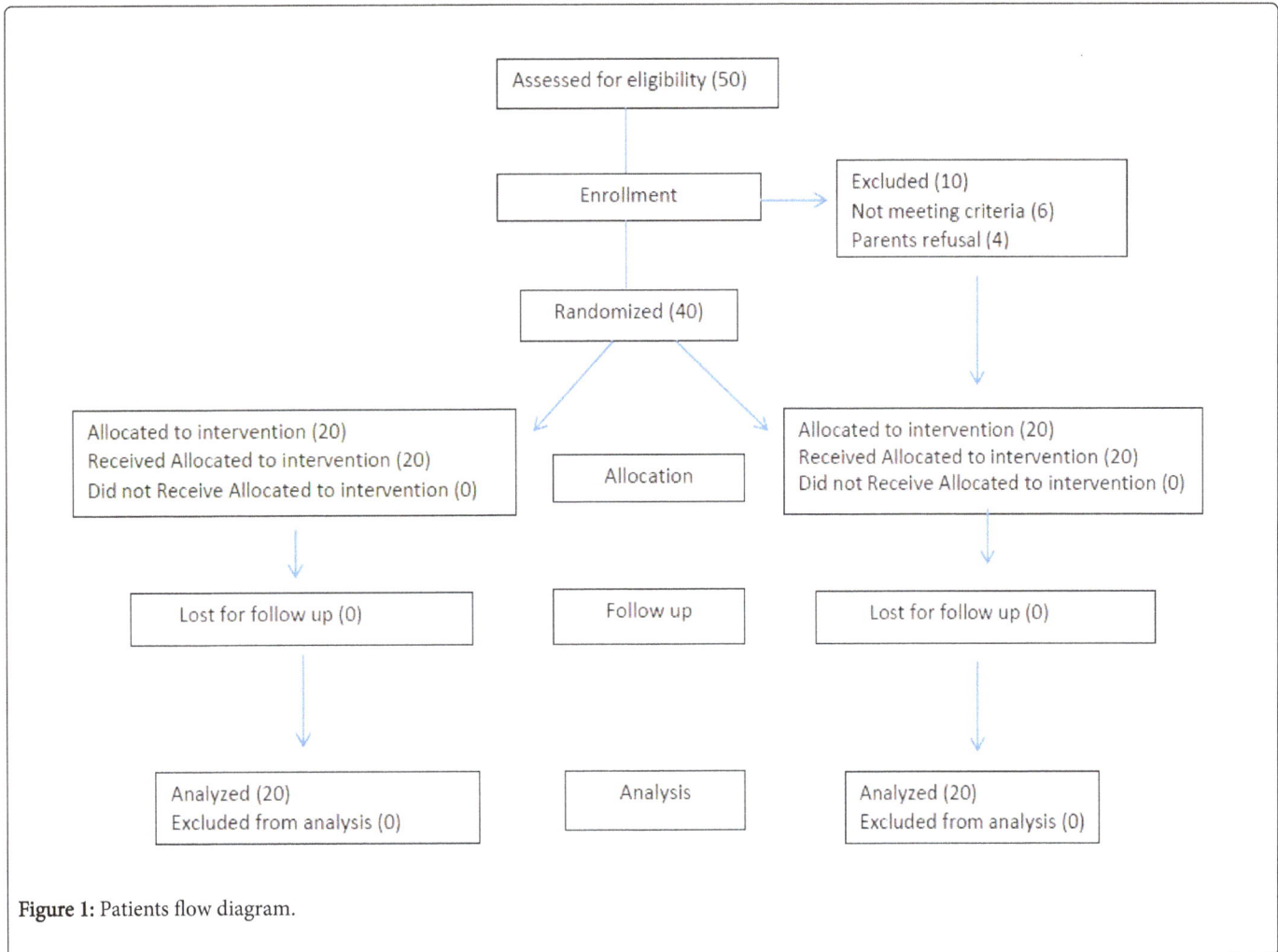

Figure 1: Patients flow diagram.

In both groups, general anesthesia was induced with intravenous injection of fentanyl 1 µg/kg, sodium thiopental 5 mg/kg, and atracurium 0.5 mg/kg. After intubation, anesthesia was maintained with 1-1.5% isoflurane in oxygen and top up doses of fentanyl and atracurium were given as needed. The tidal volume and respiratory rate were adjusted to achieve $SpO_2 \geq 95\%$ and end-tidal CO_2 between 32 and 35 mmHg. Central venous catheter was inserted through right internal jugular vein for fluids, drugs infusion and measure the central venous pressure, urinary catheter was placed for monitoring of urine output and arterial line was inserted for blood sampling and blood gas analysis.

During skin closure, intravenous (IV) infusion of diclofenac sodium (75 mg diluted in 100 ml of normal saline), and 1 gm of paracetamol were given intravenously combined with infiltration of wound with 20 ml of bupivacaine 0.5% in both groups. At the end of surgery metoclopramide 0.15 mg/kg and dexamethasone 0.15 mg/kg were administered for prophylaxis of postoperative nausea and vomiting (PONV). Ondansetron 0.1 mg/kg was administered for treatment of PONV. After completion of surgery, inhalational anesthesia was stopped and muscle relaxant was reversed with atropine and neostagmine and the patient allowed to breathe spontaneously. The ETT was removed when the patients fulfilled the criteria of extubation (spontaneous eye opening, purposeful movement, intact reflex) and

the patients were transferred to postanesthesia care unit for further follow up.

The pain intensity was assessed by a person who was blind to study by using Numeric Rating Scale (NRS) with 10 cm length (starting from 0, no pain, to 10, worst pain) at 2 h, 4 h, 6 h, 8 h, 12 h, 18 h, and 24 h after recovery. If Numeric Rating Scale (NRS) value more than 4, pethedine 0.5 mg/kg was given intravenously and can be repeated every 3 h till the NRS less than 4. The time to first dose of analgesia and total 24 h of pethedine consumption postoperatively recorded in all patients.

Measurements

- Demographic data.
- HR and MABP as base line and every 5 min till end of surgery.
- Intraoperative fentanyl, atracurium, and isoflurane consumption was recorded
- Operative time was measured from skin incision to skin closure.
- The duration of anesthesia.
- Postoperative Numeric Rating Scale (NRS).
- Time to first analgesic request.
- Total 24 h pethedine consumption.
- Side-effects such as nausea, vomiting, and shivering were noted.

Shivering scale

- Grade 0-no sign of shivering
- Grade 1-vasoconstriction, cyonosis and piloerection
- Grade 2-visible tremor only in one muscle group
- Grade 3-visible tremor in more than one muscle group
- Grade 4-intense shivering, tremor of the head and arms and piloerection

Patients were discharged postoperatively when they had no or mild pain (NRS<3), and had no bleeding and or nausea or vomiting.

Statistical analysis

The sample size was calculated using the following assumption: the reduction in opioid consumption in the first 24 h postoperatively was the main response variable. Power analysis identified 20 patients per group, required to detect 20% reduction in postoperative opioid consumption between both groups with a power 80% and a significant level of 0.05.

Comparison of demographic data, time of surgery was done by Student's t-test. Two way analysis of variance with correction for repeated measurements was used for heart rate and blood pressure comparison. Pain score was analyzed with Mann-Whitney-U test nonparametric measurements (expressed as median (range).

Results

This study was carried out on 40 adult patients divided into two groups, 20 patients in each group. There were no statistically significant differences as regards to age, weight, duration of surgery, and the duration of anesthesia between both groups (Table 1).

Characters	Group I=Magnesium sulfate group (n=20)	Group II = Transversus Abdominis Plane Block group (n=20)
Age (years)	48 ± 5	52 ± 7
Weight (kg)	68 ± 8	72 ± 7
Duration of surgery (min)	160 ± 35	155 ± 32
Duration of anesthesia (min)	168 ± 5	165 ± 6
Male/Female	15/5	16/4
Time to first analgesic request (h)	4 ± 2	4 ± 1

Data are expressed as mean ± SD (standard deviation), n= Numbers of the patients. No statistically significant differences between the 2 groups

Table 1: Demographic data, duration of surgery, duration of anesthesia and time to first analgesia.

There were no statistically significant differences in the baseline heart rates and mean arterial blood pressure in the patients in both groups. The HR and MABP were increased significantly in group II 5min, 10min, and 30 min after intubation and while it maintained stable in group I (Tables 2 and 3).

HR	Group I = Magnesium sulfate group (n=20)	Group II = Transversus Abdominis Plane Block group (n=20)
Base line	82 ± 4	84 ± 5
T1	88 ± 7	98 ± 5*
T2	86 ± 5	100 ± 7*
T3	88 ± 7	96 ± 6*
T4	80 ± 6	82 ± 8
T5	82 ± 7	84 ± 9
T6	84 ± 6	82 ± 8
At end of operation	86 ± 7	84 ± 9

Data are expressed as mean ± SD, n= Numbers of the patients, T1=5 min after induction, T2=10 min after induction, T3=30 min after induction, T4=60 min after induction, T5=90 min after induction, T6=120 min after induction. *P<0.05 denotes statistically significance between the 2 groups(the heart rate was increased significantly in transversus abdominis plane block group compared to magnesium sulfate group).

Table 2: Heart rate (beats/minute) changes in both groups.

There were no statistically significant differences in the time of the first analgesic request in both groups (Table 1). There were no statistically significant differences between both groups as regards to fentanyl, atracurium and isoflurane requirement during anesthesia (Table 4).

MABP	Group I = Magnesium sulfate group (n=20)	Group II = Trans versus Abdominis Plane Block group (n=20)
Base line	85 ± 9	84 ± 8
T1	80 ± 7	96 ± 8*
T2	84 ± 8	100 ± 10*
T3	86 ± 7	96 ± 8*
T4	86 ± 8	88 ± 7
T5	80 ± 9	86 ± 9
T6	82 ± 8	90 ± 7
At end of operation	85 ± 9	88 ± 8

Data are expressed as mean ± SD, n= Numbers of the patients, T1=5 min after induction, T2=10 min after induction, T3=30 min after induction, T4=60 min after induction, T5=90 min after induction, T6=120 min after induction. *P<0.05 denotes statistically significance between the 2 groups (the mean arterial blood pressure was increased significantly in transversus abdominis plane block group compared to magnesium sulfate group).

Table 3: Mean Arterial Blood Pressure (mmHg) changes in both groups.

Pain score was statistically insignificant between both groups at 2 h, 4 h, 6 h, 8 h, 12 h, 18 h, and 24 h postoperatively (Table 5).

Variables	Group I = Magnesium sulfate group (n=20)	Group II= Transversus Abdominis Plane Block group (n=20)
Intraoperative Fentanyl (μg/kg)	2 ± 0.6	2 ± 0.5
Atracurium (mg/kg)	0.6 ± 0.03	0.6 ± 0.04
*Dial set of isoflurane (%)	1	1
24 h Pethidine consumption (mg)	55 ± 17	56 ± 16

Data are expressed as mean ± SD, n= Numbers of the patients, *Data are expressed as (%). No statistically significant differences between the 2 groups.

Table 4: Fentanyl, Atracurium, Isoflurane and 24 h Pethidine consumption in both groups.

Variables	Group I = Magnesium sulfate group (n=20)	Group II = Transversus Abdominis Plane Block group (n=20)
2h	2	2
4 h	3	4
6h	3	2
8 h	4	3
12 h	3	3
18h	5	4
24 h	2	2

Data are expressed as median, n=Numbers of the patients. No statistically significant differences between the 2 groups.

Table 5: Postoperative Numeric Rating Scale in both groups.

There were no statistically significant differences between both groups as regards to 24 h pethidine consumption (Table 5). The incidences of postoperative nausea, vomiting and shivering were more in group II than group I (Table 6).

Characters	Group I = Magnesium sulfate group (n=20)	Group II = Trans versus Abdominis Plane Block group (n=20)
Nausea and Vomiting	2 (10%)	4 (20%)*
Shivering	1 (5%)	6 (30%)*

Data are expressed as number (%), n=Numbers of the patients. *P<0.05 denotes statistical significance between the 2 groups. The incidences of postoperative nausea, vomiting and shivering were significantly higher in transversus abdominis plane block group compared to magnesium sulfate group.

Table 6: The incidence of postoperative adverse events.

Discussion

Our study demonstrated that, preoperative administration of single dose of magnesium sulfate 50 mg/kg or performing preoperative ultrasound guided bilateral TAP block was associated with stable hemodynamic, the time of first analgesic request was prolonged, and postoperative analgesic consumption was reduced in patients undergoing colorectal surgery.

However, Magnesium sulfate administration preoperatively was associated with les postoperative nausea, vomiting and shivering.

Preemptive analgesia is a method in which the intervention was given before start of noxious stimulus so, prevents the central sensitization caused by tissue damage and inflammatory mediators which associated with decreased intraoperative and postoperative analgesic consumption and reduce the change of acute postoperative pain to chronic one. But there were conflicting results about the efficacy of preemptive analgesia in reducing the severity, and chronicity of acute postoperative pain and this could explained by the fact that, there are many factors affecting the postoperative pain as the presence of preoperative pain, genetic factors, painful intraoperative stimulations as retraction, skin incision, cutting viscera, muscle or tendon cutting and postoperative release of inflammatory mediators [19,20].

Preventive analgesia is appropriate term which utilize preemptive analgesia and multimodal techniques, began before operation and continued in the operative and postoperative time, it combines multiple analgesics regimen which reduce the dose of each drugs, reduce or eliminate the unwanted side effects, enhance recovery and reduce the hospital stay and associated with early discharge from hospital, increased duration of action of analgesic drugs to decrease long-term pain sensitivity at the peripheral and central levels [21-23].

Magnesium sulfate was considered the fourth most common cation in the body and plays an important role in many physiologic processes [24].

Our study demonstrated that, the preoperative administration of single dose magnesium sulfate was associated with prolonged time to first analgesic request and decreased the pethedine consumption postoperatively with less incidences of postoperative nausea, vomiting and shivering.

Our study was in line with Seyhan et al. [25] they concluded that, preoperative magnesium sulfate infusion was associated with reduced the 24 h postoperative morphine consumption in patients undergoing gynecologic surgery.

Additionally Gupta et al. [26] reported that, preoperative administration of magnesium sulfate in patients undergoing spinal surgeries was associated with stable hemodynamics.

Moreover, Taheri et al. [27] concluded that preoperative infusion of 50 mg/kg magnesium sulfate 15 min before surgery significantly decrease the postoperative pain and opioid consumption in patients undergoing total abdominal hysterectomy under general anesthesia without any adverse effects.

Also Ryu et al. [28] reported that, preoperative magnesium sulfate 50 mg/kg was associated with significant decrease in the postoperative pain and decrease postoperative opioid consumption.

Asadollah et al. [29] found that, preoperative and continuous infusion of magnesium sulfate was associated with significant decrease in pain score postoperatively with reduced the need to opioid analgesia in patients undergoing lower abdominal laparotomy.

Postoperative shivering was associated with undesirable effects as it increases plasma catecholamine concentrations threefold, increase oxygen consumption and requirements which may precipitate myocardial ischemia in cardiac patients and also associated with less patient's satisfaction, increase hospital cost, and were remembered as bad event and worst aspects of surgery [30].

Prevention of postoperative shivering is considered one of the most important functions of magnesium sulfate [31]. Administration of magnesium sulfate decreases the incidence of shivering by up to 70-90% [28,32].

Our study in agreement with previous studies [28,33] they concluded that intraoperative magnesium sulfate infusion was associated with less incidences of PONV and less postoperative shivering.

The main cause of postoperative pain after colorectal surgeries was the abdominal wall incision. Injection of local anesthetics into the transversus abdominis plane will result in block the nerves of the anterior abdominal wall before they pierce the musculature to innervate the abdomen wall [4].

The transverse abdominis plane (TAP) block is a peripheral nerve block which was used to block the nerves supplying the anterior abdominal wall (T6 to L1). It reduces the severity and chronicity of perioperative pain, reduces the opioid consumption in the postoperative period and reduces the side effects of opioids as sedation and postoperative nausea and vomiting [34,35].

In our study, pre-incisional ultrasound guided bilateral transversus abdominis plane block was associated with significant improved in postoperative pain score, reduced postoperative analgesic consumption, and increased in the time to first analgesic request with no reported complications.

This in agreements with Amr et al. [36] they concluded that a pre-incisional TAP was reported to be safe procedure, decrease acute postoperative pain, reduce the analgesic requirements, prolong the time to first analgesic administration with no recorded side effects.

Also, Belavy et al. [37] reported that TAP block reduced opioid consumption after cesarean section when used as a part of multimodal analgesic therapy.

Moreover, Peteren et al. [38] demonstrated that there is a clinically significant reductions of post-operative opioid requirements and pain, as well as some effects on opioid-related side effects (sedation and post-operative nausea and vomiting) in patients received TAP block.

In controversy to our study Costello et al. [39] concluded that, TAP block did not improve the quality of postoperative pain after cesarean section delivery.

Also Ghisi et al. [40] found that, TAP block did not reduce morphine consumption during the first postoperative 24 h after elective total laparoscopic hysterectomy.

The limitations of our study include the following: no control group, we did not measure the depth of anesthesia, the sample size may be small and postoperative magnesium sulfate and calcium levels were not measured.

Conclusion

Preoperative administration of a single dose of magnesium sulfate (50 mg/kg) versus preoperative ultrasound guided bilateral transversus abdominis plane block in patients undergoing colorectal surgery was

associated in both groups with reduction in the analgesic requirements postoperatively, with less postoperative nausea, vomiting and shivering in the magnesium group.

References

1. Soave PM, Conti G, Costa R, Arcangeli A (2009) Magnesium and anaesthesia. Curr Drug Targets 10: 734-743.

2. Ng A, Swami A, Smith G, Davidson AC, Emembolu J (2002) The analgesic effects of intraperitoneal and incisional bupivacaine with epinephrine after total abdominal hysterectomy. Anesth Analg 95: 158-162.

3. Kim TK, Yoon JR (2010) Comparison of the neuroendocrine and inflammatory responses after laparoscopic and abdominal hysterectomy. Korean J Anesthesiol 59: 265-269.

4. Ejlersen E, Andersen HB, Eliasen K, Mogensen T (1992) A comparison between preincisional and postincisional lidocaine infiltration and postoperative pain. Anesth Analg 74: 495-498.

5. Woolf CJ (1989) Recent advances in the pathophysiology of acute pain. Br J Anaesth 63: 139-146.

6. Leung CC, Chan YM, Ngai SW, Ng KF, Tsui SL (2000) Effect of pre-incision skin infiltration on post-hysterectomy pain--a double-blind randomized controlled trial. Anaesth Intensive Care 28: 510-516.

7. Cohen SP, Raja SN (2013) Prevention of chronic postsurgical pain: the ongoing search for the holy grail of anesthesiology. Anesthesiology 118: 241-243.

8. Shibata Y, Sato Y, Fujiwara Y, Komatsu T (2007) Transversus abdominis plane block. Anesth Analg 105: 883.

9. Tran TM, Ivanusic JJ, Hebbard P, Barrington MJ (2009) Determination of spread of injectate after ultrasound-guided transversus abdominis plane block: a cadaveric study. Br J Anaesth 102: 123-127.

10. Rafi AN (2001) Abdominal field block: a new approach via the lumbar triangle. Anaesthesia 56: 1024-1026.

11. Hebbard P, Fujiwara Y, Shibata Y, Royse C (2007) Ultrasound-guided transversus abdominis plane (TAP) block. Anaesth Intensive Care 35: 616-617.

12. Tramer MR, Schneider J, Marti RA, Rifat K (1996) Role of magnesium sulfate in postoperative analgesia. Anesthesiology 84: 340-347.

13. Hwang JY, Na HS, Jeon YT, Ro YJ, Kim CS, et al. (2010) I.V. infusion of magnesium sulfate during spinal anaesthesia improves postoperative analgesia. Br J Anaesth 104: 89-93.

14. Mostafa S, Baharestani B, Farsad BF, Hooman B, Touraj B, et al. (2011) Intraoperative magnesium sulfate can reduce narcotic requirement after coronary bypass surgery. The Iranian Journal of Cardiac Surgery 12: 32-35.

15. Haryalchi K, Ghanaie MM, Yaghoubi Y, Milani F, Faraji R (2013) An assessment of changes in Magnesium level during gynecological abdominal surgeries. Journal of Basic and Clinical Reproductive Sciences 2: 98-102.

16. Kara H, Sahin N, Ulusan V, Aydogdu T (2002) Magnesium infusion reduces perioperative pain. Eur J Anaesthesiol 19: 52-56.

17. Koinig H, Wallner T, Marhofer P, Andel H, Horauf K, et al. (1998) Magnesium sulfate reduces intra- and postoperative analgesic requirements. Anesth Analg 87: 206-210.

18. Levaux Ch, Bonhomme V, Dewandre PY, Brichant JF, Hans P (2003) Effect of intra-operative magnesium sulphate on pain relief and patient comfort after major lumbar orthopaedic surgery. Anaesthesia 58: 131-135.

19. Kissin I (2000) Preemptive analgesia. Anesthesiology 93: 1138-1143.

20. Katz J, Seltzer Z (2009) Transition from acute to chronic postsurgical pain: risk factors and protective factors. Expert Rev Neurother 9: 723-744.

21. Buvanendran A, Kroin JS (2009) Multimodal analgesia for controlling acute postoperative pain. Curr Opin Anaesthesiol 22: 588-593.

22. Møiniche S, Kehlet H, Dahl JB (2002) A qualitative and quantitative systematic review of preemptive analgesia for postoperative pain relief: the role of timing of analgesia. Anesthesiology 96: 725-741.

23. Katz J, McCartney CJ (2002) Current status of pre-emptive analgesia. Curr Opin Anaesthesiol 15: 435-441.

24. Fawcett WJ, Haxby EJ, Male DA (1999) Magnesium: physiology and pharmacology. Br J Anaesth 83: 302-320.

25. Seyhan TO, Tugrul M, Sungur MO, Kayacan S, Telci L, et al. (2006) Effects of three different dose regimens of magnesium on propofol requirements, haemodynamic variables and postoperative pain relief in gynaecological surgery. Br J Anaesth 96: 247-252.

26. Gupta K, Vohra V, Sood J (2006) The role of magnesium as an adjuvant during general anaesthesia. Anaesthesia 61: 1058-1063.

27. Taheri A, Haryalchi K, Ghanaie MM, Arejan NH (2015) Effect of Low-Dose (Single-Dose) Magnesium Sulfate on Postoperative Analgesia in Hysterectomy Patients Receiving Balanced General Anesthesia. Anesthesiol Res Pract 2015: 306145.

28. Ryu JH, Kang MH, Park KS, Do SH (2008) Effects of magnesium sulfate on intraoperative anaesthetic requirements and postoperative analgesia in gynaecology patients receiving total intravenous anaesthesia. Br J Anaesth 100: 397-403.

29. Asadollah S, Vahdat M, Yazdkhasti P, Nikravan N (2015) The effect of magnesium sulfate on postoperative analgesia requirements in gynecological surgeries. J Turk Soc Obstet Gynecol 1: 34-37.

30. Frank SM, Higgins MS, Breslow MJ, Fleisher LA, Gorman RB, et al. (1995) The catecholamine, cortisol, and hemodynamic responses to mild perioperative hypothermia. A randomized clinical trial. Anesthesiology 82: 83-93.

31. Alfonsi P (2001) Postanaesthetic shivering: epidemiology, pathophysiology, and approaches to prevention and management. Drugs 61: 2193-2205.

32. Tramer MR, Glynn CJ (2007) An evaluation of a single dose of magnesium to supplement analgesia after ambulatory surgery: randomized controlled trial. Anesth Analg 104: 1374-1379.

33. Apfel CC, Kranke P, Katz MH, Goepfert C, Papenfuss T, et al. (2002) Volatile anaesthetics may be the main cause of early but not delayed postoperative vomiting: a randomized controlled trial of factorial design. Br J Anaesth 88: 659-68.

34. McDonnell JG, Curley G, Carney J, Benton A, Costello J, et al. (2008) The analgesic efficacy of transversus abdominis plane block after cesarean delivery: a randomized controlled trial. Anesth Analg 106: 186-191.

35. Siddiqui MR, Sajid MS, Uncles DR, Cheek L, Baig MK (2011) A meta-analysis on the clinical effectiveness of transversus abdominis plane block. J Clin Anesth 23: 7-14.

36. Amr YM, Amin SM (2011) Comparative study between effect of pre-versus post-incisional transversus abdominis plane block on acute and chronic post-abdominal hysterectomy pain. Anesth Essays Res 5: 77-82.

37. Belavy D, Cowlishaw PJ, Howes M, Phillips F (2009) Ultrasound-guided transversus abdominis plane block for analgesia after Caesarean delivery. Br J Anaesth 103: 726-730.

38. Petersen PL, Mathiesen O, Torup H, Dahl JB (2010) The transversus abdominis plane block: a valuable option for postoperative analgesia? A topical review. Acta Anaesthesiol Scand 54: 529-535.

39. Costello JF, Moore AR, Wieczorek PM, Macarthur AJ, Balki M, et al. (2009) The transversus abdominis plane block, when used as part of a multimodal regimen inclusive of intrathecal morphine, does not improve analgesia after cesarean delivery. Reg Anesth Pain Med 34: 586-589.

40. Ghisi D, Fanelli A, Vianello F, Gardini M, Mensi G, et al. (2016) Transversus Abdominis Plane Block for Postoperative Analgesia in Patients Undergoing Total Laparoscopic Hysterectomy: A Randomized, Controlled, Observer-Blinded Trial. Anesth Analg 123: 488-492.

26

The Effect of Combined Intrathecal Morphine and Clonidine on Stress Response, Extubation Time and Postoperative Analgesia after Cardiac Surgery

Mona Mohamed Mogahed*, Jehan Mohammad Ezzat Hamed and Mohamed Shafik Elkahwagy

Faculty of Medicine, Tanta University, Egypt

*Corresponding author: Mona Mohamed Mogahed, Faculty of Medicine, Tanta University, Tanta, Egypt, E-mail: monamogahedfr@hotmail.com

Abstract

Background: Pain is a major complication after cardiac surgery, if it is poorly controlled, it will lead to more complication as respiratory depression, myocardial ischemia, delayed extubation, and more ICU stay, with the more analgesic consumption and patients suffering. Intrathecal morphine produces intense and prolonged analgesia and can be useful adjunct for controlling postoperative pain and facilitating early extubation after cardiac surgery. The addition of intrathecal clonidine to morphine allows the dose of intrathecal morphine to be reduced and reduces the risk of respiratory depression while maintaining good analgesia and allows early extubation. This randomized controlled study was carried out on 40 patients undergoing open cardiac surgery and was divided into two groups; group (I): is the control group (n=40) and group (II): is the morphine clonidine group (n=40), patients received intrathecal morphine 4 mcg/kg and clonidine 1 mic/kg. The aim of this study was to evaluate the effects of combined intrathecal morphine and clonidine on stress response, time of extubation, and postoperative analgesia after cardiac surgery. The results of our study revealed that, there was no statistical significant changes in CVP (central venous pressure), Sao_2 (Oxygen saturation) and lactate level in both group, but there was a decrease in HR after induction and before bypass in the intrathecal morphine clonidine group compared with the control one, also there was a significant reduction in MAP after induction, before bypass and after bypass in morphine clonidine group *vs.* control group. Cortisol level was decreased after sternotomy, after ICU admission and after extubation in the morphine group *vs.* control group. Time to extubation, vas, and morphine consumption in 24 h were all decreased in the morphine group compared with the control one, with no significant differences in post-operative complication in both studied groups.

Conclusion: In patients with well-preserved ventricular and respiratory function scheduled for fast-track cardiac surgery, the use of combined intrathecal morphine 250 µg and clonidine provides good postoperative analgesia and early extubation without side effects.

Keywords: Intrathecal; Morphine; Clonidine; Cardiac surgery

Introduction

The intensity of sternotomy incision pain after cardiac surgery, is often severe, and is worsened by coughing, deep breathing, moving or turning in bed and mobilization [1-4].

Severe pain leads to impairment of pulmonary function, and severe respiratory [5,6] and other [7] complications which is the leading cause of postcardiac surgical morbidity [8,9]. Early extubation should be the goal after cardiac surgery, as it may reduce postoperative complications and decrease ICU stay and costs [10].

Adequate control of pain leads to early extubation and rapid transfer to the ward and is mostly applied to patients who have well-preserved pulmonary and ventricular function [11]. The addition of intrathecal clonidine to morphine allow the dose of intrathecal morphine to be reduced and reduces the risk of respiratory depression while maintaining good analgesia and allows early extubation [12]. Intrathecal and epidural anesthesia have been shown to decrease stress response to surgery, improve postoperative respiratory function, and provide excellent postoperative pain relief after cardiac surgery [13].

Regional anesthetic techniques are gaining popularity in cardiac surgery and have been implemented as an integral part of some fast-track cardiac anesthesia [14].

This study investigated the effect of pre-operative intrathecal 250 µg morphine administration of combined with clonidine in patients undergoing cardiac surgery on opioid consumption and duration of controlled ventilation.

Patients and Methods

This study was carried out on forty patients (submitted to cardiac surgery CABG or valve replacement). An informed consent was taken from all patients. The patients were randomly allocated into 2 groups:

Group I (40 patients): control group.

Group II (40 patients): received intrathecal morphine and clonidine preoperatively.

Inclusion criteria: Patients undergoing cardiac surgery CABG or valve replacement with age between 25 and 60 years old.

Exclusion criteria: Emergency surgery: combined valve replacement and CABG surgery, redo CABG, patients with left ventricular ejection fraction less than 40%, patients with platelets count less than

100000/dL, patients with significant renal impairment, Patients with significant neurological impairment, patients with liver disease, patients with bleeding disorder, current anticoagulant therapy, patients with chronic cardiac or respiratory failure and patients who received corticosteroids within 24 h preoperatively. All patients underwent routine examinations as determined by age, sex and type of surgery. Clinical examination was performed to assess the ASA physical status of the patients and to exclude any contraindication. Electrocardiogram (ECG), Chest radiograph, echocardiography, liver function, Hb and Ht, renal function, prothrombin time and activity, partial thromboplastin time and complete blood picture.

All patients were premdicated with midazolam 15-20 μg/kg intravenously to facilitate the placement of the central line and arterial cannula.

The patients in group (II) were placed in sitting position and the back of the patients were sterilized with povidone-iodine (betadine). The skin was anesthetized with 3 ml of 1% lidocaine, lumber puncture was done at L2-L3 or L3-L4 interspace with a 25-gauge needle. The patients received 4 μg/kg morphine with 1 μgm/kg clonidine intrathecaly one hour before induction of anesthesia. General anesthesia was induced by fentanyl 7-10 μg/kg, etomidate 0.25 mgkg, cisatracurium 0.2 mg/kg to facilitate intubation and maintained by isoflurane 0.25-1%, cisatracurium 0.03 mg/kg, fentanyl 5-10 mcg/kg and propofol 0.1-0.2 mg/kg.

Non-invasive and invasive blood pressure, heart rate, oxygen saturation, tidal carbon dioxide and electrocardiogram (ECG). CVP, arterial blood gases and urine output.

In the ICU before extubation, pain was controlled by PCA morphine 1 mg at a lockout period of 10 min with a maximum dose of 28 mg/4 h.

Measurements: Heart rate (HR), Mean arterial pressure (MAP), Central venous pressure, Oxygen saturation, Acid-base changes (pH, Pco_2, HCO_3).

The above parameters were recorded before induction of anesthesia, after induction of anesthesia, before bypass, after bypass, before shift to ICU. On arrival to ICU. These measurements were recorded every 2 h until the patients extubated, then 15, 30, 60 min and then hourly for 4 h after extubation.

Plasma lactate level (mg/dL), plasma cortisol was measured preoperatively, poststernotomy, on admission to ICU, after extubation, after 8, 24, 48 h after ICU admission.

After extubation pain was assessed by visual analogue score (VAS) 0 no pain to 10 (worset pain imaginable) every 30 min for 1st 4 h in ICU; then every one hour for the next 4 h; then every 2 h for 20 h and finally after 24 h. When VAS equal or more than 4 morphine 2 mg was given IV.

Total dose of intravenous morphine was recorded in 1st 24 h in both group. Sedation was assessed by Ramsay sedation score.

In the ICU, Patients were extubated when they have the following criteria:

Patients awake and obey commands.

SpO_2>92% on ≤ 50% oxygen, Maximum inspiratory pressure ≥ -25 cm H_2O, Core temperature >36°C, Chest tube drainage 100 ml/h for 2 consecutive h.

Postoperative hypertension (SBP 140 mmHg) was treated with nitroglycerin infusion, Postoperative hypotension (SBP 75 mmHg) was treated by vasoactive drugs.

Side effects of intrathecal morphine were recorded such as pruritus, nausea, vomiting and respiratory depression if respiratory rate <10/ min. Time from admission to ICU up to extubation was recorded.

Assuming that mean (SD) morphine consumption would be about 50 (25) mg per 24 h, we calculated that a sample of 40 patients would be enough to detect such a difference with a type I error of 0.05 and a type II error of 0.10. Results were collected, tabulated and statistically analyzed by an IBM compatible personal computer with SPSS statistical package version 20 (SPSS Inc. Realesed 2011. IBM SPSS statistics for windows, version 20.0, Armnok, NY: IBM Corp.). Two types of statistical analysis were done: a) Descriptive statistics: e.g. was expressed in: Number (No), percentage (%) mean ($\bar{x}$) and standard deviation (SD). b) Analytic statistics: e.g. Student's t-test is a test of significance used for comparison of quantitative variables between two groups of normally distributed data, while Mann Whitney's test was used for comparison of quantitative variables between two groups of not normally distributed data. 2 Chi-square test ($\chi2$) was used to study association between qualitative variables. Whenever any of the expected cells were less than five Fischer's Exact test with Yates correction was used. P value of <0.05 was considered statistically signifcant. Logistic regression was not done as prediction was not an aim of this work; however, the 2 groups were matched at the beginning of the study for gender, age and ASA (Table 1).

Demographic Data		Group I	Group II	T-test	
				t	P-value
Age (years)		25	26		
	Range	59	58		
	Mean	38.55	37.75		
	SD	13.081	11.229	0.756	0.863
Weight (kg)	Range	60	60		
		75	78		
	Mean	65.55	65.8		
	SD	4.98	5.083	0.853	0.956
Height (cm)	Range	165	167		
		182	182		
	Mean	174.1	174.45		
	SD	5.119	5.246	-0.214	0.896
Sex M/F		11/9	12/8	P value -0.749	
*statistically significant difference at P<0.05.					

Table 1: Comparison of demographic data in both groups.

Results

There was a statistically significant decrease in HR in group II at time after induction (T1) and before bypass (T2) in comparison with group I (P<0.05) (Figure 1), While there was a statistically significant decrease in MABP in group II at time after induction (T1), before bypass (T2) and after bypass (T3) in comparison with group I (P<0.05) (Figure 2).

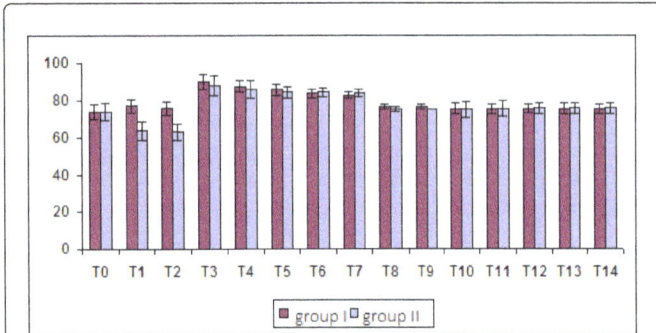

Figure 1: Comparison of HR (beats/min) changes in both groups.

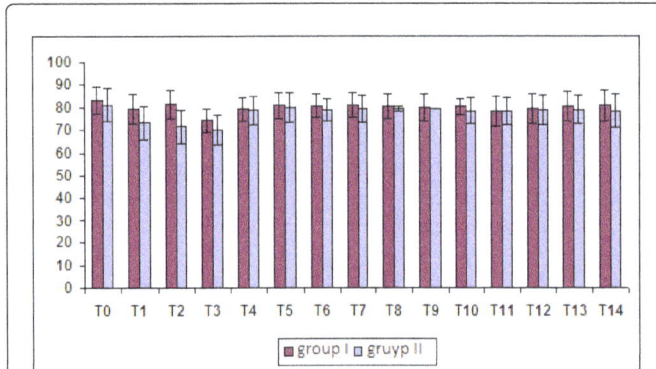

Figure 2: Comparison of MAP (mmHg) changes in both groups.

No statistically significant difference in both groups as regards to plasma lactate level (mg/dl) (P>0.05) (Figure 3), However, there was a statistically significant lower plasma cortisol level (µg/dl) in group II at time of poststernotomy (T1), on admission to ICU (T2) and following tracheal extubation (T3) in comparison with group I (P<0.05) (Figure 4).

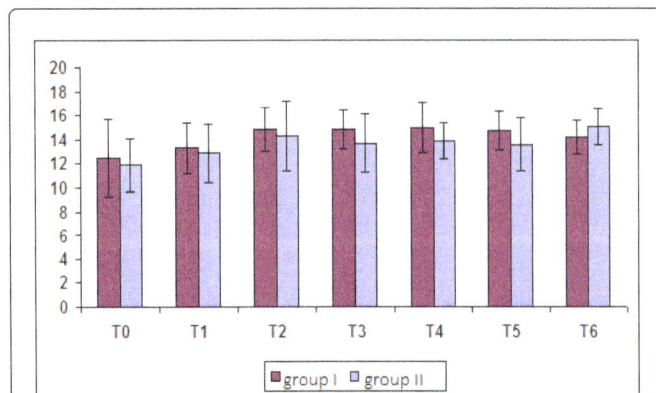

Figure 3: Comparison plasma lactate level (mg/dL) in both group.

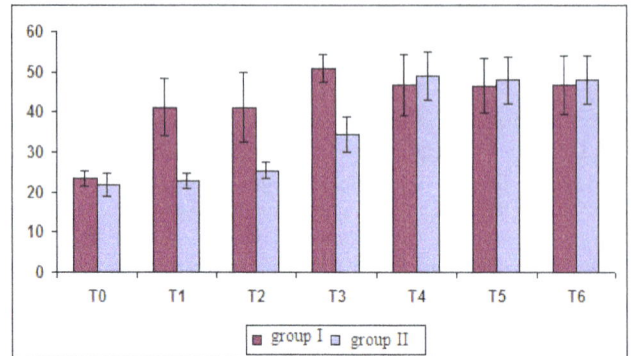

Figure 4: Comparison of changes in plasma cortisol level (µg/dL) in both groups.

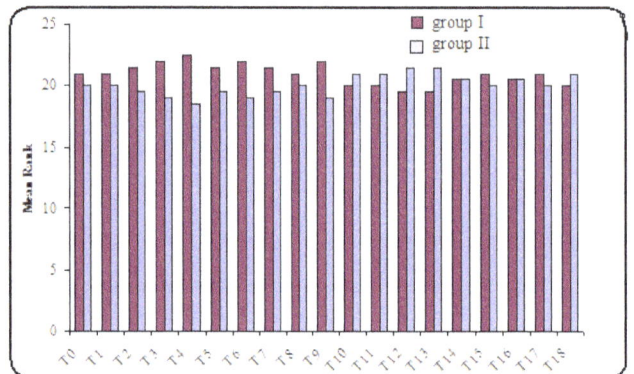

Figure 5: Comparison of changes in postoperative sedation score in both groups.

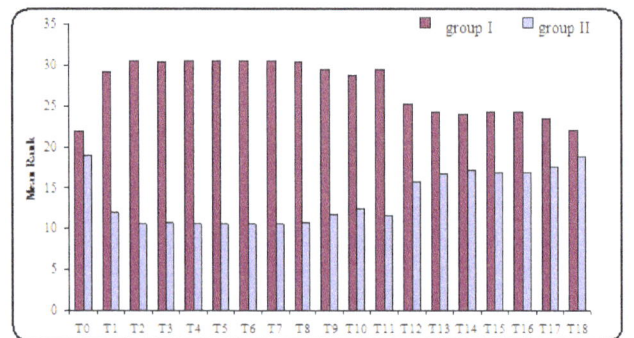

Figure 6: Comparison of changes in visual analogue score (VAS) in both groups.

Sedation score in both groups showed no statistically significant difference between both groups (p>0.05) (Figure 5) While the visual analogue score (VAS) in both groups showed statistically significant higher pain score in group I after one h in ICU (T1) and onward to time 20 h in ICU (T17) in comparison with group II (P<0.05) (Figure 6).

The amount of morphine consumption in 24 h in both groups was statistically significant lower in group II with mean value was 6 ± 1.2, in comparison to group I with mean value was 14 ± 1.2 (p<0.05) (Figure 7).

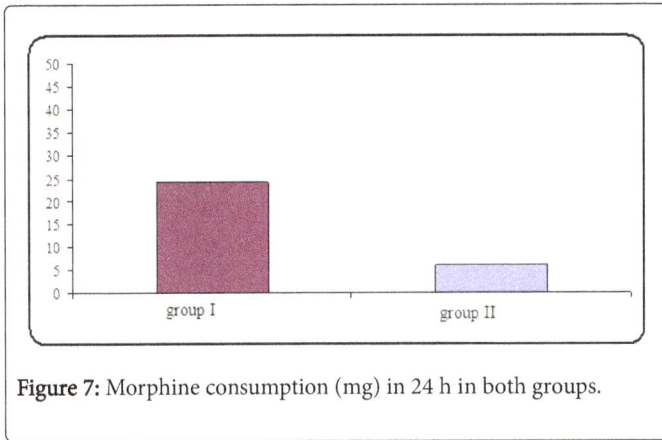

Figure 7: Morphine consumption (mg) in 24 h in both groups.

The mean time of extubation in (group II) 293.2 ± 54.6 was statistically less significant in comparison to the mean time to extubation in group I 339.00 ± 29.6 (P>0.05). (Figure 8). No significant difference in both groups as regards to frequencies of postoperative complication (Table 2).

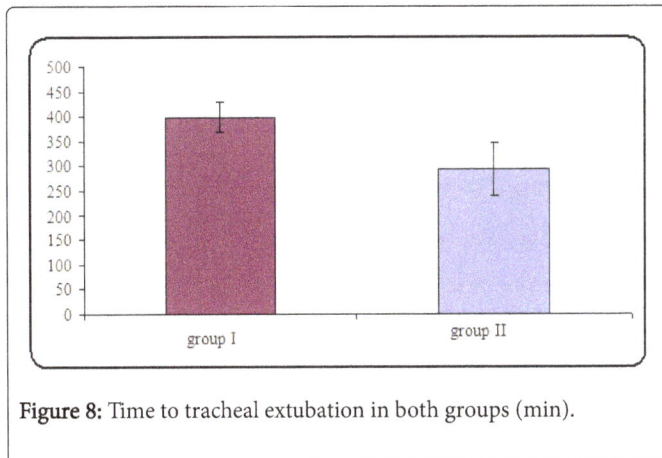

Figure 8: Time to tracheal extubation in both groups (min).

Type of complications	Group I (n=20)	Group II (n=20)	P
Opoid related complications			
Nausea	6	7	0.99
Vomiting	3	4	0.99
Purities	0	2	0.99
Urinary retention	0	2	0.99
Respiratory depression	0	0	0.99
Spinal anesthesia complications			
Post-spinal tap headache	0	0	0.99
Central neuroaxial haematoma	0	0	0.99
Cardiac complications			
Postoperative myocardial infarctions	0	0	0.99
Atrial fibrillation	2	2	0.99
Ventricular tachycardia	1	1	0.99
Stroke	0	0	0.99
Death	0	0	0.99
*statistically significant difference at P<0.05.			

Table 2: Frequencies of post-operative complication in both groups.

Discussion

The quality of postoperative analgesia and its relationship has recently received much attention [15]. There are various methods for postoperative pain management ranging from regional blocks with local anesthetics to systemic administration of synthetic opioids [16]. Inadequate analgesia during the postoperative period may lead to many adverse hemodynamics (tachycardia, hypertension, vasoconstrictor-ion), respiratory (tachypnea, decreased tidal volume), metabolic (increased catabolism), immunologic (impaired immune response), and haemostatic (platelet activation) alteration. Aggressive control of postoperative pain has been shown to decrease morbidity and mortality in high risk patients after noncardiac surgery [17].

Driven by economic reasons, it is better in cardiac surgery to extubate patients during the immediate postoperative period [18]. However, in patients undergoing cardiac surgery, perioperative myocardial ischemia (diagnosed by electrocardiography and/or transesophageal echocardiography) is most commonly observed during this time (25%-38% incidence) and is likely related to outcome [19]. For this and other reasons, early extubation may be associated with risk and is not appropriate in certain patients [20]. When early extubation is planned, aggressive control of pain is essential to decrease morbidity and mortality [8,9].

In the present study the central venous pressure, oxygen saturation, arterial blood gases and plasma lactate level remained almost constant throughout the study period with no statistical significant differences in both groups, there was a decrease in heart rate (HR) after induction and before bypass in relation to the baseline values in the morphine group and this decrease was statistically significant when compared with the control group, the mean arterial pressure (MAP) showed a decrease after induction, before bypass and after bypass in morphine group, in comparison with the baseline values, whereas in control group, this decrease was limited to after bypass time. Intrathecal opioid has been shown to provide effective analgesia following non-cardiac surgery [21] and cardiac surgery [22].

Our study agrees with Chiari et al. [23] in a study on analgesic and hemodynamic effects of intrathecal clonidine as the sole analgesic agent, showed that mean arterial pressure decreased significantly from baseline in all groups after injection of 50 µg, 100 µg, 200 µg, intrathecal clonidine onset time of this decrease was dose dependent. Heart rate decreased after injection of 100 µg, 200 µg intrathecal clonidine. However Ferreira C et al. injected subarachnoid in patients undergoing cardiac surgery with cardiopulmonary bypass and showed that the use of clonidine at the spinal dose of 1 µg/kg [1] was not able to reduce the intensity of response to surgical trauma [24].

Our study showed that plasma levels of cortisol in morphine group were lower than in control group, on admission to ICU and at the time of tracheal extubation.

Roediger et al. [25,26] who studied the use of pre-operative intrathecal morphine for analgesia following coronary bypass surgery, showed that catecholamines plasma concentration were significantly lower in the intrathecal group, plasma and urinary cortisol concentration were similar in both groups.

Our study also in agreement with Chaney et al. [26] who studied the effect of large-dose intrathecal morphine for coronary artery bypass grafting and found that norepinerphine and epinerphine levels tended to be lower in intrathecal morphine group patients than those in placebo, the difference was not statistically significant.

As regard extubation time, our study showed that patients who were tracheally extubated during the postoperative period, mean time to extubation was less after intrathecal morphine+clonidine (Group M) compared with the control group (Group C).

Our results go in hand with the work of Dominique et al. [27] in a study to compare the effect of combined intrathecal morphine and sufentanil with low-dose iv sufentanil during propofol anesthesia for fast-track cardiac surgery. The results of that study showed that intrathecal sufentanil and morphine allowed shorter duration of intubation.

In contrast to our result, Chaney et al. [26] found no difference in extubation times with either 4.0 mg or 10 ug/kg of intrathecal morphine compared with placebo. A relatively high dose of intraoperative fentanyl (50 and 20 μg/kg) may have a significant contributing factor for delayed extubation in these studies.

Our results are agreed with the work done by Chaney et al. [26] who investigated the use of large-dose intrathecal morphine for cardiac surgery and its effects on postoperative analgesic requirements. Patients were randomized to receive either 4.0 mg of intrathecal morphine or intrathecal saline placebo. The results of this study showed that patients in the intrathecal morphine group required significant less postoperative intravenous morphine than in intrathecal saline placebo, and was not surprisingly that they found that the analgesia produced from the dose (4.0 mg) lasted approximately 48 h (morning of operative day to morning of postoperative day 2).

Zarate et al. [14] who evaluate the use of remifentanil combined with intrathecal opioid on extubation time, analgesia, and intensive intrathecal morphine as an alternative to sufentanil during desflurane anesthesia. They concluded that intrathecal morphine provided superior pain control after cardiac surgery compared with a sufentanil general anesthetic technique.

Bowler et al. [28] who studied a combination of intrathecal morphine and remifentanil (RITM) for fast-track cardiac anesthesia and surgery. Patients in the RITM group exhibited significantly lower visual pain scores during the first 2 h after surgery, sedation score were significantly lower in the RITM during the first 3 h after extubation and postoperative morphine requirements during the 24 h were significantly lower in RITM than in the control group.

In our results as regard the side effects of intrathecal morphine, the incidence of nausea and vomiting was similar in both groups. Nausea and vomiting were controlled with standard antiemetic therapy. The pruritus experienced by 2 of the patients in the intrathecal morphine

group was only mild and did not need treatment. Other cardiac postoperative complications were similar in both groups.

Our results are in accordance with Zarare et al. [14] who found that, the incidence of postoperative, opioid-related side effects (e.g., nausea and vomiting, pruritus, and urinary retention) were small, and no differences were noted between the two groups.

The safety of an intrathecal injection immediately prior systemic heparinization required for CPB; It has been recommended that the technique should not be used in patients who demonstrate known preoperative coagulopathy from any cause, surgery should be delayed 24 h if a bloody tap occurs, and the time from lumbar puncture to systemic heparinization should exceed 60 min [29]. An analysis estimates the risk of spinal hematoma in patients receiving spinal blockade for cardiac surgery is in the range of 1:220,000 to 1:3600, with 95% confidence [30].

Conclusion

1. In conculsion, pre-operative intrathecal morphine administration of 250 μg in patients undergoing cardiac surgery improved analgesia and reduced opioid consumption, without increasing incidence of opioid related-side effects.

2. 250 μg intrathecal morphine appears to be the optimal dose of intrathecal morphine to provide significant postoperative analgesia without delaying tracheal extubation.

3. Low-dose ITM offer an alternative anesthetic technique, which appears to have some benefits over general anesthesia alone for cardiac surgery.

4. The combination of intrathecal morphine and clonidine allow the dose of morphine to be reduced, reduces the risk of respiratory depression, gives effective control of postoperative pain in cardiac patients and reduce the duration of controlled ventilation.

5. In patients with well-preserved ventricular and respiratory function scheduled for fast-track cardiac surgery, the use of combined intrathecal morphine and clonidine provides superior postoperative analgesia and early extubation.

6. Intrathecal morphine partially ameliorated the stress response to cardiac surgery.

References

1. Mueller XM, Tinguely F, Tevaearai HT (2000) Pain location, distribution, and intensity after cardiac surgery. Chest 118: 391-396.

2. Milgrom LB, Brooks JA, Qi R (2004) Pain levels experienced with activities after cardiac surgery. Am J Crit Care 13: 116-125.

3. Lahtinen P, Kokki H, Hynynen M (2006) Pain after cardiac surgery: a prospective cohort study of 1-year incidence and intensity. Anesthesiology 105: 794–800.

4. Mazzeffi M, Khelemsky Y (2011) Poststernotomy pain: a clinical review. J Cardiothorac Vasc Anesth 25: 1163-1178.

5. Baumgarten MC, Garcia GK, Frantzeski MH (2009) Pain and pulmonary function in patients submitted to heart surgery via sternotomy. Rev Bras Cir Cardiovasc 24: 497-505.

6. Sasseron AB, Figueiredo LC, Trova K (2009) Does the pain disturb the respiratory function after open heart surgery? Rev Bras Cir Cardiovasc 24: 490-496.

7. Bigeleisen PE, Goehner N (2015) Novel approaches in pain management in cardiac surgery. Curr Opin Anaesthesiol 28: 89-94.

8. Filsoufi F, Rahmanian PB, Castillo JG (2008) Predictors and early and late outcomes of respiratory failure in contemporary cardiac surgery. Chest 133: 713-721.

9. Ubben JF, Lance MD, Buhre WF (2015) Clinical strategies to prevent pulmonary complications in cardiac surgery: an overview. J Cardiothorac Vasc Anesth 29: 481-490.

10. Badenes R, Lozano A, Belda FJ (2015) Postoperative pulmonary dysfunction and mechanical ventilation in cardiac surgery. Crit Care Res Pract 2015: 420513.

11. Scott NB, Turfrey DJ, Ray DA (2001) A prospective randomized study of the potential benefits of thoracic epidural anesthesia and analgesia in patients undergoing coronary artery bypass grafting. Anesth Analg 93: 523-525.

12. Ossipov MH, Harris S, Lioyd P, Messineo E (1990) An isobolographic analysis of the antinociceptive effect of systemically and intrathecally administered combinations of clonidine and opiates. J Pharmacol Exp Ther 255: 1107-1116.

13. Liem TH, Booij LH, Gielen MJ (1992) Coronary artery bypass grating using two different anesthetic techniques: part 3 Adrenergic responses. J Cardiothorac Vasc Anesth 6: 162-167.

14. Zarate E, Latham P, White PF (2000) Fast- track cardiac anesthesia Use of remifentanil combined with intrathecal morphine as an alternative to sufentanil during desflurane anesthesia. Anesth Analg 91: 283-287.

15. Liu S, Carpenter RL, Neal JM (1995) Epidural anesthesia and analgesia their role in postoperative outcome. Anesthesiology 82: 1474-1506.

16. Scott LJ, Perry CM (2000) Tramadol: a review of its use in perioperative pain. Drugs 60: 139-176.

17. Tuman KJ, McCarthy RJ, March RJ (1991) Effects of epidural anesthesia and analgesia on coagulation and outcome after major vascular surgery . Anesth Analg 73: 696-704.

18. Cheng DCH (1995) Pro. Early extubation after cardiac surgery decreases intensive care unit stay and cost. J Cardiothorac Vasc Anesth 9: 460-464.

19. Smith RC, Leung JM, Mangano DT (1991) Postopertive myocardial ischemia in patients undergoing coronary artery bypass graft surgery. Anesthesiology 74: 464-473.

20. Guenther CR (1995) Early extubation after cardiac surgery decreases intensive care unit stay and cost. Con: early extubation after cardiac surgery dose not decrease intensive care unti stay and cost. J Cardiothorac Vasc Anesth 9: 465-467.

21. Derrode N, Lebrun F, Levron JC (2003) Influence of peroperative opioid on postoperative pain after major abdominal surgery: sufentanil TCI versus remifentanil TCI. A randomised, controlled study. British Journal of Anaesthesia 91: 842-849.

22. Fleron MH, Weiskopf RB, Bertrand MA (2003) Comparison of intrathecal opioid and intravenous analgesia for the incidence of cardiovascular, respiratory, and renal complications after abdominal aortic surgery. Anesthesia and Analgesia 97: 2-12.

23. Chiari A, Lober C, Eisenach JC (1999) Analgesic and hemodynamic effects of intrathecal clonidine as the sole analgesic agent during first stage of Labor: a dose response study. anesthesiology 91: 388-396.

24. Ferreira C, Tenório S (2014) Subarachnoid clonidine and trauma response in cardiac surgery with cardiopulmonary bypass. Rev Bras Anestesiol 64: 395-399.

25. Roediger L, Senard JJ, Larbuisson MR (2006) The use of pre-operative intrathecal morphine for analgesia following coronary artery bypass surgery. Anesthesia 61: 838-844.

26. Chaney MA, Smith KR, Barclay JC, Slogoff S (1996) Large dose intrathecal morphine for coronary artery bypass grafting. Anesth Analg 83: 215-222.

27. Dominique A, Schimidlin D (2002) Intrathecal sufentanil-morphine shortens the duration of intubation and improves analgesia in fast-track cardiac surgery. Can J Anesth 49: 711-717.

28. Lena P, Balarac N, Arnulf JJ (2005) Fast –track coronary artery bypass grafting surgery under general anesthesia with remifentanil and spinal analgesia with morphine and clonidine. J Cardiothorac Vasc Anesth 19: 49-53.

29. Vandermeulen EP, Van Aken H, Vermylen J (1994) Anticoagulantsand spinal epidural anesthesia. Anesth Analg 79: 1165-1177.

30. Ho AM, Chung DC, Joynt GM (2000) Neuraxial blockade and haematoma in cardiac surgery Estimating the risk of a rare adverse event that has not (yet) occurred. Chest 117: 551-555.

27

The Effects of Dexmedetomidine or Remifentanil Continuous Infusion on End-Tidal Sevoflurane Concentration in Patients Undergoing Laparoscopic Cholecystectomies, Monitored by Bispectral Analysis

Mona Mohamed Mogahed* and **Atteia Gad Anwar**

Faculty of Medicine, Tanta University, Tanta, Egypt

*Corresponding author: Mogahed MM, Anesthiology and Surgical Intensive Care, El Moatasem St, Faculty of Medicine, Tanta University, Tanta, Egypt, E-mail: monamogahedfr@hotmail.com

Abstract

Background and Objective: Owing to the hemodynamic response to pneumoperitoneum, laparoscopic is not devoid of risk; adjuvants have been used to decrease the dose of volatile agents and their side effects and to blunt the hemodynamic response. This study was designed to compare the effect of dexmedetomidine and remifentanil on sevoflurane expired fraction concentration (EF sevo) in general anesthesia, monitored by BIS. Hemodynamic response, postoperative recovery profile, analgesic requirements and PONV were also recorded.

Patients and methods: General anesthesia induction with propofol 2.5 mg/kg rocuronium bromide 0.6 mgkg and sevoflurane 1-1.5 MAC. Tracheal intubation was performed and patients were mechanically ventilated. Patients were allocated to Groups D or R. Group D (≤ 40) was the dexmedetomidine group, they received dexmedetomidine diluted with 0.9% NaCl to a concentration of 4 ugmL in 50 mL (an initial loading dose of 0.7 ug/kg given for a 10 min period followed by 0.5 ug/kg/h). Group D (n=40) was the dexmedetomidine group, they received dexmedetomidine (Precedex, 200 ug per 2 mL; Abbott, USA) (an initial loading dose of 0.7 ug/kg given for a 10 min period followed by 0.4 ug/kg/h). Group R (n=40) was the remifentanil group and received an intravenous (i.v.) remifentanil (an initial loading dose of 0.7 ug/kg given for a 10 min period followed by 0.2 ug/kg/h). The infusion was stopped 15 min before the end of surgery. sevoflurane concentration adjusted to maintain BIS between 40 and 60. The parameters evaluated (BIS, SBP, DBP, MAP, HR, and EF sevo) were expressed as mean and standard deviation at 15 min before induction, during induction of anesthesia, 15 min later, during pneumperitonium, after release of insufflation and 15 min after release of insufflation.

Statistical analysis: Student's t-test is a test of significance used for comparison of quantitative variables between two groups of normally distributed data, while Mann Whitney's test was used for comparison of quantitative variables between two groups of not normally distributed data. Chi-square test ($\chi2$) was used to study association between qualitative variables. Whenever any of the expected cells were less than five, Fischer's Exact test with Yates correction was used. P-value of <0.05 was considered statistically significant.

Results: No patients had marked hypotension MAP less than 60 mmHg or bradycardia HR less than 45 in both groups but there were significant decrease in HR and MAP between the two groups during induction, 15 min after induction, during pneumperitonium, aftert release of insufflation and 15 min after release of insufflation, extubation time, spontaneous eye movement, eye movement to verbal stimuli, spontaneous arm movement, purposeful movement and time of discharge to recovery room were significantly lower in group R than group D, However group R showed significantly higher EF sevo 15 min after induc, BSI during insufflation of CO_2, EF sevo during insufflation of CO_2, BSI after release. CO_2, EF sevo after release of CO_2, BSI before end of surgery and EF sevo before end of surgery than group D.

Conclusion: Both dexmedetomidine and remifentanil reduce the anesthetic requirement and depress the hemodynamic response during pneumoperitoneum with more significant decrease in EF sevo in the D group, however dexmedetomidine provides better postoperative analgesia and less incidence of PONV.

Keywords: Bispectral index; Dexmedetomidine; Remifentanil; Sevoflurane

Introduction

Laparoscopic cholecystectomy (LC) procedure is a more preferable technique than open cholecystectomy in the treatment of symptomatic cholelithiasis; [1] it reduces postoperative pain, with faster recovery and more rapid return to normal activities and lesser hospital stay [2].

Several adjuvants have been used to decrease the dose of inhalational agents and to provide better sedation, hypnosis, and analgesia [3].

Dexmedetomidine is a potent alpha-2 adrenoreceptor agonist and reduces the volatile anesthetics requirements. It has beneficial properties when used in anesthesia as it provides better hemodynamic and adrenergic stability *via* its sympatholytic action, sedation and decreased anesthetic and analgesic consumption without marked ventilatory depression [4]. Remifentanil is an analogue of fentanyl its rapid onset and half time of nearly three to five min make it an easy drug to control for achieving the desired depth of anesthesia and its rapid offset provides optimal analgesia without any delayed recovery [5].

The most common method of titration of volatile anesthetics is the minimum alveolar concentration (MAC) but, this includes chiefly the immobilizing potency (prevention of movement to skin incision in 50% of patients) of the anesthetic agent [6].

The dose of the hypnotic agent used to maintain the patient unconscious is detected by bispectral index (BIS) which is EEG-derived parameter. Many studies have shown that BIS has a great correlation with the brain metabolism and with hypnotic and sedative effects of various anesthetic agents as isoflurane, sevoflurane, midazolam and propofol [7,8].

The aim of this study was to evaluate the influence of either dexmedetomidine or remifentanil continuous infusion on expiratory fraction sevoflurane concentration (EF sevo) during general anesthesia, monitored by bispectral index (BIS).

Methods

After institutional review board approval and written informed consent, 80 ASA I-II patients their ages were between 40 and 50 years old and their weight were between 80 and 90 Kg scheduled for elective Videolaparoscopic cholecystectomy were included in a prospective, randomized, double-blind study and equally divided into two groups, Dexmedetomidine (D group) and Remifentanil (R group). Patients were excluded if they had severe cardiac disease, chronic obstructive lung disease, renal and hepatic insufficiency, endocrine, metabolic or central nervous system disorders, a-2-agonist or antagonist therapy taken, and active upper respiratory infection, those receiving medications known to affect MAC, or having a history of alcohol or drug abuse; and women who were lactating or pregnant. One of the anesthetists participating into the study randomized patients into one of the two study groups, using a computer- generated random number table. Study drugs (dexmedetomidine and remifentanil) were prepared by a nurse without any marks on the syringes. The same nurse who knew the study protocol adjusted the perfused dose and the perfuser's syringe and screen were covered to enable double blindness throughout the operation, and no change of the dose was allowed. The anesthetist blinded to the drug continued with the anesthesia process and recorded the study parameters.

All patients had general anesthesia induction, after previous oxygenation for 3 min, at anesthesia induction with propofol 2.5 mg/kg rocuronium bromide 0.6 mgkg and sevoflurane 1-1.5 MAC. Tracheal intubation was performed and patients were mechanically ventilated with 100% oxygen inspired fraction (FiO_2), 2.5 L/min fresh gas flow and 8 mL/kg tidal volume, with respiratory rate adjusted to maintain ET CO^2 between 35 and 40 mmHg, using circle system with CO_2 absorber.

In this double-blind study, patients were allocated to Groups D or R. Group D («=40) was the dexmedetomidine group, they received dexmedetomidine (Precedex, 200 ug per 2 mL; Abbott, USA) (an initial loading dose of 0.7 ug/kg given for a 10 min period followed by

0.4 ug/kg/h). Group R (n=40) was the remifentanil group and received an intravenous (i.v.) remifentanil (an initial loading dose of 0.7 ug/kg given for a 10 min period followed by 0.2 ug/kg/h). Dexmedetomidine or remifentanil was prepared and administered using a syringe pump (Fresenius-Vial-Pilot A2 perfuser; Homburg, Germany) by the same nurse and the infusion was stopped 15 min before the end of surgery.

Anesthetic depth was controlled by varying sevoflurane concentration to maintain BIS between 40 and 60. Muscle relaxation was achieved by rocuronium bromide 0.3 mgkg for maintenance of neuromuscular blockade but no intraoperative narcotics were used in both groups. During the perioperative period, both groups received i.v lactated ringer solution at 4 mL/kg.

In the operating room, routine monitoring (Cardiocaps/5; Datex-Ohmeda, Helsinki, Finland) included five lead electrocardiogram (ECG), pulse oximeter, non-invasive blood pressure (BP) measurement. Electrodes for monitoring the Bispectral Index (BISTM, model A-2000s; Aspect Medical Systems, Norwood, MA, USA) were attached to the head and an iv. line was sited. End-tidal CO_2 ($ETCO_2$) concentration and end-expiratory concentration of sevoflurane were also recorded (Cardiocaps/5) from the time of anesthesia induction to the time of extubation.

The parameters evaluated (BIS, SBP, DBP, MAP, HR, and EF sevo) were expressed as mean and standard deviation in moments at 15 min before induction, during induction of anesthesia, 15 min later, during pneumperitonium, after release of insufflation and 15 min after release of insufflation. Twenty min before the end of surgery, all patients received, dexamethasone 8 mg, ondansetron 4 mg for the prevention of postoperative nausea and vomiting (PONV). Infusion drugs were turned off 15 min before the completion of surgery and patients were ventilated with 100% oxygen at 5 L/min. Following a spontaneous recovery, a combination of atropine 0.02 mg/kg and neostigmine 0.05 mg/kg was administered i.v. to reverse the neuromuscular block. The endotracheal tube was removed when the patient was fully awake. Patients were kept in the post-anesthesia care unit for 2 h.

Sedation was assessed using Ramsay Sedation Scale (RSS) by a blinded nurse, at 5, 15 and 30 min following tracheal extubation. Pain were assessed using a Visual Analog Scale (VAS) from 0 to 10, where 0 no pain and 10 the worst imaginable pain. The predetermined analgesia level was set as a VAS, 4 and rescue i.v. bolus doses of fentanyl (25 mg) were administered if the initial regimen failed to achieve or maintain this goal or if the patient asked for additional analgesics. The presence of PONV and the need for additional analgesics or antiemetics were recorded.

Statistical analysis of the collected data

Results were collected, tabulated and statistically analyzed by an IBM compatible personal computer with SPSS statistical package version 20 (SPSS Inc. Realesed 2011. IBM SPSS statistics for windows, version 20.0, Armnok, NY: IBM Corp.).

Two types of statistical analysis were done:

a) Descriptive statistics: e.g. was expressed in: Number (No), percentage (%) mean ($\bar{x}$) and standard deviation (SD).

b) Analytic statistics: e.g. 1-Student's t-test is a test of significance used for comparison of quantitative variables between two groups of normally distributed data, while Mann Whitney's test was used for comparison of quantitative variables between two groups of not normally distributed data. 2 Chi-square test ($\chi2$) was used to study association between qualitative variables. Whenever any of the expected cells were less than five, Fischer's Exact test with Yates correction was used. P value of <0.05 was considered statistically significant.

We planned a study of a continuous response variable from independent control and experimental subjects with 1 control (s) per experimental subject. In a previous study (Paventi et al.) [9], the response within each subject group was normally distributed with standard deviation 0.7. If the true difference in the experimental and control means is 0.5, we will need to study 36 experimental subjects and 36 control subjects (which we rounded to 40) to be able to reject the null hypothesis that the population means of the experimental and control groups are equal with probability (power) 0.85. The Type I error probability associated with this test of this null hypothesis is 0.05.

Logistic regression was not done as prediction was not an aim of this work , however, the 2 groups were matched at the beginning of the study for gender, age and ASA (Table 1).

Results

Variable	No.	%
Gender		
Male	17	21.3
Female	63	78.8
ASA		
I	58	72.5
II	22	27.5
Mean ± SD		
Age	42.7 ± 3.43	
Weight	88.78 ± 4.13	
Surgical time	85.96 ± 6.11	

Table 1: Socio-demographic data of the studied group.

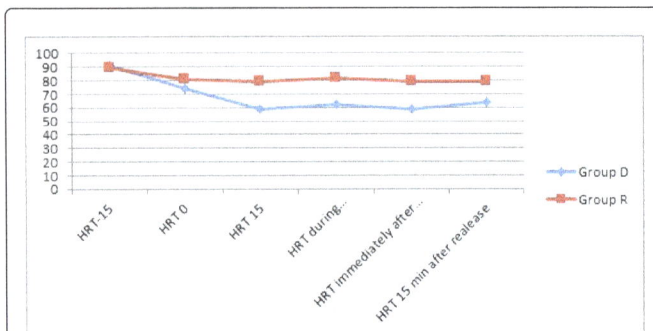

Figure 1: Heart rate (HRT) at different times readings in the 2 studied groups.

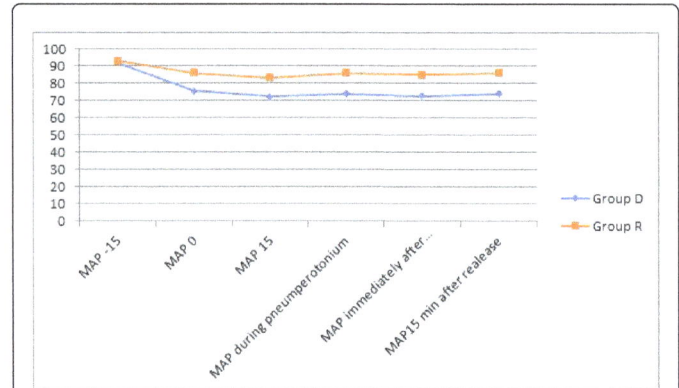

Figure 2: Mean arterial blood pressure (MAP) at different times readings in the 2 studied groups.

No patients had marked hypotension MAP less than 60 mmHg or bradycardia HR less than 45 in both groups but there were significant decrease in HR and MAP between the two groups during induction, 15 min after induction, during pneumperitonium, aftert release of insufflation and 15 min after release of insufflation (Figures 1 and 2).

	Group D (n=40) Mean ± SD	Group R (n=40) Mean ± SD	t-test	P value
Extubation time:	18.80 ± 2.69	4.40 ± 0.90	32.09	<0.001
Spontaneous eye move.	7.57 ± 1.41	2.36 ± 0.65	21.20	<0.001
Eye movement to verbal:	8.92 ± 1.50	3.31 ± 0.76	20.98	<0.001
Spontaneous arm movement:	4.67 ± 0.47	2.46 ± 0.65	17.31	<0.001
Purposeful movement:	6.60 ± 0.81	1.97 ± 0.72	7.86*	<0.001
Time of discharge to recovery room:	21.30 ± 2.78	6.27 ± 0.98	32.16	<0.001
*Mann Whitney test				

Table 2: This table shows that extubation time, spontaneous eye movement, eye movement to verbal stimuli, spontaneous arm movement, purposeful movement and time of discharge to recovery room were significantly lower in group R than group D.

Table 2 shows that extubation time, spontaneous eye movement, eye movement to verbal stimuli, spontaneous arm movement, purposeful movement and time of discharge to recovery room were significantly lower in group R than group D.

	Group D (n=40) Mean ± SD	Group R (n=40) Mean ± SD	t-test	P value

VAS at 5 min	2.05 ± 0.74	1.57 ± 0.63	3.05	0.003
VAS at 15 min	3.32 ± 0.72	4.37 ± 0.49	7.55	<0.001
VAS at 30 min	4.02 ± 0.83	4.90 ± 0.78	5.06	<0.001

Table 3: Mean visual analogue score (VAS) score at different times in both groups.

VAS score at 5 min was significantly higher in group D than group Rhowever it turned to be significantly higher in group R than group D at 15 and 30 min (Table 3).

	Group D (n=40) Mean ± SD	Group R (n=40) Mean ± SD	t-test	P value
Sedation score at 5 min	3.67 ± 0.47	1.50 ± 0.50	19.82	<0.001
Sedation score at 15 min	2.50 ± 0.50	1.07 ± 0.26	15.74	<0.001
Sedation at 30 min	1.22 ± 0.42	1.00 ± 0.00	3.36	0.002

Table 4: Mean sedation score at different times in both groups.

Sedation score was significantly higher in group D than group R at 5 min, 15 min and 30 min (Table 4).

	Group D (n=40) No. %		Group R (n=40) No. %		χ^2	P value
Need for analgesia						
No	24	60.0	12	30.0	7.27	0.007
Yes	16	40.0	28	70.0		
Nausea 1 h						
No	36	90.0	31	9	2.29	0.13
Yes	4	10.0	77.5	22.5		
Nausea 2 h						
No	38	2	35	5	0.63*	0.42
Yes	95.0	5.0	87.5	12.5		
Vomiting 1 h						
No	39	1	36	4 10.0	0.85*	0.35
Yes	97.5	2.5	90.0			
Vomiting 2 h						
No	40	100.0	38	2	0.51*	0.47
Yes	0	0.0	95.0	5.0		
*Fisher's Exact test						

Table 5: The need for analgesia and postoperative nausea and vomiting at 1 and 2 hours postoperatively.

The need of analgesia was significantly higher in group R than group D, however nausea and vomiting at 1 and 2 h were not statistically significantly different (Table 5).

	Group D (n=40) Mean ± SD	Group R (n=40) Mean ± SD	t-test	P value
BSI base line	97.97 ± 0.15	97.97 ± 0.15	0.00	1.00
BSI 15 min after induc	50.67 ± 2.41	51.52 ± 3.12	1.36	0.17
EF sevo 15 min after induc	2.00 ± 0.10	2.09 ± 0.16	3.08	0.003
BSI during insuf CO_2	53.55 ± 2.64	55.02 ± 2.09	2.76	0.007
EF sevo during insuf CO_2	1.46 ± 0.15	1.61 ± 0.19	3.97	<0.001
BSI after release of CO_2	53.12 ± 2.66	55.42 ± 2.06	4.32	<0.001
EF sevo after release of CO_2	0.82 ± 0.10	0.92 ± 0.17	2.97	0.004
BSI before end of surgery	54.80 ± 2.38	56.30 ± 1.80	3.17	0.002
EF sevo before end of surgery	0.23 ± 0.07	0.61 ± 0.12	16.29	<0.001

Table 6: BSI and EF sevo at different times in the two groups.

BSI : Bispectral index.

EF sevo : Expiratory fraction of sevoflurane.

Group R showed significantly higher EF sevo 15 min after induc, BSI during insufflation of CO_2, EF sevo during insufflation of CO_2, BSI after release CO_2, EF sevo after release of CO_2, BSI before end of surgery and EF sevo before end of surgery than group D (Table 6).

Discussion

In this study, we compared dexmedetomidine and remifentanyl in hemodynamic stability, the dose of inhalational anesthetics, Recovery parameters and post-operative analgesic requirements in patients undergoing laparoscopic cholecystectomy. This study demonstrates that both drugs blunted the smpathoadrenal responces during surgery, however dexmedetomidine had superior postoperative pain control efficacy and reduced the analgesic requirement and PONV incidence compared to remifentanil. Dexmedetomidine is an ideal sedative as it is a highly selective alpha-2-agonist, with a shorter duration of action than clonidine, [10] it produces a state of hypnosis similar to normal sleep, it doesn't depress the respiration. [11] It has a good analgesic effect by suppression of the nociceptive neurotransmission and inhibition of pain signals propagation. Its sympatholytic effect causes reduction of blood pressure and heart rate; that help in attenuation of the stress response of surgery [12]. It also attenuates the sympathoadrenal effects of tracheal intubation [12]. The ultra-short acting mu opioids receptor agonist, remifentanil [5] is a potent opioid and has predictable controllability owing to its short half-life and rapid elimination; thus make it has an ultrashort duration of analgesia [13,14].

Some studies [15-17] have shown the role of dexmedetomidine both loading and maintenance dose in reducing the dose of inhalational anesthetics and other studies [18,19] have shown the role of remifentanil in reducing the dose of inhalational anesthetics. In our study, BIS monitoring was allowed for maintaining anesthetic depth within a standard variation to avoid unnecessary deep anesthesia or awareness, we noticed that the sevoflurane requirements were decreased in both groups as the intraoperative BIS-guided sevoflurane alteration led to decrease in the fraction of exspired concentration of sevoflurane (EF sevo). Thus, the EF sevo became significantly lower in group D than in group R 15 min after induction, during pneumperitonium, after release of insufflation and before the end of surgery.

Shin et al. [15] gave preanaesthetic dexmedetomidine 1µg/kg single infusion and found that patients had the end-tidal concentration and total sevoflurane consumption were significantly reduced in dexmedetomidine group more than in control group. Ozcengiz et al. [20] noted in minor surgeries in children that end-tidal sevoflurane concentration was significantly lower in dexmedetomidine group prior to incision, after incision, and after the surgery than in control group. Ohtani et al. [21] made a study in patients undergoing lower abdominal surgeries and found that dexmedetomidine decreased the anesthetic requirements needed to keep BIS of 45 by 20–30%, reducing sevoflurane from $1.1 \pm 0.2\%$ to $0.8 \pm 0.2\%$ and propofol from 4.4 ± 0.8 mg/kg/h to 3.1 ± 1 mg/kg/h. Keniya et al. 13 found that dexmedetomidine has significant opioid and anesthetic sparing property. It significantly reduces the sympathoadrenal response to tracheal intubation. Ni W et al. [22] showed that remifentanil effectively decreased the sympathetic adrenergic response to CO_2 pneumoperitoneum stimulus, and decreased the end-tidal sevoflurane concentration needed during anesthesia.

In our study the pain stimuli included a small skin incision and the distension of the peritoneum by CO_2 pneumoperitoneum expected to induce a violent sympathetic adrenergic response but both dexmedetomidine and remifentanil are effective to blunt hemodynamic responses all over the surgery.

During the maintenance of anesthesia in group D, we observed significant decrease in HR and MABP values, this is may be due to the combined effect of vasodilatation and myocardial depression with volatile agents. statistically significant hypotension and bradycardia was reported by Patel et al. [23] in patients received dexmedetomidine throughout the intraoperative period with partial blunting of response to intubation and reduction of sevoflurane consumption. While group R showed no significant changes all over the surgery in the hemodynamics. These desirable effects of remifentanil on hemodynamic stability has been shown in previous studies using different doses of remifentanil [24-27].

Our study also showed that patients in group D had a prolonged extubation time than patients in group R. Also Spontaneous eye move, Eye movement to verbal stimli, Spontaneous arm movement, Purposeful movement and Time of discharge to recovery room were more delayed in group D as shown in Table 3 and the postoperative sedation was significant in group D.

Song D et al. [27] found that awakening and extubation times decreased on using of remifentanil (0.05-0.2 µg/kg/min) in obese patients had sevoflurane anesthesia undergoing a laparoscopic cholecystectomy.

Patel et al. [23] in their study observed that postoperatively dexmedetomidine group showed a significant sedation at 2 h compared to control group. Shin et al. reported similar findings [15]. Ebert TJ et al. explained this by the 2 h elimination half-life of dexmedetomidine [11].

In our study as compared to remifentanil, dexmedetomidine also reduced the analgesic requirements; in group D 40% (16 patients) while in group R 70% (28 patients) needed analgesia in the postoperative period. Damian J et al. showed that an alternative analgesic should be given before discontinuation of remifentanil [18]. Previous studies have shown the postoperative analgesic effect of dexmedetomidine [28,29]. and other studies have demonstrated that dexmedetomidine had superior efficacy compared to remifentanil in pain management during a PACU stay [30,31].

Our results showed that PONV incidence was lower in group D; as the incidence of nausea and vomiting during the first 2 h were lower in group than in group R. This was in consistence with Hwang W et al. who compared dexmedetomidine and remifentanil as adjuvants in propofol-based TIVA and found that dexmedetomidine produced more efficient pain control and lesser incidence of PONV [30].

Conclusion

We conclude that any of the two anesthetic techniques are acceptable for in laparoscopic cholecystectomy, both groups are effective in reducing sevoflurane requirement and blunt hemodynamic response during pneumoperitoneum with more significant decrease in EF sevo with dexmedetomidine. Remifentanil provides earlier recovery but with less postoperative analgesia and more incidence of PONV than dexmedetomidine.

References

1. Vivek MA, Augustine AJ, Rao R (2014) A comprehensive predictive scoring method for difficult laparoscopic cholecystectomy. J Minim Access Surg 10: 62-67.

2. Gerges FJ, Kanazi GE, Jabbour-Khoury SI (2006) Anesthesia for laparoscopy: a review. J Clin Anesth 18: 67-78.

3. Ebert TJ, Schmid PG (2001) Inhalation anaesthesia. In: Barash PG, Cullen BF, Stoelting RK, editors. Clinical Anaesthesia. Philadelphia: Lippincott Williams and Wilkins 2000: 377-417.

4. Shin H, Yoo HN, Kim DH, Lee H, Shin HJ, et al. (2013) Preanaesthetic dexmedetomidine 1µg/kg single infusion is a simple, easy and an economic adjuvant for general anaesthesia. Korean J Anaesthesiol 65: 114-120.

5. Beers R, Camporesi E (2004) Remifentanil update: clinical science and utility. CNS Drugs 18: 1085-1104.

6. Rampil IJ, Mason P, Singh H (1993) Anesthetic potency (MAC) is independent of Forebrain structures in threat. Anesthesiology 78: 707-712.

7. Glass PS, Bloom M, Kearse L, Rosow C, Sebel P, et al. (1997) Bispectral analysis measures sedation and memory effects of propofol, midazolam, isoflurane, and alfentanil in healthy volunteers. Anesthesiology 86: 836-847.

8. Song D, Joshi GP, White PF (1997) Titration of volatile anesthetics using bispectral index facilitates recovery after ambulatory anesthesia. Anesthesiology 87: 842-848.

9. Paventi S, Santevencchi A, Sollazzi L (2002) Effect oe remifentanil infusion bispectral titrated in early recoveryfor obese outpatients undergoing laparoscopic cholecystectomy. Minerva Anesthesiologica 68: 351-357.

10. Kaur M, Singh PM (2011) Current role of dexmedetomidine in clinical anesthesia and intensive care. Anesth Essays Res 5: 128-133.

11. Ebert TJ, Hall JE, Barney JA, Uhrich TD, Colinco MD (2000) The effects of increasing plasma concentrations of dexmedetomidine in humans. Anesthesiology 93: 382-394.

12. Grewal A (2011) Dexmedetomidine: New avenues. J Anaesthesiol Clin Pharmacol 27: 297-302.

13. Keniya VM, Ladi S, Naphade R (2011) Dexmedetomidine attenuates sympathoadrenal response to tracheal intubation and reduces perioperative anaesthetic requirement. Indian J Anaesth 55: 352-357.

14. Fan Q, Hu C, Ye M, Shen X (2015) Dexmedetomidine for tracheal extubation in deeply anesthetized adult patients after otologic surgery: a comparison with remifentanil. BMC Anesthesiology 15: 106-107.

15. Shin H, Yoo HN, Kim DH, Lee H, Shin HJ, et al. (2013) Preanaesthetic dexmedetomidine 1μg/kg single infusion is a simple, easy and an economic adjuvant for general anaesthesia. Korean J Anaesthesiol 65: 114-120.

16. Ghodki PS, Thombre SK, Sardesai SP, Harnagle KD (2012) Dexmedetomidine as an anesthetic adjuvant in laparoscopic surgery: An observational study using entropy monitoring. J Anaesthesiol Clin Pharmacol 28: 334-338.

17. Reshma B Muniyappa, Geetha C Rajappa, Suresh Govindswamy, Prathima P (2016) Effect of dexmedetomidine bolus dose on isoflurane consumption in surgical patients under general anesthesia. Anesth Essays Res 10: 649-654.

18. Damian J, William M, Natalie A (2005) Remifentanil decreases sevoflurane requirements in children. Can J Anaesth 52: 1064–1070.

19. Albertin A, Casati A, Bergonzi P, Fano G, Torri G (2004) Effects of two target-controlled concentrations (1 and 3 ng/ml) of remifentanil on MACBAR of sevoflurane. Anesthesiology 100: 255–259.

20. Ozcengiz D, Unlügenç H, Günes Y, Karacaer F (2012) The effect of dexmedetomidine on bispectral index monitoring in children. Middle East J Anaesthesiol 21: 613-618.

21. Ohtani N, Kida K, Shoji K, Yasui Y, Masaki E (2008) Recovery profiles from dexmedetomidine as a general anesthetic adjuvant in patients undergoing lower abdominal surgery. Anesth Analg 107: 1871-1874.

22. Ni WG, Zhong TD (2007) Effects of different target concentrations of remifentanil onMAC-BAR of sevoflurane in patients during abdominal surgery. Chin J Anesthesiol 27: 588-590.

23. Patel CR, Engineer SR, Shah BJ, Madhu S (2013) The effect of dexmedetomidine continuous infusion as an adjuvant to general anesthesia on sevoflurane requirements: A study based on entropy analysis. J Anaesthesiol Clin Pharmacol 29: 318-322.

24. Park BY, Jeong CW, Jang EA, Kim SJ, Jeong ST, et al. (2011) Dose-related attenuation of cardiovascular responses to tracheal intubation by intravenous remifentanil bolus in severe pre-eclamptic patients undergoing Caesarean delivery. Br J Anaesth 106: 82-87.

25. Yoo KY, Kang DH, Jeong H, Jeong CW, Choi YY, et al. (2013) A dose-response study of remifentanil for attenuation of the hypertensive response to laryngoscopy and tracheal intubation in severely preeclamptic women undergoing caesarean delivery under general anaesthesia. Int J Obstet Anesth 22: 10-18.

26. Li C, Li Y, Wang K, Kong X (2015) Comparative Evaluation of Remifentanil and Dexmedetomidine in General Anesthesia for Cesarean Delivery. Med Sci Monit 21: 3806-3813

27. Song D, Whitten CW, White PF (2000) Remifentanil infusion facilitates early recovery for obese outpatients undergoing laparoscopic cholecystectomy. Anesth Analg 90: 1111-1113.

28. Gurbet A, BasaganMogol E, Turker G, Ugun F, Kaya FN, et al. (2006) Intraoperative infusion of dexmedetomidine reduces perioperative analgesic requirements. Can J Anaesth 53: 646-652.

29. Feld JM, Hoffman WE, Stechert MM, Hoffman IW, Ananda RC (2006) Fentanyl or dexmedetomidine combined with desflurane for bariatric surgery. J Clin Anesth 18: 24-28.

30. Hwang W, Lee J, Park J, Joo J (2015) Dexmedetomidine versus remifentanil in postoperative pain control after spinal surgery: a randomized controlled study. BMC Anesthiol 15: 21.

31. Sahoo J, Sujata P, Sahu M (2016) Comparative Study Betweeen Dexmedetomidine and Remifentanyl for Efficient Pain and Ponv Management. Int J Pharm Sci Rev Res 38: 212-216.

28

The Efficacy of Non Inflatable Cuff (I-gel and SLIPA) Versus Inflatable Cuff (Soft Seal LMA) Supraglottic Airways in Paralyzed Adult Patients

Mona Mohamed Mogahed* and Atteia Gad Anwar

Faculty of Medicine, Tanta University, Tanta, Egypt

***Corresponding author:** Mogahed MM, Anesthiology and Surgical Intensive Care, El Moatasem St, Faculty of Medicine, Tanta University, Tanta, Egypt, E-mail: monamogahedfr@hotmail.com

Abstract

Aim: To compare the efficacy of non-inflatable cuff supraglottic airways (I-gel and SLIPA) to inflatable cuff soft seal Laryngeal mask airway (SSLMA) in patients requiring general anesthesia and controlled ventilation during elective surgical procedures.

Patients and methods: An experimental study design was used, with comparison of three groups of patients using i-gel, SLIPA and SSLMA. Patients with risk of gastro esophageal reflux were excluded. Ease of insertion, quality of seal, effective ventilation, hemodynamic responses, side effects and surgical time were assessed. . An Oropharyngeal sealing pressure or 'leak' test was performed with the airway devices to quantify the efficacy of the seal with the patient airway. Airway sealing pressure tests claimed to be excellent for clinical purposes.

Results: Overall success of insertion was 100% in i-gel, 97.5% and 95% in SSLMA and SLIPA respectively. The i-gel permitted ventilation with a significantly high tidal volume (485 ± 82 ml) at a significantly low peak airway pressure (12 ± 3 cmH$_2$O) and a significantly high leak pressure (26 ± 6.3 cmH$_2$O). All groups show stable hemodynamic responses to insertion and removal of the devices. Insertion time was significantly shorter with i-gel (15 ± 2.5 sec.) compared to SLIPA and SSLMA, 22 ± 4.6 sec. and 19 ± 3.85 sec, respectively. Sore throat was significantly high in SSLMA 30%. Whereas, blood traces on the device and gastric air insufflations were highly significant with SLIPA 8% and 10% respectively.

Conclusion: The three disposable SGAs proved to be suitable for controlled ventilation during elective short surgical operations. The i-gel provides effective ventilation with minimal side effects. Whereas, SLIPA is associated with a high incidence of gastric air insufflations, The Soft Seal LMA provides high leakage volume and incidence of sore throat postoperatively.

Keywords: Laryngeal masks; i-gel; SLIPA; SSLMA; Comparison

Introduction

The supraglottic airway devices (SGAs) are devices that designed to be inserted above the level of the vocal cord for ventilation during spontaneous or intermittent positive pressure ventilation [1]. SGAs provide a possible alternative technique to the use of tracheal tubes during elective surgical procedures. Blind insertion and effective positive pressure ventilation are the advantages of SGAs. The The supraglottic airways are established devices during general anesthesia, for difficult airway management and for airway management during cardiopulmonary resuscitation [2]. SGAs with non-inflatable cuff include The i-gel (Intersurgical Ltd., Wokingham, Berkshire, UK) which is a single-use supraglottic airway device provides a seal without cuff inflation. Its drain tube prevents both gastric insufflations and aspiration, facilitates gastric tube insertion [3]. And the streamlined liner of the pharynx airway (SLIPA Medical Ltd, Douglas, Isle of Man, UK) which is a disposable SAD made of plastic material. It is a hollow boot shaped chamber similar to the contour of the pharynx [4]. SLIPA is designed to decrease the risk of aspiration during positive pressure ventilation [5]. This relates to the large capacity of its hollow structure (50 mL) which is almost double the volume of the stomach contents (26 mL) in fasted patients [6]. The LMA challenged the gold standard of endotracheal intubation with a cuffed tube to maintain a clear airway and provide positive pressure ventilation with a lower risk of trauma [7]. A new single-use disposable supraglottic airway device, the Soft Seal LM (Portex Ltd., Hythe Kent, United Kingdom), has been introduced recently. It is fabricated from latex-free medical-grade plasticized polyvinyl chloride (PVC) [8].

Patients and Methods

A total of 120 patients scheduled for elective general surgery were consecutively recruited in the study. Only patients classified as ASA I and II were eligible for inclusion. The exclusion criteria were high risk for pulmonary aspiration: diabetic, obese and pregnant women. Patients having lung disease, difficult airway, surgery performed in non supine position, oral or nasal surgery and preoperative sore throat were also excluded.

Approval was given by the Hospital Ethics Committee prior to study commencement. Informed signed consent was obtained from each patient participating in the study. The maneuvers and medications used are not harmful to the patients when professionally used, and have been used in the management of similar cases.

During pre-anesthetic evaluation, the patient's age, gender, heights, weights, Mallampati grade mouth opening and thyromental distance were recorded. After placement of pulse oximeter (SPO$_2$), electrocardiogram (ECG) and non-invasive blood pressure (NIBP) monitor, intravenous 1 µg/kg fentanyl was given. Following pre-oxygenation for 3 min, anesthesia was induced with 3 mg/kg propofol and 0.5 mg/kg rocuronium. The lungs were ventilated manually with sevoflurane (2%-3%) and O$_2$ 100% via a facemask with or without the use of an oral airway. One minute later a single anesthesiologist inserted the airway device as out-lined in the manufacturer's instructions. Before insertion, a water-soluble lubricant was applied to all devices. The i-gel was grasped along the integral bite block and was introduced into the mouth towards the hard palate until resistance was felt. The SLIPATM was introduced into the pharynx. The SSLMA was introduced with the cuff partially inflated till a definite resistance was felt as the tip entered the hypopharynx. The cuff was inflated to a 'just seal' pressure, defined as no leak on gentle manual ventilation. If substantial leakage occurred despite optimal placement another 10 ml of air was added. Then the SGA was secured after successful placement.

Successful placement and adequate ventilation was confirmed by clinically observing bilateral chest wall movement, square capnogram waveform during manual ventilation, and silent epigastrium by auscultation. An Oropharyngeal sealing pressure tests were performed using continuous fresh gas flow of 3 L/min was set with the adjustable pressure-limiting valve closed and the circuit connected to the reservoir bag. Stopping ventilation, keeping the patient apneic, and recording the airway pressure at which equilibrium was achieved. At this time, air leak can be detected at the mouth by hearing an audible noise coming from the mouth or by putting a stethoscope just lateral to the thyroid cartilage The leak volume was calculated as the difference between the inspired and the expired tidal volumes [9]. Intermittent positive pressure ventilation with tidal volume 8ml/kg and respiratory rate of 10/min, then started. Tidal volume and respiratory rate were adjusted to maintain ETCO$_2$ between 35 and 40 mmHg. Anesthesia was maintained with sevoflurane (2%-3%). Intraoperative analgesia was maintained with intravenous infusion of diclofenac sodium 75 mg in 100 ml normal saline, with supplementary fentanyl 25-50 µg iv given as required. Rocuronium 0.1mg every 20 min was given.

If the first insertion was unsuccessful, the patient received a supplementary dose of propofol up to 1 mg/kg and the head was repositioned to permit another attempt. If the third attempt was unsuccessful, it was to be recorded as a failure and the patient had an endotracheal tube inserted. An unsuccessful attempt of insertion was defined as placement of the device into the mouth and withdrawal from the mouth. Insertion time was noted i.e. the time (in sec) taken from opening the patient's mouth to successful SGAs insertion. The size of the SSLMA and i-gel were chosen, based upon body weight, according to the manufacturer's recommendations. The SLIPA size was chosen by matching the width across the thyroid cartilage with that of the bridge of the SLIPA. Blood pressure, heart rate and O$_2$ saturation were measured before anesthesia, immediately before airway

placement, and five minutes after placing the airway. Gastric air insufflations were monitored by auscultation of the patient's stomach, immediately after insertion of the airway, after positioning, and at the end of surgery. After surgery, muscle relaxant was reversed by atropine and neostigmine. Once consciousness is regained and protective reflexes have returned, gentle suction around the airway device in the pharynx and hypopharynx, by asking the patient to open his/her mouth wide, was done. SGA was removed and replaced with oxygen facemask. The blood or gastric fluids on SGA devices were noted. In the recovery room, the patient continued to breathe oxygen and was monitored for 30 minutes. Presence of sore throat was enquired at 2 and 24 hours after surgery.

Thereafter, the single anesthesiologist who inserted the devices gave a subjective assessment of the insertion procedure and the handling of each device. The overall performance was rated as high, moderate, low and poor.

Results

Table 1 shows the demographic data of the patients. All groups were similar as regards age and sex distribution. No statistically significant differences were revealed regarding their body weight and height, ASA classification, predictors of difficult airway and duration of surgeries.

	i-gel (n _40)	SLIPA (n _40)	SSLMA (n_40)	P value
Height (cm)	165 ± 5	169 ± 5	170 ± 6	0.214
Weight (kg)	786	75 ± 4	74 ± 6	0.986
Age (yr)	55 ± 10	49 ± 13	52 ± 12	0.241
Sex (M – F)	30-Oct	25/15	21/19	0.112
ASA I/II	23/17	25/15	22/18	0.78
Mallampati I/II/III /IV	20/16/4/0	21/16/3/0	19/18/3 /0	-
Mouth opening (mm)	49 ± 10	50 ± 9	44 ± 10	0.542
Thyromental Distance(mm)	64 ± 14	70 ± 12	69 ± 13	0.754
Duration of surgery (min)	32.20 ± 5.36	33.25 ± 6.87	31 ± 4.36	0.639

Table 1: Description of patients in the three study groups.

As shown in Table 2 The seal quality in all devices ('I-gel', SLIPA^{TM} and the SSLMA) permitted the use of low flows tidal volumes , 485 ± 82 and 451 ± 30 and 402 ± 23 mL (P=0.2) respectively. The peak pressure was significantly high in the SLIPA group (16 ± 3 cm H$_2$O), while leak pressure was significantly high in i-gel group (26 ± 6.3 cm H$_2$O). End tidal CO$_2$ was significantly higher in SSLMA group (40 ± 3 mm Hg).

	i-gel (n _40)	SLIPA (n _40)	SSLMA (n _40)	p value
Tidal volume (mL)	485 ± 82	451 ± 30	402 ± 23	0.028*
Respiratory rate (bpm)	11 ± 1	13 ± 2	11 ± 2	0.079

End-tidal CO$_2$ (mm Hg)	36 ± 4	38 ± 2	40 ± 3	**0.022***
Peak pressure (cm H$_2$O)	12 ± 3	16 ± 3	14 ± 4	**0.041***
Leak volume (ml)	20 ± 2	24 ± 1.5	26 ± 6.3	**0.044***
Oropharyngeal sealing pressure (cm H$_2$O)	28 ± 3	24 ± 7	19 ± 2	**<0.001***
(*)Significant p. value <0.05				

Table 2: Ventilation parameters, peak pressure and leak pressure.

There were no significant differences in hemodynamic variables and oxygen saturation percent (S$_p$O$_2$) values between the three groups at any time (Figure 1).

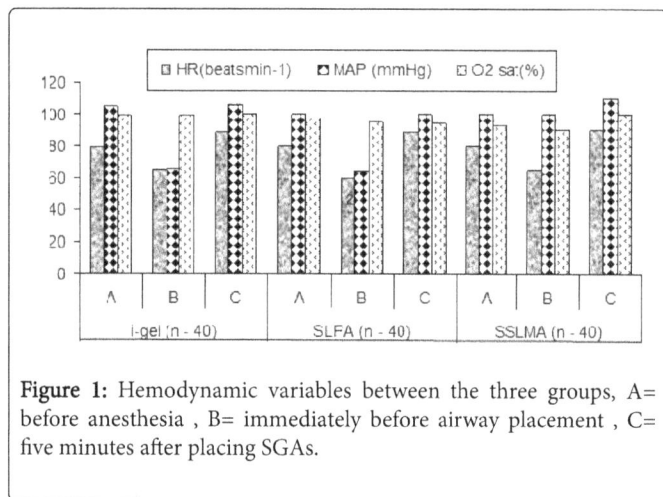

Figure 1: Hemodynamic variables between the three groups, A= before anesthesia , B= immediately before airway placement , C= five minutes after placing SGAs.

In the i-gel group, a significantly high successful placement was established in 38 patients (95%) on the first attempt and in the remaining 2 patients (100%) on the second attempt. In the SLIPA group, device insertion was successful in 34 patients (85%) on the first attempt, in four patients (95%) on the second attempt and in two patient (5%) failed attempts. In LMA group, insertion was successful in 35 patients (87.5%) on the first attempt, in three patients (95%) on the second attempt, in one patient (97.5%) after three attempts and one failed (2.5%). Time of insertion was comparable with the SLIPA (22 ± 4.6 sec.) and the SSLMA (19 ± 3.85 sec.), it was significantly (p=0.033) shorter in the i-gel group (15 ± 2.5 sec) (Table 3).

Insertion of the airway device was generally easier in the i-gel and SSLMA groups compared to the SLIPA. A high performance was noted in the i-gel group 26 patients compared with 22,24 in the SLIPA and SSLMA group respsectively (Figure 2).

	i-gel	SLIPA	SSLMA	P value
1st attempt success rate	95%	85%	87.50%	0.038*
Overall success rate	100%	95%	97.50%	0.248
Insertion time (sec.)	15 ± 2.5	22 ± 4.6	19 ± 3.85	0.033*

(*) Significant p. value <0.05

Table 3: Success rate (%) and insertion time: I-gel , SLIPA and SSLMA.

Maximum airway sealing pressure was 28 ± 3 cm H2O , 24 ± 7 cmH2O and 19 ± 2 cmH$_2$O in the i-gel and the SLIPA and SSLMA groups, respectively. No major adverse event occurred during the perioperative period in any patient in our study. However, one patient in the SLIPA and two in the SSLMA groups experienced bronchospasm and airway obstruction two min. after device insertion. In second attempt, airway was replaced by a smaller device in two patients in the SLIPA group and in three patients in the SSLMA group. The airway was replaced by a larger device in two patients in the SLIPA group and in one patient in the SSLMA group.

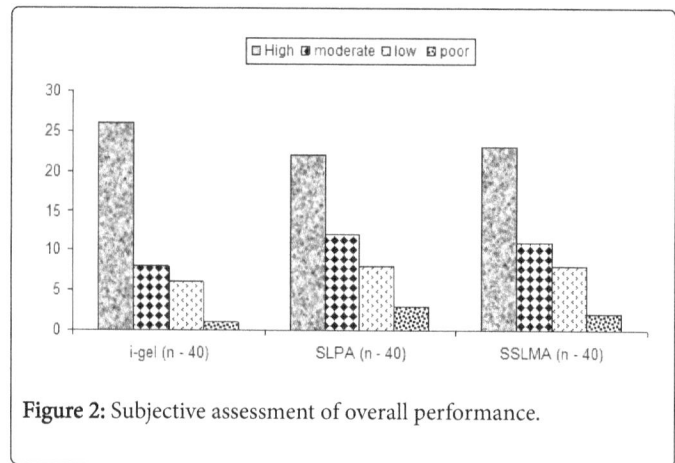

Figure 2: Subjective assessment of overall performance.

Group	i-gel	SLIPA	SSLMA	p value
Gastric air insufflations (%)	0	10	5	0.042*
Blood traces on airway device (%)	4	8	6	0.033*
Incidence of sore throat (%)	8	20	30	0.028*
(*)Significant p. value <0.05				

Table 4: Side effects associated with i-gel, SLIPA and SSLMA.

Side effects associated with i-gel, SLIPA and SSLMA are shown in (Table 4). Gastric air insufflations and blood trace were significantly high in the SLIPA group (10, p=0.042 and 8, p=0.033 respectively). No gastric fluids were found. Sore throat in the postoperative period was significantly high in SSLMA group (30, p=0.028) after 2 hours. No complain was recorded after 24 h in the three groups.

Discussion

SGA devices have become widely used in the anesthesia practice and airway management as an alternative to tracheal intubation during spontaneous or controlled ventilation [10].

In our study, the overall success rates were 100% of patients using i-gel, 97.5% using LMA and 95% using the SLIPA and in a relatively high number of patients, insertion of the supraglottic airway devices was successful on first attempt (95%, 85% and 87.5% in i-gel, SLIPA and SSLMA respectively). Although these results are lower than the findings of Jeon et al. [11] who reported a first insertion success rate of 100% with both PLMA and I-gel devices on the first insertion attempt, and other studies that reported insertion success rates of 84-100% for the i-gel [12] and 96-100% for the SLIPA [13].

A high performance was noted with the i-gel group patients compared with supraglottic devices including SLIPA [14] on the other hand SSLMA was more likely to be rated inferior regarding handling [15].

Castl et al. in their study comparing the I-gel with LMA and showed that the I-gel had shortest insertion time [16]. Gatward et al. found that I-gel was inserted approximately 50% faster than the other devices as PLMA manikin during resuscitation [17]. Xu et al. compared SLIPA, PLMA, and standard endotracheal intubation and recorded a first insertion success rate of 96% and 98% for the PLMA and SLIPA respectively [18]. In the opposite of our result Chio et al. compared SLIPA with PLMA in 60 patients undergoing surgeries under general anesthesia. And found that, the first insertion success rates for PLMA and SLIPA were 93.3% and 73.3%, respectively. This variation in results might be due to the relative experience of the anesthesiologist who has selected inappropriate size of SLIPA airway. Hence correct size selection is necessary for successful insertion [19]. Atef et al. showed that insertion of I-gel was significantly faster than insertion of LMA [20]. Goyal et al. on comparing size 2 i-gel with PLMA and cLMA in spontaneously breathing children undergoing elective surgery, showed that the success rate for first attempt was 95% for the i-gel group and 90% for the two laryngeal mask airway groups [21].

Time of insertion was with the SLIPA (22 ± 4.6 sec.) and the SSLMA (19 ± 3.85 sec). It was significantly (p=0.033) shorter in i-gel group (15 ± 2.5 sec.). Time of insertion of SSLMA was almost similar to other study (median of 20 sec.) [22] Meanwhile, time of insertion of SLIPA and i-gel were longer than other studies 10.5 ± 6.7 sec and 8.5 ± 6.3 sec. respectively [23].

Although, we used optimal conditions for easy SGAs insertion, we had higher incidence of low successful first attempts and longer insertion time. Frequently, we encountered difficulty in passing the SGAs between the patient front incisors, which was attributed to ethnic characters. In addition, choosing the correct size of SGAs is very important. Matching of the thyroid cartilage width to the SLIPA bridge was reliable indicator of right size, though there were still errors in choosing size (4/40) [24]. Choosing SSLMA size according to body weight resulted in few errors (4/40), probably because of cumbersome size of the semi-inflated cuff during insertion and the wide, stiff tube which restrict oral manipulation leading to impaction at the back of the mouth and more malposition [25], optimal insertion, adequate lubrication, optimal cuff inflation, proper patient's head and neck

position and the device insertion until a definitive resistance is felt [26].

In our study SSLMA, contrary to other study [27], has significantly low leak volume compared to i-gel and SLIPA. Moreover, SSLMA provided our patients with significantly low tidal volume resulted in significantly high end tidal volume CO_2. Peak airway pressure was, also, significantly higher than i-gel. Our results can be attributed to the fact that volume cycled modes cannot ventilate effectively and constantly in the presence of airway leaks. Moreover, rising airway pressure can force compressible air volume in the circuit to rise and effective tidal volume to fall [28].

The i-gel, in our study, provided effective ventilation with significantly high leak volume. The gel like cuff seems to create a perfect fit to peri-laryngeal structures, though enables reliable application [28].

Theoretically a supraglottic airway device with higher sealing pressures should better protect the airway from aspiration, however, the use of SGA devices equipped with an additional esophageal lumen often prevents tracheal aspiration of gastric content .So Pulmonary aspiration of gastric contents remains a major concern when using SGA devices [29].

Zanfaly et al. found in their study that the mean airway sealing pressure was lower in the i-gel group (24.8 ± 5.8 cmH_2O) than in the LMA group (27.33 ± 6.5 cmH_2O) and the ETT group (28.5 ± 5.7 cmH_2O), but the difference was statistically nonsignifcant [30].

No regurgitation of gastric contents was observed in any group in our study. Contrary to our results, in some paralysed patients reflux occurred during maintenance and emergence without clinical consequences [24]. The tendency to reflux is related to lower esophageal sphincter (LOS) pressure and the barrier pressure (BrP), which is the difference between gastric and sphincter pressures. Patient factors, operation factors, anesthesia factors, and device factors affect LOS tone and predispose the patient to insufflations, regurgitation and aspiration [31].

The i-gel has a drainage tube that allows escape of both ventilating gases and regurgitated fluid. The i-gel appears to be an improvement on the standard LMA for preventing aspiration. However, studies on Pro-Seal LMA imply that its effectiveness varies with the flow rate of regurgitated fluid, with greater probability of aspiration at higher flow rates [24]. Thus, risk of aspiration using i-gel might be similar to that for the standard LMA, but with smaller volumes actually aspirated.

The absence of inflatable cuff might increase the risk of gastric insufflations [6]. However, the ability of the SLIPA to protect against aspiration is limited to the storage capacity of the device, which exceeds the volume of gastric contents of fasted patients [6].

Although blood traces were significantly high in SLIPA group, postoperative sore throat was significantly higher in SSLMA group. The rigid material of the SLIPA appears to be more traumatic to the pharynx. The pressure-induced mucosal trauma resulted from SSLMA inflatable cuff seems to be more prevalent.

The postoperative sore throat percent was (30%). A systematic review and meta-analysis of the i-gel_ vs laryngeal mask airway in adults also showed a reduced the rate of postoperative sore throat [32].

Conclusion

The three disposable SGAs proved to be suitable for controlled ventilation during elective short surgical operations. The i-gel provides effective ventilation with minimal side effects and provide the best sealing quality, and the least leakage volume . Whereas, SLIPA is associated with a high incidence of gastric air insufflations, However, SSLMA associated with mild sore throat postoperatively.

References

1. Ueki R, Komasawa N, Nishimoto K, Sugi T, Hirose M, et al. (2014) Utility of the Aintree Intubation Catheter in fiberoptic tracheal intubation through the three types of intubating supraglottic airways: a manikin simulation study. J Anesth 28: 363–367.

2. Miller DM, Youkhana I, Karunaratne WU (2001) Presence of protein deposits on 'cleaned' re-usable anesthetic equipment. Anesthesia 56: 1069–1072.

3. Uppal V, Gangaiah S, Fletcher G, Kinsella J (2009) Randomized crossover comparison between the i-gel and the LMA-Unique in anaesthetized, paralysed adults. Br J Anaesth 103: 882–885.

4. Woo YC, Cha SM, Kang H, Baek CW, Jung YH, et al. (2011) Less perilaryngeal gas leakage with SLIPATM than with LMAProSealTM in paralyzed patients. Can J Anaesth. 58: 48–54.

5. Miller DM, Lavelle MA (2002) A Streamlined Pharynx Airway Liner: pilot study in 22 patients in controlled and spontaneous ventilation. Anesth Analg 94: 759–761.

6. Lange M, Smul T, Zimmermann P, Kohlenberger R, Roewer N, et al. (2007) The Effectiveness and Patient Comfort of the Novel Streamlined Pharynx Airway Liner (SLIPA®) Compared with the Conventional Laryngeal Mask Airway in Ophthalmic Surgery. Anesth Analg 104: 431-434.

7. Nicholson A, Cook TM, Smith AF, Lewis SR, Reed SS (2013) Supraglottic airway devices versus tracheal intubation for airway management during general anaesthesia in obese patients. Cochrane Database Syst Rev 9: CD010105.

8. Van Zundert AA, Fonck K, Al-Shaikh B, Mortier EP (2004) Comparison of cuff-pressure changes in LMAClassic® and the new Soft Seal® laryngeal masks during nitrous oxide anaesthesia in spontaneous breathing patients. Eur J Anaesthesiol 21: 547-552.

9. Keller C, Brimacombe JR, Keller K, Morris R (1999) Comparison of four methods for assessing airway sealing pressures with the laryngeal mask airway in adult patients. Br J Anaesth 82: 286-287.

10. Jakobsson J (2010) The airway in day surgery. Minerva Anesthesiol 76: 38–44.

11. Jeon WJ, Cho SY, Baek SJ, Kim KH (2012) Comparison of the proseal LMA and intersurgical I-gel during gynecological laparoscopy. Korean J Anesthesiol 63: 510–514.

12. Halwagi AE, Massicotte N, Lallo A, Gauthier A, Boudreault D, et al. (2012) Tracheal intubation through the I-gel supraglottic airway versus the LMA Fastrach: a randomized controlled trial. Anesth Analg 114: 152–156.

13. Woo YC, Cha SM, Kang H, Baek CW, Jung YH, et al. (2011) Less perilaryngeal gas leakage with SLIPATM than with LMA ProSealTM in paralyzed patients. Can J Anaesth 58: 48– 54.

14. Jackson KM, Cook TM (2007) Evaluation of four airway training manikins as patient simulators for the insertion of eight types of supraglottic airway devices. Anaesthesia 62: 388–393.

15. Orlikowski CE (2004) An audit of the Single Use Portex Laryngeal Mask. Anaesth Intensive Care 32: 693–696.

16. Castle N, Owen R, Hann M, Naidoo R, Reeves D (2010) Assessment of the speed and ease of insertion of three supraglottic airway devices by paramedics: a manikin study. Emerg Med J 27: 860–863.

17. Gatward JJ, Thomas MJ, Nolan JP, Cook TM (2008) Effect of chest compressions on the time taken to insert airway devices in a manikin. Br J Anaesth 100: 351–356.

18. Xu J, Zhong TD (2010) Comparison and superiority of streamlined liner of the pharynx airway to laryngeal mask airway or tracheal tubes for gynecological laparoscopy. Zhonghua yi xue za zhi 90: 49–52.

19. Chio YM, Cha SM, Kang H, Baek CW, Jung YH, et al. (2010) The clinical effectiveness of the streamlined liner of pharyngeal airway (SLIPA) compared with the laryngeal mask airway Proseal during general anesthesia. Korean J Anesthesiol 58: 450–457.

20. Atef HM, Helmy AM, El-Taher EM, Henidak AM (2012) Comparative study between I-gel, a new supraglottic airway device, and classical laryngeal mask airway in anesthetized spontaneously ventilated patients. Middle East J Anesthesiol 21: 583–590.

21. Goyal R, Shukla RN, Kumar G (2012) Comparison of size 2 i-gel supraglottic airway with LMA-ProSeal™ and LMA-Classic™ in spontaneously breathing children undergoing elective surgery, Paediatr Anaesth 22: 355–359.

22. Dörges V, Francksen H, Bein B, Obermöller T, Steinfath M (2005) LMA Unique™ vs. Soft Seal Laryngeal Mask: An Evaluation during Routine Surgical Procedures. Anesthesiology 103: A1171.

23. Keijzer C, Buitelaar DR, Efthymiou KM, Sramek M, Cate J, et al. (2009) A Comparison of Postoperative Throat and Neck Complaints After the Use of the i-gel_ and the La Premiere_ Disposable Laryngeal Mask: A Double-Blinded, Randomized, Controlled Trial. Anesth Analg 109: 1092–1094.

24. Miller DM, Light D (2003) Laboratory and clinical comparisons of the streamlined liner of the pharynx airway (SLIPA) with the laryngeal mask airway. Anesthesia 58: 136–4211.

25. Brimacombe J, Goedecke A, Keller C, Brimacombe L, Brimacombe M (2004) The Laryngeal Mask Airway Unique™ versus the Soft Seal™ Laryngeal Mask: A Randomized, Crossover Study in Paralyzed, Anesthetized Patients. Anesth Analg 99: 1560–1563.

26. Chapman D (2009) Phenomenon with I-Gel airway: a reply. Anaesthesia 64: 216–229.

27. Natalini G, Pacchetti P, Dicembrini MA, Lanza G, Rosano A, et al. (2001) Pressure controlled versus volume controlled ventilation with laryngeal mask airway. J Clin Anesth 13: 436-439.

28. Levitan RM, Kinkle WC (2005) Initial anatomic investigations of the i-gel airway: a novel supraglottic airway without inflatable cuff. Anaesthesia 60: 1022-1025.

29. Verghese C, Berlet J, Kapila A, Pollard R (1998) Clinical assessment of the single use laryngeal mask airway – the LMA-unique. Br J Anaesth 80: 677–679.

30. Zanfaly H, Ali M, Hassan A (2015) I-gel against proseal laryngeal mask airway and endotracheal tube during minor surgical procedures: a comparative study. Ain-Shams J Anesthesiol 08: 521–528.

31. De Leon A, Thorn SE, Wattwil M (2010) High-Resolution Solid-State Manometry of the Upper and Lower Esophageal Sphincters During Anesthesia Induction: A Comparison Between Obese and Non-Obese Patients. Anesthesia Analgesia 111: 149-153.

32. De Montblanc J, Ruscio L, Mazoit JX, Benhamou D (2014) A systematic review and meta-analysis of the i-gel vs laryngeal mask airway in adults. Anaesthesia 69: 1151–1162.

29

The Hidden Features of Breathing

Aynur Şahin[1], **Serkan Doğru**[1], **İsmail Okan**[2], **Fatih Altıparmak**[1] and **Mustaffa Süren**[1]*

[1]*Department of Anesthesiology and Reanimation, Tokat, Turkey*

[2]*Department of General Surgery, Gaziosmanpaşa University, Tokat, Turkey*

*Corresponding author:** Mustaffa Süren, Department of Anesthesiology and Reanimation, Tokat, Turkey, E-mail: drmustafasuren@gmail.com

Abstract

Purpose: Humans have two types of breathing pattern, abdominal and thoracic, which show physiological differences. The primary goal of the present study is to assess the spirometric variability of breathing patterns in individuals, and secondary goal is to elucidate the influence of age and gender differences on breathing types.

Methods: Patients aged between 18 and 40 years were asked to participate in the study, and spirometry using the Spirodoc® (MIR-Medical International Research-Srl, Roma, Italy) was preoperatively performed on subjects. Age, gender, weight, height, body-mass index, the American Society of Anesthesiologists score, the observed breathing pattern (thoracic or abdominal) while standing, and the spirometric measurements were recorded into a standardized data sheet.

Results: A total of 126 subjects were included in the study. The mean age of the patients was 29.90 ± 6.76, and the mean body-mass index value was 26.20 ± 5.84. Sixty-seven subjects were female and 59 were male. The forced expiratory time value of spirometry was found to be significantly higher in patients with abdominal breathing (5.94 ± 1.01) compared to thoracic (4.47 ± 1.32; p=0.007). The Forced inspiratory vital capacity measurement in patients with abdominal breathing pattern (4.26 ± 1.01) was higher than in thoracic (3.61 ± 1.04; p=0.063). The thoracic breathing pattern was observed at a rate of 84.7% (n=50) among subjects of the 18-29-year age group, and 73.8% (n=45) in subjects of the 30-40-year age group (p=0.139).

Conclusion: The present study revealed that abdominal breathing is superior in some aspects of spirometric measurements compared to thoracic breathing.

Keywords: Spirometry; Breathing; Abdominal wall; Thoracic wall; Vital capacity; Abdominal breathing; Thoracic breathing

Introduction

Undoubtedly, one of the critical life-support systems of the body is the respiratory system. The respiratory system is composed of various mechanical structures including the lungs, thoracic wall and diaphragm, inthe abdominal rib cage compartment. The main function of this system is the "breathing" which provides gas exchange with the environment through the continual muscle action of the thoracic wall [1]. According to the current knowledge, the two basic patterns of breathing are diaphragmatic (abdominal) and thoracic. Thoracic breathing is defined as the filling of the middle and upper portion of the lungs, whereas diaphragmatic breathing is described as inflating all three parts of the lungs including the lower parts, which is considered to be the most efficient due to the increased amount of blood to receive oxygen. A third pattern, clavicular breathing, is defined as pulling up the clavicles or collar bones to raise the intake of air [2,3]. Furthermore, chest and abdominal wall mobility is a significant factor in the evaluation of respiratory functional status. Breathing pattern and thoracal/abdominal wall motion can be affected by various factors including an individual's position, age, gender, respiratory overload, neuromuscular diseases, increased airway resistance, and chronic obstructive pulmonary disease [3-6]. The loss of any wall mobility may be a predictor of forthcoming respiratory complication [7]. It is reported that there is less abdominal movement observed in females compared to males [8].

Spirometry is the most useful technique to obtain quantitative measurements of lung volume and flow, thus allowing comparable results among individuals. It is a physiological test that evaluates an individual's inhaled and exhaled volumes of air. The outcome of spirometry, which has well-validated normal values, is very effective and accurate in diagnosing and monitoring upper and lower airway disorders. In this context, we hypothesized that thoracal and abdominal breathing patterns may reveal significant differences in spirometric measurements.

Therefore, the primary goal of the present study is to assess the spirometric variability of breathing patterns in individuals, and the secondary goal is to elucidate the influence of age and gender differences on breathing types.

Materials and Methods

After approval of Gaziosmanpasa University Clinical Trials Ethics Committee (14-KAEK-194), this prospective study was conducted from 2014 to 2015. Patients aged between 18 and 40 years with an American Society of Anesthesiologists score (ASA) of I or II, who were admitted to the outpatient unit of the Department of Anesthesiology,

Medical Faculty, Gaziosmanpasa University for preoperative assessment to undergo elective surgery requiring general anesthesia, were invited to participate in the study. The following parameters were the exclusion criteria: patients scheduled for ear-nose-throat surgery, cardiovascular surgery, or those with an upper airway pathology (eg: maxillofacial fractures and tumors), a history of head/neck surgery or maxillofacial surgery, obstructive or restrictive pulmonary disease, and a history of smoking (tobacco and tobacco products). In the outpatient unit, spirometry using the Spirodoc® (MIR-Medical International Research-Srl, Roma, Italy) was preoperatively performed on subjects, after obtaining written informed consent. The age, gender, weight, height, body-mass index (BMI), the ASA score, the observed breathing type (thoracic or abdominal) while standing, and the measurements (FVC (Forced Vital Capacity), FEV_1 (Forced Expiratory Volume in 1st second), FEV_3 (Forced Expiratory Volume in 3 seconds), FEV_6 (Forced Expiratory Volume in 6 seconds), FEV_1/FVC, FEV_3/FVC, PEF (Peak Expiratory Flow), FEF_{25} (Forced Expiratory Flow 25%), FEF_{50} (Forced Expiratory Flow 50%), FEF_{75} (Forced Expiratory Flow 75%), $FEF_{25/75}$, FET (Forced Expiratory Time), FIVC (Forced Inspiratory Vital Capacity), FIV_1 (Forced Inspiratory Volume in 1st second), FIV_1/FVC and PIF (Peak Inspiratory Flow)) belonging to all subjects were recorded into a standardized data sheet. All variables were dichotomized in terms of thoracic or abdominal breathing pattern.

Statistical analysis

Normality and variance were tested using the one-Sample Kolmogorov-Smirnov test for each variable. Quantitative data were presented as means and standard deviation, and qualitative data as frequency and percentage. Associations were performed by using the Spearman's correlation coefficient (ρ). The comparisons were carried out by using the Mann-Whitney U test. Analyses were completed by using the Statistical Package for the Social Sciences (SPSS Inc., Chicago, IL) version 20.0 program. The statistical significance for all analyses was set at P<0.05.

Results

A total of 126 subjects were included in the study. Demographical data is presented in Table 1.

	Thoracic Breathing	Abdominal Breathing	p
Age (years)	29.33 ± 6.72	31.16 ± 7.13	0.252
Gender (F/M)	51/44	11//14	0.389
Height (cm)	167.57 ± 8.75	168.36 ± 14.98	0.175
Weight (kg)	73.31 ± 14.26	72.56 ± 17.46	0.936
BMI (kg/m2)	26.14 ± 5.19	26.13 ± 8.35	0.665
F: Female; M: Male; BMI: Body Mass Index. Mann-Whitney U test.			

Table 1: Demographic characteristics.

The mean age of the patients was 29.90 ± 6.76, and the mean BMI value was 26.20 ± 5.84. Sixty-seven subjects were female and 59 were male. A total of 51 (82.3%) females and 44 (75.9%) males had thoracic breathing. The relationship between breathing pattern and spirometric outcomes is displayed in a correlation matrix (Table 2).

	Thoracic/Abdominal breathing pattern	
	P	P
FVC	0.104	0.258
FEV_1	0.117	0.203
FEV_3	0.098	0.287
FEV_6	0.108	0.242
FEV_3/FVC	−0.134	0.145
FEV_1/FEV_6	−0.019	0.837
FEV_1/FVC	−0.025	0.785
PEF	0.132	0.149
FEF_{25}	0.11	0.232
FEF_{50}	0.135	0.14
FEF_{75}	0.062	0.5
$FEF_{25/75}$	0.117	0.203
FET	0.249*	0.006*
FIVC	0.246	0.063
FIV_1	0.171	0.2
FIV_1/FVC	−0.131	0.326
PIF	0.056	0.681

FVC, Forced Vital Capacity; FEV_1, Forced Expiratory Volume in 1st second; FEV_3, Forced Expiratory Volume in 3 seconds; FEV_6, Forced Expiratory Flow in 6 seconds; PEF, Peak Expiratory Flow, FEF_{25}, Forced Expiratory Flow 25%; FEF_{50}, Forced Expiratory Flow 50%; FEF_{75}, Forced Expiratory Flow 75%; FET, Forced Expiratory Time; FIVC, Forced Inspiratory Vital Capacity; FIV_1, Forced Inspiratory Volume in 1st second; PIF, Peak Inspiratory Flow.

Spearman's correlation analysis. *p<0.05

Table 2: Correlation matrix.

The FET value of spirometry was found significantly higher in patients with abdominal breathing (5.94 ± 1.01) compared to thoracic (4.47 ± 1.32; p=0.007; Table 3). The FIVC measurement in patients with abdominal breathing pattern (4.26 ± 1.01) was higher than in thoracic (3.61 ± 1.04; p=0.063). The thoracic breathing pattern was observed at a rate of 84.7% (n=50) among subjects of the 18-29 year age group, and 73.8% (n=45) in subjects of the 30-40-year age group (p=0.139).

	Thoracic Breathing	Abdominal Breathing	p
FVC	3.92 ± 0.96	4.38 ± 0.96	0.257
FEV_1	3.14 ± 0.74	3.53 ± 0.87	0.202
FEV_3	3.79 ± 0.91	4.21 ± 0.91	0.285
FEV_6	3.90 ± 0.96	4.37 ± 0.95	0.241
FEV_3/FVC	96.90 ± 3.62	96.27 ± 2.27	0.144
FEV_1/FEV_6	80.93 ± 6.72	80.27 ± 6.96	0.836

FEV$_1$/FVC	80.69 ± 7.06	80.02 ± 6.90	0.784
PEF	5.22 ± 1.58	6.05 ± 2.12	0.149
FEF$_{25}$	4.92 ± 1.42	5.67 ± 1.99	0.231
FEF$_{50}$	3.61 ± 0.96	4.30 ± 1.56	0.14
FEF$_{75}$	1.60 ± 0.59	1.77 ± 0.72	0.497
FEF$_{25/75}$	3.35 ± 0.94	3.78 ± 1.27	0.202
FET	4.47 ± 1.32	5.94 ± 1.01	0.007*
FIVC	3.61 ± 1.04	4.26 ± 1.01	0.063
FIV$_1$	2.93 ± 1.15	3.45 ± 1.20	0.198
FIV$_1$/FIVC	82.01 ± 21.17	79.34 ± 15.20	0.322
PIF	3.00 ± 1.05	3.39 ± 1.52	0.678

FVC, Forced Vital Capacity; FEV$_1$, Forced Expiratory Volume in 1st second; FEV$_3$, Forced Expiratory Volume in 3 seconds; FEV$_6$, Forced Expiratory Volume in 6 seconds; PEF, Peak Expiratory Flow, FEF$_{25}$, Forced Expiratory Flow 25%; FEF$_{50}$, Forced Expiratory Flow 50%; FEF$_{75}$, Forced Expiratory Flow 75%; FET, Forced Expiratory Time; FIVC, Forced Inspiratory Vital Capacity; FIV$_1$, Forced Inspiratory Volume in 1st second; PIF, Peak Inspiratory Flow.

Mann-Whitney U test. *p<0.05

Table 3: Comparison of spirometric measurements.

Discussion

The present study showed that the forced expiratory time is longer in abdominal breathing, and also the forced inspiratory vital capacity has a tendency to be higher in patients with the abdominal breathing pattern. In addition, advanced age leads to a slight shift from thoracic to abdominal breathing. Abdominal breathing, which has been described as the typical adult breathing pattern, has a respiration rate of 12 to 20 times per minute with a physiological sinus arrhythmia, and also includes shallow thoracic movements. The tidal volume generally ranges between 750 and 2000 ml per inhalation. Abdominal breathing depends on the rhythmic diaphragm movements, upwards during exhalation and downwards during inhalation [9,10]. It also has a longer exhalation pause time leading to a prolonged expiration phase. Abdominal breathing is defined as effortless breathing [11], whereas, thoracic breathing is a tendency to breathe using the upper chest structures of the rib cage, including pectoral muscles, scalene muscles, and trapezius muscles. The diaphragm is pulled up during inspiration and down during expiration. Therfore, thoracic breathing may lead to dyspnea, fatigue, irritation, headaches, and increased feelings of anxiety. Prolonged thoracic breathing can cause lower O$_2$ levels in the blood [10].

Abdominal breathing has been shown as useful in the treatment of various health disorders including asthma, sympathetic activation, anxiety, panic attacks, hyperventilation, and the discomfort of menopause-related hot flashes, while also increasing endurance and physical performance [10]. Abdominal breathing is a teachable and learnable technique by verbal instructions, role modeling and limitation. Tibbets et al. showed that teaching slow abdominal breathing to asthmatic adults led to an increase in inhalation volume, decreased thoracic muscle use, diminished administration of medical therapy for asthma, and fewer emergency room visits and breathless episodes. The authors also reported that the improvements remained

over 16 months [12]. In addition, breath training is considered a beneficial treatment modality for dyspnea, chronic obstructive pulmonary disease, and hypertension; however there has been littleclinical data on the benefits of teaching abdominal breathing to adults or children [13,14]. Gender differences may be seen in breathing pattern. Abdominal breathing pattern is more common in males. Females have a wider rib cage and minimal abdominal support to generate tidal volume compared to males during quiet breathing [15,16]. Recently, Kaneko et al. reported that females show more thoracic motions with less abdominal contributions than male subjects in the supine position. They also indicated that thoracic movement decreased with age [8]. Similarly, Verschakelen et al. demonstrated that males over 50 years of age showed less movement with their rib cages [3]. The present study revealed that a higher percentage of both females and males had thoracic breathing; however, females had a greater tendency toward thoracic breathing than males, and we also showed that abdominal breathing pattern with advanced age increased at a rate of 10% compared to thoracic, which was consistent with the outcomes of previous studies mentioned above.

Moreover, spirometry has been a widely used method to evaluate the pulmonary functions of an individual. Forced expiratory time is one of the components of outcomes obtained from spirometry. A recent study by Tsai et al., on a population of 37 normal and 65 obstructive patients, found that longer forced expiratory time was associated with higher forced vital capacity and first second forced expiratory volume [17]. In addition, forced vital capacity was dependent on expiratory time [18]. The present study showed that forced expiratory time is shorter in subjects with thoracic breathing; however, forced inspiratory vital capacity instead of the associated parameter, forced vital capacity, displayed a significant correlation with forced expiratory time. Forced inspiratory vital capacity is defined as the maximal volume of gas that can be inhaled during a forced and complete inspiration from a position of full expiration. It is closely associated with FEV$_1$, the volume of air inhaled in one second during the performance of the forced inspiratory vital capacity [19]. In this context, the amount of inhaled volume of air may lead to longer exhalation times during spirometry. This study showed that FIVC and FEV$_1$ comparisons of the individuals in have a tendency to be higher in abdominal breathing compared to thoracic breathing. It can be suggested that abdominal breathing may provide a higher volume of air intake compared to thoracic breathing, leading to a time difference during expiration. The chief muscle of inspiration during abdominal breathing is the diaphragm. Individuals with thoracic breathing show less diaphragm movement. Indeed, diaphragm paralysis leads to mild to severe restrictive findings on pulmonary function tests. The forced expiratory volume in one second (FEV$_1$) is decreased approximately 70% of predicted values in unilateral paralysis and 50% of predicted values in bilateral paralysis. The forced vital capacity is lowered to 75% of predicted, in unilateral paralysis and 45% of predicted, in bilateral paralysis [20]. In relation, abdominal breathing mostly associated with the diaphragm movement holds most of the functions of lungs and have significant effects on pulmonary volumes and flows.

The present study has several limitations. First, our results are limited by the relatively small sample size. Therefore, definitive results such as how demographic factors might influence spirometric measurements must await further studies with a larger population. Second, most subjects performed a maximum of three loops, hence no interpretation can be made on subsequent trends in the performance of spirometric measurements. Third, the age groups of the study consisted of young adults, which restricts the application of results to other settings and patient populations.

In conclusion, this is the first study presented on the quantitative differences between abdominal and thoracic breathing in the English literature. It revealed that abdominal breathing, which can be learned and used to cope with various significant breathing disorders in adults, is superior in some aspects of spirometric measurements compared to thoracic breathing. The findings of the present study suggest that the abdominal breathing pattern is efficient in terms of inhalation, and increased age leads to a tendency toward the abdominal breathing type. However, further studies demonstrating the increase in tissue oxygenation by improving preoperative pulmonary functions in patients to undergo elective operations are required.

Acknowledgements

We wish to express our gratitude to Alkan Karakış, Yakup Borazan, Seval Ekerer, Sevdiye Şıvgın, Hümeyra Astan, Olcayto Uysal, İbrahim Kızıldağ, Tuğrul Şahin, Selim Adatepe and Ali Koçman. There was no financial support or sponsorship and the authors declare that there are no conflicts of interest.

References

1. Macklem PT (1988) Clinical assessment of the respiratory muscles. Pneumonol Pol 56: 249-253.

2. Zimberoff D, Hartmann D (1999) Exploring the Frontier of "Being" and "Doing". J Heart-centered Ther 2: 3-52.

3. Verschakelen JA, Demedts MG (1995) Normal thoracoabdominal motions. Influence of sex, age, posture, and breath size. Am J Respir Crit Care Med 151: 399-405.

4. Kiciman NM, Andréasson B, Bernstein G (1998) Thoracoabdominal motion in newborns during ventilation delivered by endotracheal tube or nasal prongs. Pediatr Pulmonol 25: 175-181.

5. Maynard V, Bignall S, Kitchen S (2000) Effect of positioning on respiratory synchrony in non-ventilated pre-term infants. Physiother Res Int 5: 96-110.

6. Perez T, Becquart LA, Stach B, Wallaert B, Tonnel AB (1996) Inspiratory muscle strength and endurance in steroid-dependent asthma. Am J Respir Crit Care Med 153: 610-615.

7. Bockenhauer SE, Chen H, Julliard KN, Weedon J (2007) Measuring thoracic excursion: reliability of the cloth tape measure technique. Am J Respir Crit Care Med 107: 191-196.

8. Kaneko H, Horie J (2012) Breathing Movements of the Chest and Abdominal Wall in Healthy Subjects. Respir Care 57: 1442-1451.

9. Yuan G, Drost NA, McIvor RA (2013) Respiratory Rate and Breathing Pattern. MUMJ 10: 23-25.

10. Kajander R, Peper E (1998) Teaching diaphragmatic breathing to children. Biofeedback 26: 14-17.

11. Peper E, Crane-Gockley V (1990) Towards effortless breathing. Med Psychother 3: 135-140.

12. Tibbetts V, Peper E (1993) The effects of therapist breathing style on subject's inhalation volumes. Biofeedback Self Regul 18: 115-120.

13. Estève F, Blanc-Gras N, Gallego J, Benchetrit G (1996) The Effects of Breathing Pattern on Ventilatory Function in Patients with COPD. Biofeedback Self Regul 21: 311-321.

14. Ley R (1995) Highlights of the 13th International Symposium on Respiratory Psychophysiology Held at the Inaugural Meeting of the International Society for the Advancement of Respiratory Psychophysiology. Biofeedback Self Regul 20: 369-379.

15. Binazzi B, Lanini B, Bianchi R, Romagnoli I, Nerini M, et al. (2006) Breathing pattern and kinematics in normal subjects during speech, singing and loud whispering. Acta Physiol (Oxf) 186: 233-246.

16. Bellemare F, Jeanneret A, Couture J (2003) Sex differences in thoracic dimensions and configuration. Am J Respir Crit Care Med 168: 305-312.

17. Tsai AG, Christie JD, Gaughan CA, Palma WR Jr, Margolis ML (2006) Change in forced expiratory time and spirometric performance during a single pulmonary function testing session. Respir Care 51: 246-251.

18. Swanney MP, Jensen RL, Crichton DA, Beckert LE, Cardno LA, et al. (2000) FEV6 is an acceptable surrogate for FVC in the spirometric diagnosis of airway obstruction and restriction. Am J Respir Crit Care Med 162: 917-919.

19. Quanjer PH, Tammeling GJ, Cotes JE, Pedersen OF, Peslin R, et al. (1993) Lung volumes and forced ventilatory flows. Report Working Party Standardization of Lung Function Tests, European Community for Steel and Coal. Official Statement of the European Respiratory Society. Eur Respir J Suppl 16: 5-40.

20. Qureshi A (2009) Diaphragm Paralysis. Semin Respir Crit Care Med 30: 315-320.

30

The Validity and Reliability of the Arabic Version of FLACC Scale: A Clinical Trial

Rahaf DA*, Hisham Shakhashero and Mohamad Basier Al-Monaqel

Damascus University, Syrian Arab Republic

***Corresponding author:** Rahaf Dak Albab, Damascus University, Syrian Arab Republic, E-mail: rahaf.dds@hotmail.com

Abstract

Introduction and aim: It is difficult to determine pain level using (patient-based-pain) scales in children. Hence, there is a need to translate (Arabizate) of an international non-self-pain scale (FLACC) as an alternativeclinician-basedpain scale, and test its psychometric properties (validity and reliability).

Materials and methods: The study was carried out on (250) children who needed dental treatments, aged (6-14) years, their behavior were valuated as definitely positive or positive (according to Behavior Frankl Scale) in Damascus-University. Each child has received local injection in one side and a placebo (touching the oral mucosa with covered needle) in the other side. Children were filmed with a digital camera to record pain reaction. The reactions were evaluated by two examiners (blinded-injection type) using; FLACC (Face-Legs-Activity-Cry-Consolability) and SEM (Sound-Eye-Motor) scales.

Results: About 2000 non-self-assessments were obtained. FLACC scale showed high Construct Validity because of the rising of pain intensity from (0.13) with placebo into (3.6) with injection. Criterion Validity was good between FLACC and SEM. The scale showed high Internal Consistency Validity where values of correlation coefficients ranged (0.723-0.792) between scale items and its total degree. FLACC showed good reliability; correlation coefficient between external evaluators (r=0.805), Cronbach's alpha value was high (0.809), and Kappa value reached (0.952) for the first evaluator and (0.893) for the other. These positive values pointed to high reliability of the (FLACC) scale.

Conclusion: The Arabic version of (FLACC) scale characterized by validity and reliability, and it is recommended to use.

Literature Review

Children's Pain assessment can be conducted by three means: self-evaluating, selfless-evaluating by behaviour observation and recording, Physiological measurements [1]. However, according to some scientists; the ideal evaluation is the combined evaluation which includes self-evaluating for pain associated with one of the methods stated above [2], but this approach can be considered unpractical, inapplicable and useless for children in the phase before talking or whom are unable to talk, or those have perceptual problems, so some of scientists said that it is better to evaluate pain by selfless methods that depends on watching Child's reaction against pain alarm and registering it. The demand for using self-pain evaluating as "The gold standard" is a clear exaggeration due to the complications and factors that contribute in prejudicing the rather for himself when he asked to evaluate his pain by his self [3-5].

And FLACC scale, this scale was developed by Merkel et al in 1997, consists of five clauses, each clause's value ranges between (0-2) so the whole scale has a value between (0-10) [6], it is convenient for young children; their ages below 3 years, and it is used for low perceptual ability's children [7], and it has chosen with CHEOPS scale as the best pain evaluating scales by Von Baeyer and Spagrud systematic review [8]. FLACC scale was translated into four languages (Chinese, Thai, Swedish, and Brazilian Portuguese) [9-12].

SEM (Sound-Eye-Motor) scale has been used in many recent studies [13-17] and Baghdadi study in Syria [18], this scale concentrates on the changes in patient's sound, eyes and movement to evaluate patients relax or pain during treatment [19].

Aim of Study

To study the Psychometric properties (validity and reliability) of the Arabic version of selfless pain measurement FLACC.

Materials and Methods

An ethical approval was obtained from the local ethics committee prior to the commencement of the study, CONSORT Statement was followed when the current study was designed and conducted.

Current study had started On February 2014, and ended on March 2015. The sample included (250) children from the Department of Pediatric Dentistry of the Dentistry-Faculty of Damascus University. Their ages ranged between 6 and 14 years. Each of them needed intraoral local anesthesia for various treatment purposes (e.g: pulptomy, dental extraction, restorative treatment). Informed consent from one of the parents or the guardian of the child has been taken after the current study and its purposes had been explained. The included children were fit and healthy with no nervous disturbances, cooperative and classified as (absolute positive or positive) on Frankel's classification scale. All children needed treatments that require intraoral anesthesia. None received any sedative or analgesic drugs in the last three hours prior to intraoral injection, and there was no abscess (acute or chronic) in the site of injection.

Randomisation

The randomization was conducted in this study by alternating the order of injection and placebo (see below) on the child according to the randomization distributing tables.

The injections

A local anesthetic injection has been given to each child after drying the oral mucosa by sterilized cotton sticks and applying Benzocaine gel (20%) for two minutes, traditional local anesthetic has been given on the side that needed the dental treatment.

The operator has also pretended to give the child another "placebo" local anesthesia injection by touching lightly the oral mucosa by the injection site (while the injection needle was capped) without any pressure. So, the child has received one local intraoral injection, whereas he thought he has received two injections.

Hiding local anesthesia syringe from child's sight pattern has been applied on all sample's children in all ages, that because of the positive effects of hiding the syringe on the child's behaviour, those effects were approved by many global recent and old studies [20-23].

Recording

The child reaction was recorded during the injection procedure (in both groups) using a high definition digital camera (14 Mega pixel). The recordings were then edited to mask the type of injection given and therefore blind the assessors. All edited recordings were evaluated by external raters, each independently completes two clinician-based pain evaluation scales (SEM and FLACC).

Arabisation (Translation) of the FLACC scale

The FLACC pain scale has been Arabized using foreword-backward translation, and was used for the first time in Arabic in the current study.

Methods of studying the psychological properties of measurement scale:

Validity

The content and construct validities were tested as follows:

Content validity: This has been checked by a number of experts in the field of pain and education to ensure the content safety, language fluency, and the measurement ability to reflect its parts and purpose; which is defining the pain level.

Construct validity: This was examined by testing rising pain intensity during injection in comparison with placebo. The internal consistency between the scale's five elements was examined by checking their individual relation with the whole measurement. The construct validity was tested also by detecting Discrimination validity

and the measurement ability on retrieving differences between children who suffered from the maximum pain level relatively with their companions who suffered from minimum pain level, and the criterion validity was detected by exploring the convergent validity, which conducted by detecting the engagement level of FLACC scale with other scales that applied.

Reliability: The reliability has been checked by: the method of testing and retesting, and calculating Cronbach's alpha factor, and inter-rater reliability, so the raters were tested (inter-rater reliability) to ensure their ability on evaluating pain trustfully, and to study the reliability of FLACC scale in selfless pain evaluating.

Results

The sample included (250) children, and the pain level was evaluated selflessly on selfless scales by external raters, which means there was (1000) selfless evaluation for pain for both in injection and placebo, so they were (2000) selfless pain evaluation in total, as shown in Table 1.

Content validity study's result suggested making no adjustments on test clauses and instructions because its clearance, and appropriateness for the purpose that they have been put for.

Construct validity for the Arabic version of FLACC scale was studied by testing the rising pain level during injection procedure in comparison with Placebo, and the results of this kind of validity was gained by calculating the degree of pain intensity in both procedures (injection, and placebo) then compared between these two values using t-student test.

Table 2 shows the result of that statistical test, it is clear from the previous table that the value of pain intensity was raised with injections into (3.6) in comparison with placebo (0.13) which was significant statistically on the significance level (0.05), which means FLACC test measures what it was put for, that indicates on Construct validity of FLACC test.

Internal Consistency Validity showed correlation between every clause of FLACC scale clauses, those correlations ranged between (0.792-0.723) as shown in Table 3, and it is positive and statistically significant on the significance level (0.01) which indicates high Internal Consistency for FLACC scale.

External Criterion Validity study (convergent validity) showed strong correlation between FLACC and SEM selfless scales.

Table 4 shows FLACC scale's correlation factor with SEM scale (external criterion) which was (0.799), that indicates criterion validity for FLACC scale.

Reliability study by testing and retesting method, which has been conducted through external raters examining the same investigated people at the same time independently, has shown strong correlation which indicates good reliability for FLACC scale, as shown in Table 5 rater's correlation coefficient value has reached (0.805).

Cronbach's Alpha factor has been calculated for FLACC scale and its value was high and reached (0.809), as shown in Table 6.

Research sample (250) child	Selfless pain scales the number of rates using

	First rater		Second rater		Total rates	
	SEM scale	FLACC scale	SEM scale	FLACC scale	SEM scale	FLACC scale
placebo	250	250	250	250	500	500
injection procedure	250	250	250	250	500	500
total rates	1000		1000		2000	

Table 1: shows the sample's distribution according to pain assessments by the external raters using selfless pain scales.

Correlation coefficient	0.233
significance level	0.579
the decision	insignificant

Table 2: Shows the correlation coefficient between pain level during placebo and injection procedure according to FLACC scale.

Internal consistency of FLACC parts			
The part	Part significant	Correlation coefficient value	Dicision
1	F	0.723**	significant
2	L	0.729**	significant
3	A	0.792**	significant
4	C	0.764**	significant
5	C	0.757**	significant
**significant on the significance level of 0.01			

Table 3: correlation coefficients between each part and the total grade of FLACC scale.

Inter-rater reliability test for each rater showed high and positive Kappa's factors for both raters as shown in Table 7. They were close to complete one and reached (0.952) for the first one and (0.893) for the second rater, which means high compatibility for both raters, and indicates high inter-rater reliability for FLACC scale.

Correlation coefficient	0.799**
significance level	0
decision	Significant
**significant on the significance level of 0.01	

Table 4: shows correlation coefficient's values between FLACC and SEM scales (external criterion).

Correlation coefficient value for the FLACC scale between the external raters	
correlation coefficient	0.805**
significance level	0
Decision	significant
**significant on the significance level of 0.01	

Table 5: shows the correlation coefficient value between the first and the second ratters.

Total level	Cronbach's Alpha factor
	0.809

Table 6: reliability factors for FLACC scales using Cronbach's Alpha factor.

Inter-rater reliability study	Rater	Compatibility factor's value	Significance levels value	The significance of compatibility	Compatibility intensity
	First rater	0.952	0	there is significant compatibility	excellent
	Second rater	0.893	0	there is significant compatibility	excellent

Table 7: Inter-rater reliability of FLACC scale using Kappa compatibility factor's method.

Discussion

FLACC scale has been chosen as the best, first, easiest and the most compatible scale with self-evaluating scales, which their grades ranges between 0 and 10 simultaneously with FLACC scale, and that was according to von Baeyer's systematic review [8].

FLACC scale has been appointed as a standard scale for convergent validity investigations for some common scales [24], or recently innovate [25,26] so the researcher tries to approve its innovated scale's convergence or exceeding in comparison with FLACC scale, to get the acceptance and propagation for his scale [27].

In the current study, FLACC scale has fulfilled the construct validity, due to the rising of pain level during injection procedure in comparison with placebo, which agreed with many studies like Voepel-Lewis et al., Tsze et al., and Tomlinson et al. [6,28-30].

According to this study's results, FLACC showed criterion validity, so it converged to SEM scale, and this validity was assured according to various studies like Tomlinson et al. in 2010 who indicated to the correlation between FLACC scale and parent's scale, correlation coefficient value ranged between (0.65-0.87), Malviya in 2006 also registered strong correlation for FLACC scale with self-pain evaluating for the sample's children and their parents, the correlation coefficient ranged between (0.65-0,87), Voepel-Lewis et al. registered the value of (0.84) for FLACC scale's correlation coefficient with selfless COMFORT scale, and that study indicated good criterion convergent validity [6,27,28,31].

In the way of studying the reliability of FLACC scale by testing and retesting, the correlation value between the external raters, who defined the pain level in this study, has reached (0.805), this value converged with the value that Gomez et al. has gained in 2013, which was (0.95) [32]. Nevertheless, an indicator of the scale reliability was Cronbach's alpha factor's value, which was (0.809), and its convergence with many studies like Voepel-lewis et al. their factor's value was (0.882) [6], it was higher than Cronbach's alpha factor in Fathi et al. study in 2010, which was (0,85) [28].

Internal consistency validity study cleared high values for each part of the scale, those values ranged between (0.723-0.792), and it was convergent to the values registered by Tomlinson et al. in 2010, which ranged (0.76-0.9) [31].

Summary

The Arabic version of FLACC scale showed good psychometric properties, so the scale was valid and reliable, which made it applicable scale in selfless pain level assessment.

Acknowledgment

The authors gratefully acknowledge Damascus University and Prof. Adel Moufti for great help and support.

References

1. Walco GA, Conte P, Labay L, Engel R, Zeltzer L (2005) Procedural distress in children with cancer: self-report, behavioral observations, and physiological parameters. Clin J Pain 21: 484-490.

2. Champion GD (1998) Self-report measures of pain in children. Measurement of pain in infants and children. Pain Res Manag 10: 123-160.

3. de C Williams AC, Davies HT, Chadury Y (2000) Simple pain rating scales hide complex idiosyncratic meanings. Pain 85: 457-463.

4. Hodgins M (2001) Interpreting the meaning of pain severity scores. Pain Res Manag 7: 192-198.

5. Anand K, Craig KD (1996) New perspectives on the definition of pain. Pain 67: 3-6.

6. Voepel-Lewis T, Zanotti J, Dammeyer JA, Merkel S (2010) Reliability and validity of the face, legs, activity, cry, consolability behavioral tool in assessing acute pain in critically ill patients. Am J Crit Care 19: 55-61.

7. Puntillo KA (1997) Relationship between behavioral and physiological indicators of pain, critical care patients' self-reports of pain, and opioid administration. Crit Care Med 25: 1159-1166.

8. von Baeyer CL, Spagrud LJ (2007) Systematic review of observational (behavioral) measures of pain for children and adolescents aged 3 to 18 years. Pain 127: 140-150.

9. Bai J, Hsu L, Tang Y, van Dijk M (2012) Validation of the COMFORT Behavior scale and the FLACC scale for pain assessment in Chinese children after cardiac surgery. Pain Manag Nurs 13: 18-26.

10. Suraseranivongse S, Santawat U, Kraiprasit K, Petcharatana S, Prakkamodom S, et al. (2001) Cross-validation of a composite pain scale for preschool children within 24 hours of surgery. Br J Anaesth 87: 400-405.

11. da Silva FC, Santos Thuler LC, de Leon-Casasola OA (2011) Validity and reliability of two pain assessment tools in Brazilian children and adolescents. J Clin Nurs 20: 1842-1848.

12. Johansson M, Kokinsky E (2009) The COMFORT behavioural scale and the modified FLACC scale in paediatric intensive care. Nurs Crit Care 14: 122-130.

13. Lee SH, Lee NY (2013) An alternative local anaesthesia technique to reduce pain in paediatric patients during needle insertion. Eur J Paediatr Dent 14: 109-112.

14. Kreider KA, Stratmann RG, Milano M, Agostini FG, Munsell M (2001) Reducing children's injection pain: lidocaine patches versus topical benzocaine gel. Pediatr Dent 23: 19-23.

15. Nayak R, Sudha P (2006) Evaluation of three topical anaesthetic agents against pain: A clinical study. Indian J Dent Res 17: 155.

16. Asl Aminabadi N, Mostofi Zadeh Farahani R (2008) Correlation of parenting style and pediatric behavior guidance strategies in the dental setting: preliminary findings. Acta Odontologica 66: 99-104.

17. Aminabadi NA, Ghoreishizadeh A, Ghoreishizadeh M, Oskouei SG (2011) Can drawing be considered a projective measure for children's distress in paediatric dentistry? Int J Paediatr Dent 21: 1-12.

18. Baghdadi ZD (1999) Evaluation of electronic dental anesthesia in children. Oral Surg Oral Med Oral Pathol Oral Radiol Endod 88: 418-423.

19. Kotb RM, Abdella AA, El Kateb MA, Ahmed AM (2009) Clinical evaluation of Papacarie in primary teeth. J Clin Pediatr Dent 34: 117-123.

20. Maragakis G, Musselman R, Ho C (2007) Reaction of 5 and 6 year olds to Dental Injection after Viewing the Needle: pilot study. Journal of Clinical Pediatric Dentistry 31: 28-31.

21. Munshi A, Hegde A, Bashir N (2002) Clinical evaluation of the efficacy of anesthesia and patient preference using the needle-less jet syringe in pediatric dental practice. Journal of Clinical Pediatric Dentistry 25: 131-136.

22. De Menezes Oliveira Maria Angélica H, Bonfim OCR (2010) Device for covering a syringe and needle in order to alleviate the fear and anxiety experienced during pediatric medical and odontological procedures, such as the administration of anesthetics and the like.

23. Glassman P, Peltier B (1995) Guidelines for the administration of local anesthesia in fearful dental patients. J Calif Dent Assoc 23: 23.

24. Armfield JM, Milgrom P (2011) A clinician guide to patients afraid of dental injections and numbness. SAAD Dig 27: 33-39.

25. Schnakers C, Chatelle C, Vanhaudenhuyse A, Majerus S, Ledoux D, et al. (2010) The Nociception Coma Scale: a new tool to assess nociception in disorders of consciousness. Pain 148: 215-219.

26. Nuttall NM, Gilbert A, Morris J (2008) Children's dental anxiety in the United Kingdom in 2003. J Dent 36: 857-860.

27. Beyer JE, McGrath PJ, Berde CB (1990) Discordance between self-report and behavioral pain measures in children aged 3-7 years after surgery. J Pain Symptom Manage 5: 350-356.

28. Fathi A, Al-Sharabasy AA (2012) Threshold of Pain Perception to Intraoral Anesthetic Injections among Egyptian Children. Life Science Journal 9: 1480-1483.

29. Tomlinson D, von Baeyer CL, Stinson JN, Sung L (2010) A systematic review of faces scales for the self-report of pain intensity in children. Pediatrics 126: e1168-1198.

30. Tsze DS, von Baeyer CL, Bulloch B, Dayan PS (2013) Validation of self-report pain scales in children. Pediatrics 132: e971-979.

31. Malviya S, Voepel-Lewis T, Burke C, Merkel S, Tait AR (2006) The revised FLACC observational pain tool: improved reliability and validity for pain assessment in children with cognitive impairment. Pediatric Anesthesia 16: 258-265.

31

Timing of Prophylactic Antibiotic Administration in Elective Surgical Patients at Jimma University Teaching Hospital

Hunduma Jisha*

Department of Anesthesiology, Jimma University, Ethiopia

*Corresponding author: Hunduma Jisha, Department of Anesthesiology, Jimma University, Jimma, Ethiopia, E-mail: hunjisha@gmail.com

Abstract

Study objective: To evaluate the timing of prophylactic antibiotic administration in elective surgical patients, and anesthetists' opinion regarding this issue.

Design: Prospective, facility based cross-sectional study was employed.

Setting: Jimma university teaching hospital (JUTH)

Patient: Elective surgical patients and anesthesia professional of the hospital.

Measurement: Data were collected prospectively from all elective surgical patients (except emergency, obstetric cases) and interred in predesigned forms as per existing protocol in JUTH from February 01 to March 30, 2014. The time of antibiotic prophylactic administration in respect to incision time was analyzed and descriptive result was presented as percentages of total responses.

Main results: Prophylactic antibiotics was given before skin incision for 107 (79.9%) patients and 27 (20.1%) after skin incision. However; only 75 (56%) patients were get administered within proper time (60minutes) and the mean time of preoperative administration was 66+24 minutes. Prophylactic antibiotic medication was continued for >24 hours in 95% cases and re-dosing were not given for six surgical procedures which lasted >3 hours.

Out of 26, only 71% anesthetists could mention the recommended time of antibiotic prophylaxis administration. About 21(80.8%) of anesthetists agreed that its surgeon's responsibility for preoperative antibiotic selection and shared with nurses for preoperative administration. Anesthetists assume that they are responsible for confirmation of pre-incision administration and repeat administration during prolonged surgery. They indicated training was inadequate and deemed necessary in 77% of participants.

Conclusion: The timing of prophylactic antibiotic administration was below the standard of practice. Hospital administration and infection control officer should work to improve compliance in accordance with published evidence-based guidelines.

Keywords: Administration; Anesthetist; Prophylactic antibiotics; Timing; Training; JUTH

Introduction

Surgical site infection continue to be a major public health problem that imposes enormous impacts both on patients' life and substantially to the financial cost of patient care. Surgical site infection is the second most common hospital associated infections accounting 14-16% of all hospitalized patients; and 38% among that of surgical patients [1-3].

In developing countries, especially in sub-Saharan Africa this figure is twice or three times higher than developed countries [4].

Although information was limited, the overall SSI rate in Ethiopia was reported to be in a range of 14.8-75% in general surgical wards at different teaching hospitals [4-7].

Almost all surgical sites are contaminated with bacteria to some extent though optimal care was taken to maintain asepsis and causing surgical site infection. Although there are various ways of preventing SSIs, administering antibiotic prophylaxis at the appropriate time, (60-30 minute before surgery) contributes a lot than other methods [8].

Different researcher showed that the standard surgical precaution; proper prophylactic antibiotics administration significantly minimizes the incidence of SSI by 40-60%. Different Guideline and researcher has been promoted on three areas; proper timing of administration within 60 minutes prior skin incision, correct selection of antibiotics and correct duration of postoperative administration [9,10].

It has been documented that untimely use or omission of single dose perioperative antibiotic prophylaxis has been associated with increased incidence and severity of postoperative SSIs [11].

The selection of antibiotic should be taken into consideration for its safety, cost-effectiveness, and active against commonly encountered pathogens based on the type of procedures which will be guided by local resistance patterns [12-14]. Usually first and second-generation cephalosporins are appropriate prophylaxis for most procedures, although coverage of anaerobes is necessary for colon and some gynecologic surgery [12].

It is generally agreed that all clean wound do not need but for all procedures of clean-contaminated prophylactic antibiotics should be administered before skin incision (within 60 minutes). However, contaminated or dirty wounds are already infected and need therapeutic pre-operative antibiotics not for prophylactic purposes [12,14,15]

The intention of perioperative prophylaxis is to attain therapeutic levels of antibiotic agents in the tissues at the time of microbial contamination. Therefore timing of administration is critical in order to ensure effective drug levels, as both early and late administration are associated with increased infection rates [12,17].

A single dose of prophylactic antibiotic given prior to incision is sufficient for most surgical procedures. However, re-dosing should be considered when there is extensive hemorrhage and surgery lasting longer than 3 hours. In patients antimicrobial prophylaxis is planned to be continued postoperatively, the duration is recommended to be less than 24 hours [12,17].

Despite such timing and appropriate selection of prophylactic antibiotic administration is important for a patient safety and outcome [11], it is continuously appended and challenging as showed in many study results [18,19]. A Health Care Quality Improvement Project of New York State showed from retrospective review of 2651 patients; about 27%-54% of all patients did not receive antimicrobial prophylaxis in a timely fashion [18]. Although it's inevitably advantageous in outcome of surgical patients no attempts were made before to explore the extent of proper timing of prophylactic administration in our hospital.

As the existing trend in JUTH a list of scheduled patients posted a day before surgery on major theatre and surgical ward's board. Preoperative anesthetic evaluations performed a day before surgery by anesthetists for verification of fitness of patients for anesthesia and get prepared on each side by surgeon, anesthetists and nurses. Every medication (including antibiotics) given on the early morning usually at 6:00 am on the day of surgery if indicated; then the ward nurse took patients to operation theatre (waiting corridor) turn by turn according to list on schedule. The expected time of skin incision for the first patient is at 8:00 am for all elective cases.

Therefore this survey aimed to assess time of initial dose, re-dosing time and duration of administration in elective surgical patients. Also the opinion of anesthesia professional's regarding perioperative antibiotics administration and their role was explored.

Methods and Materials

A hospital based prospective study was conducted from February 01 to March 30, 2014 at Jimma University Teaching Hospital (JUTH) in Jimma, located 346 km away from Addis Ababa to South West Ethiopia. The hospital provides a range of health care services with a multidisciplinary team of diverse professionals; and capacity of 450 beds (from these 125 surgical beds) through its 9 medical and other clinical and diagnostic departments for approximately 15,000

inpatients and 160,000 outpatients each year and a total of more than 1448 staffs. The major departments includes: the Pediatrics, Surgery, Gynecology and Obstetrics, Internal Medicine, Ophthalmology, Dentistry, Psychiatry. More than 8000 patients get admitted in dentistry, surgical and gynecology wards per year and on average seven major operations would performed per day.

Operation room (OR) unit is one of the service units of JUTH. We have five operation theatres; of which three major tables shared in common to all departments; but ophthalmic and maternity (for caesarean section surgeries) have isolated theatre each. In the hospital different surgery were performed such as orthopedic surgery, hysterectomy, thyroidectomy, mastectomy, colostomy, herniorraphy, hemoriedectomy, laparatomy, prostatectomy and etc.

We observed 168 cases of elective major surgery who received prophylactic antibiotics as per existing practice in the hospital to determine the timing of prophylactic antibiotics administration relative to skin incision time. Pre-designed data sheet was kept in each operation theatre to be filled in by each respective anesthetists by reviewing patients' card or if any medication in the theatre. The form focused on the preoperative patient character; surgical type and procedure; time of induction, antibiotic administration drug type, dose and time, incision time, re-dosing time and duration of surgery were recorded. Those patients were followed every day post operatively until the prophylactic antibiotic administration stopped. Additional questionnaire focusing on anesthetist's opinion regarding the responsibility of selection, confirmation and administration of prophylactic antibiotics and adequacy/need of training were administered to all anesthetists of JUTH.

All elective surgery scheduled that has been administered prophylactic antibiotics was included after verbal consent obtained. Emergency surgery and obstetric cases were excluded from the study because of the physiologic difference and time constraint. Patients who have been on antibiotic treatment for any reason and not cooperated were also excluded.

Timing of administration was analyzed as in intervals before and after incision. It was considered as early preoperative administration if given before 1 hr before skin incision, preoperative if within 1hr before skin incision, perioperative if within 3hrs after skin incision and postoperative if after 3 hrs after skin incision.

After the data entered to computer; analyzed using SPSS version16 and presented as percentages of total observation and responses.

Ethical Clearance

Studies were conducted after ethical approval letter obtained from the Jimma university ethical review committee and official permission confirmed from hospital administration. All participants were asked for volunteer participation in study. Verbal consent was obtained from each participant; as this was an observational study of existing practice in the hospital.

Result

Timing of prophylactic antibiotics administration

A total of 230 patients have been underwent elective surgery during study period. Among this antibiotics were administered for 168 (73%) patients. From these 34 patients were on antibiotic treatment because they have developed infection preoperatively and excluded from study. Therefore only 134 (58 male and 76 female) patients who have given antibiotics for prophylactic purpose were included in the study. Half (49.3%) of study participants were classified in the first category of American Society of Anesthesiology (ASA I). The age of the study subjects ranges from 2½ to 75 years, with the majority aged between 41-50years. Ninety eight (73.1%) patients were from rural area and 50.7 %(68) of them did not attend formal education (Table 1).

		Sex		Total	Percentage
		Female(N)	Male (N)	(N=134)	
Age	<10 years	5	12	17	12.7
	11-20years	7	5	12	9
	21-30years	9	10	19	14.2
	31-40years	10	6	16	11.9
	41-50years	25	7	32	23.9
	51-60years	15	15	30	22.4
	>60 years	5	3	8	6
ASA class	I	41	25	66	49.3
	II	27	30	57	42.5
	III	8	3	11	8.2
Educational Status	Illiterate	37	31	68	50.7
	Literate	39	27	66	49.3
Residency	Rural	55	43	98	73.1
	Urban	21	15	36	26.9

Table 1: Preoperative characteristics of elective surgical patient; JUTH, 2014.

The study results showed that in 79.9% (46 male and 61 female) of patient prophylactic antibiotics administration was before skin incision. But only 75 (56%) and five (3.7%) patients have given within 60 minutes, and between 60 and 120 minutes respectively. Mean time of preoperative prophylactic antibiotics administration was 1.7 ± 0.8 hours. However, in 20.1% (27) patients it was administered after skin incision; of which five (3.7%) patients given within 3 hours and 22 (16.4%) patients have took 3 hours later after skin incision. The study revealed almost in all patients PA medication was continued for more than 24hrs and preponderance up to 5 days. Even though large number (>56%) of surgical procedure lasted more than two hours with mean duration of 2.1+0.8 (range from 20 to 270 minutes); re-dosing was not considered for any operations (six cases) lasted more than three hours (Table 2).

Variable	Perioperative Character	Female	Male	Total	Percentage
Timing of administration (minutes)	Before skin incision between				
	0-30	17	10	27	20.1
	30-60	23	25	48	35.8
	60-120	4	1	5	3.7
	120-180	16	8	24	17.9
	before 180	1	2	3	2.2
	After skin incision between				
	0-30	1	0	1	0.7
	30-60	1	2	3	2.2
	60-180	0	1	1	0.7
	180-240	8	7	15	11.2
	later than 240	5	2	7	5.2
Duration of surgery (hour)	<2	26	27	53	39.6
	2-3	49	26	75	56
	>3	1	5	6	4.5
Surgical type	Orthopedic surgery	14	25	39	29.1
	Gastrointestinal surgery	21	15	36	26.9
	Gynecologic surgery	23	0	23	17.2
	Urologic surgery	0	11	11	8.2
	Maxillofacial surgery	1	2	3	2.2
	Others*	17	5	22	16.4
Duration of prophylaxis administration (day)	One (24hours)	4	3	7	5.2
	Two (48hours)	5	10	15	11.2
	Three (72hours)	19	18	37	27.6
	Four	12	9	21	15.7
	Five	33	11	41	30.6
	Week	3	7	10	5.5
Timing of administration in intervals (hours)	Early preoperative	21	11	32	23.9
	Preoperative	40	35	75	56
	Perioperative	2	3	5	3.7
	Postoperative	13	9	22	16.4
	Re-dosing	0	0	0	0

*thyroidectomy, breast surgery, tissue excision

Table 2: Perioperative characteristics of surgical patients who have taken prophylactic antibiotic in JUTH; 2014.

The most procedure that has been performed during study period was open reduction and internal fixation17 (12.7%) followed by external fixation, open cholecystectomy and hysterectomy 14 (10.4%) each; bowel resection 11 (8.2%), breast surgery 10 (7.5%); herniorhaphy and laparotomy (ovarian tumor) nine (6.7%) each; thyroidectomy and prostatectomy eight (6%) each; debridement five (3.7%); amputation and tissue excision (tissue sarcoma) three (2.2%) each; mandibular correction, uretroplasty and gastroduodinal surgery two (1.5%) each; and mandibulectomy one (0.7%) each (Table 3).

Surgical type	Surgical procedure	Sex of patients		Total N=134	percentage
		Female	Male		
orthopedic surgery	ORIF	5	12	17	12.7
	Amputation	1	2	3	2.2
	Debridement	1	4	5	3.7
	External fixation	7	7	14	10.4
Gastrointestinal surgery	Hernioraphy	5	4	9	6.7
	Open cholecystectomy	14	0	14	10.4
	Surgery for intestinal obstruction	1	10	11	8.2
	Gastroduodnal surgery	1	1	2	1.5
Gynecologic surgery	Hysterectomy	14	-	14	10.4
	Laparotomy (ovarian tumor)	9	-	9	6.7
Urologic surgery	Prostatectomy (BPH)	-	8	8	6
	Uretroplasty (uriteral stricture)	-	3	3	2.2
Maxillofacial surgery	Mandibulectomy	1	0	1	0.7
	Mandibular correction	0	2	2	1.5
Others	Mastectomy (breast mass)	10	0	10	7.5
	Tissue excision (tissue sarcoma)	2	1	3	2.2
	Thyroidectomy	5	4	9	6.7

Table 3: Surgical type and procedures who have taken prophylactic antibiotics in JUTH; 2014.

Six different combinations of antimicrobial drugs were used for prophylaxis. The most frequently (51%) prescribed classes of antibiotics were cephalosporins (ceftriaxone and cefazolin) followed by penicillin 32% (amoxicillin 500 mg) and chloramphenicol (CAF) 500 mg. Fifty five percent of (74) patients received a single drug (ceftriaxone 1g) for prophylaxis while 43 patients (32.1%) received two drugs (ceftriaxone and gentamycine). Ten patients (7.5%) received three drugs (ceftriaxone, ampicillin and gentamicin) and seven received four drugs (cefotaxime, metronidazole, CAF & gentamicin) for prophylaxis.

Anesthetists' opinion and their role in the timing of prophylactic antibiotic administration

A total of 31 questionnaires were administered to anesthesia team of JUTH with response rate of 83.9% (4 female and 22 male). Most (84.6%) of participants have been provided anesthesia services for more than 3 years and 38.7% (12) them were senior Master degree holder. The participants' age ranges from 26-56 years (mean=31+1.2) with a mean experience year of 6+0.9 years (Table 4). Although they believe that prophylaxis should be administered preoperatively none of them mentioned the recommended time for prophylaxis. Also only 25.8% (8) of them were knows for which type of surgical wounds prophylactic antibiotic are indicated.

		Female	Male	
Age (year)	<30	2	10	12 (38.7)
	30-40	2	9	11 (35.5)
	41-50	0	2	2 (6.5)
	>50	0	1	1 (3.2)
qualification level	Diploma	0	2	2 (6.5)
	BSc degree	2	7	9 (29)
	MSc degree/ above	1	11	12 (38.7)
	Resident	1	2	3 (9.7)
Year of experience	<3 year	2	4	4 (15.4)
	3-5 yrs	5	13	12 (46.2)
	5-10 yrs	3	1	8 (30.8)
	>10 yrs	1	2	2 (7.7)

Table 4: Sociodemography of anesthetists who have been participated in study; JUTH, 2014.

	Sex of participants	Total N (%)

All of them do not have information when re-dosing of prophylactic antibiotic should be considered. Majority 64.5% (20) of anesthetists agreed that they are responsible for the confirmation of PA administration. However; only 9.7% (3) anesthetists were noticed that they have been checking for every patient. They consider that it's the responsibility of surgeon for the selection and nurses for administration of prophylactic antibiotics. In surgical procedures lasting more than 3 hrs, they indicate that anesthetist and surgeon should be responsible for intraoperative re-dosing (Table 5).

Activities	Responsible professionals				
	Surgeon n (%)	Ward nurse n (%)	OR nurse n (%)	Anesthetists n (%)	Total n (100%)
Selection	21(80.8%)	2(7.7%)	1(3.8%)	2(4.35%)	26
Confirmation of administration	6(23.1%)	2(7.7%)	4(15.4%)	14(53.8%)	26
Timing of administration	10(38.5%)	9(34.6%)	3(11.5%)	4(15.4%)	26

Table 5: The anesthetists' response regarding the responsibility of selection, confirmation and timing of prophylactic antibiotics administration; JUTH, 2014.

Eighteen anesthetists were feeling they are not trained adequately and it seems additional training is compulsory in 67.7% of them (Figure 1).

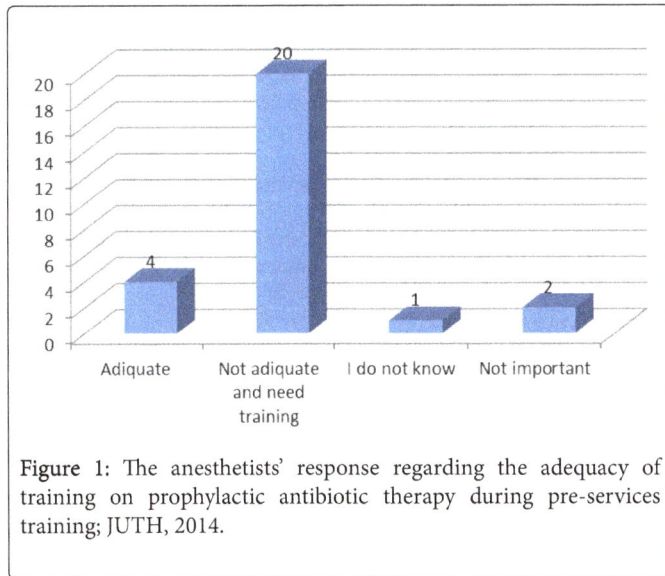

Figure 1: The anesthetists' response regarding the adequacy of training on prophylactic antibiotic therapy during pre-services training; JUTH, 2014.

Discussion

Surgical site infections (SSIs) continued causing significant morbidity, mortality and add to the cost of patient care as reports shows from different researchers [11]. Aseptic techniques alone do not eliminate bacteria, and Staphylococci aurous are often found at surgical sites. To overcome this catastrophic problem antimicrobial treatment begun prior to contamination is called antibiotic prophylaxis (AP) which is an important adjunct to control bacterial growth and significantly lower the incidence of SSIs [20].

Orthopedic (29.1%) and abdominal (22.4%) surgery was the most frequently performed surgery type and also majority of them among others took prophylaxis within the first hour.

From a total of 230 surgical cases that has been underwent elective surgery, prophylaxis was given for 73% (168 cases). Out of 168, 34 (20.2%) were for treatment purpose and 134 (79.8%) prophylactic

purposes. The age of study participants (patients) ranges from 2½ to 75 years with majority (23.9) in 41 – 50years. More than half (56.7%) of them were females. This figure goes in line with the study done in Iraq [21]. Comparable figure were obtained by other researchers [22]. Among 134, in 79.9% (107) and 27 (20.1) patients the administered was before and after skin incision respectively. However; only 75 (56%) patients were get administered within 60 minutes before skin incision, (%) within 1hours before skin incision, (%) within 3 hours after skin incision and (%) after 3 hours after skin incision. Similar finding was obtained in other study India [23], Utah (USA) [20], Iraq [21]. However, it is better than that of Shah JN et al. in Nepal [22,24].

Different guideline recommends that prophylactic antibiotics are more effective if administered as close as to skin incision time; especially with in 60minutes before skin incision [18]. We found 17.9% were administered 2 hours earlier before skin incision. Therefore, it needs an improvement of adherence to prophylactic antibiotic medication guide line in our hospital [25]. In other studies better compliance were observed [26].

Though published guide lines promote to end prophylactic administration within 24 hrs [8,27,28]. But in ours we found for more than half (50.7%) the administration continued for up to five days. In different studies comparable results were reported [22,29]. Different researchers identified prolonged use of antimicrobials may contribute to bacterial resistance; the guidelines recommend that prophylaxis better end within 24 hours of surgery except in cardiothoracic surgery up to 72 hours. The problem of adherence to guideline in prophylactic administration was also identified by study done in Athens, Greece [30].

Though different guidelines recommend single drugs with extended spectrum except some procedures like colorectal surgery [31-34]; this study revealed in more than 44% study participants, in which combinations of antimicrobials were used. However; in our study abdominal surgery represents only 26.9% of study participants [35].

From 31, 26 anesthetists were responded. Out of 26, 12 were master's degree holder and have been served for more than three years. Though they feel responsible for confirmation of administration, only two anesthetists indicated that they check for every patient whether prophylaxis was administered. Only two out of 26 anesthetists mention the proper timing of prophylaxis (within 1 hour prior skin incision).

Also we noticed majority were not felt that they have adequate knowledge regarding the selection, indication, and guidelines of prophylactic antibiotics administration. But different studies showed involvement of anesthesia staffs improve the compliance on timing of prophylaxis administration [24,32,36]. Twenty (64.5%) of anesthetists agreed that they are responsible for the confirmation of PA administration and re-dosing. However; only 9.7% (3) anesthetists were noticed that they have been checking for every patient. They consider that it's the responsibility of surgeon for the selection and nurses for administration of prophylactic antibiotics [37].

Conclusion

To my knowledge, a reliable method to ensure compliance with the appropriate timing of prophylactic antibiotics did not exist in this hospital prior to this study.

High rate of passivity with proper timing of prophylactic antibiotic administration in elective surgical patients was observed during the study period. Physician, Anesthetists and nursing management, and hospital infection control office had to work for improvement of current practice to the standard of prophylactic antibiotic administration. Continues (refresher) training should be provided for staffs every year. All operating room personnel, including the surgeons, anesthetists, and nursing staff, were committed to the concept that patients should receive antibiotics in a timely manner.

The limitations to this study include the non-response and the convenient sampling used. These preclude generalizations for a nationwide practice.

Acknowledgement

Author would like to thank the hospital administration offices and participant (patients) for their co-operation. Author's gratitude also extends to anesthesia team for their help in completing the form and nurses who helped by delivering information regarding administration of prophylactic antibiotics.

References

1. Cannon JA, Altom LK, Deierhoi RJ, Morris M, Richman JS, et al. (2012) Preoperative oral antibiotics reduce surgical site infection following elective colorectal resections. Dis Colon Rectum [Internet]. 55: 1160-1166.
2. Cziraki K, Lucas J, Rogers T, Page L, Zimmerman R, et al. (2008) Communication and relationship skills for rapid response teams at hamilton health sciences. Healthc Q 11(3 Spec No.
3. Karim R (2011) Factors Responsible for Surgical Site Infections Following Emergency Nontraumatic Abdominal Operations.
4. Mengesha RE, Kasa BG, Saravanan M, Berhe DF, Wasihun AG (2014) Aerobic bacteria in post surgical wound infections and pattern of their antimicrobial susceptibility in Ayder Teaching and Referral Hospital, Mekelle, Ethiopia. BMC Res Notes 7: 575.
5. Mulu W, Kibru G, Beyene G, Damtie M (2012) Postoperative infections and antimicrobial resistance pattern of bacteria isolates among patients admitted at felege hiwot referral hospital, bahirdar, Ethiopia. Ethiop J Health Sci 22: 7-18.
6. Amenu D, Belachew T, Araya F (2011) Surgical site infection rate and risk factors among obstetric cases of jimma university specialized hospital, southwest ethiopia. Ethiop J Health Sci 21: 91-100.
7. Godebo G, Kibru G, Tassew H (2013) Multidrug-resistant bacterial isolates in infected wounds at Jimma University Specialized Hospital, Ethiopia. Ann Clin Microbiol Antimicrob 12: 17.
8. Bratzler DW, Dellinger EP, Olsen KM, Perl TM, Auwaerter PG, et al. (2013) Clinical practice guidelines for antimicrobial prophylaxis in surgery. Am J Health Syst Pharm 70: 195-283.
9. Wacha H, Hoyme U, Isenmann R, Kujath P, Lebert C, et al. Perioperative antibiotic prophylaxis. Evidence based guidelines by an expert panel of the Paul Ehrlich Gesellschaft. Chemotherapie Journal 19: 70-84.
10. Hedrick TL, Anastacio MM, Sawyer RG (2006) Prevention of surgical site infections. Expert Rev Anti Infect Ther 4: 223-233.
11. Akalin HE (2002) Surgical prophylaxis: the evolution of guidelines in an era of cost containment. J Hosp Infect 50 Suppl A: S3-7.
12. Bratzler DW, Dellinger EP, Olsen KM, Perl TM, Auwaerter PG, et al. (2013) Clinical practice guidelines for antimicrobial prophylaxis in surgery. Am J Health Syst Pharm 70: 195-283.
13. Grabe M (2001) Perioperative antibiotic prophylaxis in urology. Curr Opin Urol 11: 81-85.
14. Enzler MJ, Berbari E, Osmon DR (2011) Antimicrobial prophylaxis in adults. Mayo Clin Proc 86: 686-701.
15. Gray SH, Hawn MT (2007) Prevention of Surgical Site Infections. Hosp Physician 2007: 41–51.
16. Clasener HL, Vollaard EJ (1991) Perioperative systemic antibiotic prophylaxis. Bailliere's Clinical Anaesthesiology 5: 123-140.
17. Bratzler DW, Houck PM (2005) Antimicrobial prophylaxis for surgery: An advisory statement from the National Surgical Infection Prevention Project. American Journal of Surgery 189: 395-404.
18. Burke JP (2001) Maximizing appropriate antibiotic prophylaxis for surgical patients: an update from LDS Hospital, Salt Lake City. Clin Infect Dis 33 Suppl 2: S78-83.
19. Codina C, Trilla A, Riera N, Tuset M, Carne X, et al. (1999) Perioperative antibiotic prophylaxis in Spanish hospitals: results of a questionnaire survey. Hospital Pharmacy Antimicrobial Prophylaxis Study Group. Infect Control Hosp Epidemiol. 20: 436-439.
20. Tan JA, Naik VN, Lingard L (2006) Exploring obstacles to proper timing of prophylactic antibiotics for surgical site infections. 15: 32-38.
21. Al-dabbagh AA, Hajy MA (2013) How Good is Compliance with Surgical Antibiotic Prophylaxis Guidelines in Erbil/ Iraq? 2nd International Conference on Medical, Biological and Pharmaceutical Sciences (ICMBPS'2013) June 17-18, 2013 London (UK).
22. AnyadohNwadike SO, Eri O, Nwaokoro JC, Nwadike PO (2011) Prevalence of Staphylococcus aureus within the Hospital Environment. Asian journal of medical sciences 2: 18-22.
23. Rehan HS, Kakkar AK, Goel S (2010) Pattern of surgical antibiotic prophylaxis in a tertiary care teaching hospital in India. Int J Infect Control 6: 1-6.
24. Silver A, Eichorn A, Kral J, Pickett G, Barie P, et al. (1996) Timeliness and use of antibiotic prophylaxis in selected inpatient surgical procedures. The Antibiotic Prophylaxis Study Group. Am J Surg 171: 548-552.
25. Setiawan B (2011) The role of prophylactic antibiotics in preventing perioperative infection. Acta Med Indones 43: 262-266.
26. Rosenberg AD, Wambold D, Kraemer L, Begley-Keyes M, Zuckerman SL, et al. (2008) Ensuring appropriate timing of antimicrobial prophylaxis. J Bone Joint Surg Am 90: 226-232.
27. Holtom PD (2006) Antibiotic prophylaxis: current recommendations. J Am Acad Orthop Surg 14(10 Spec No.
28. Széll M, Hofmann S, Pietsch M, Gerhart E, Wenisch C (2006) [Perioperative antibiotic prophylaxis. Use in orthopaedics]. Orthopade 35: 805-812, quiz 813.
29. Willemsen I (2010) Improving antimicrobial use and control of resistant micro-organisms in the hospital. Optima Grafische Communicatie, Rotterdam.

30. Apostolopoulou E, Zaxos N, Georgoudi A, Tsakona M, Nikoloudi P (2010) Adherence with guidelines of perioperative antibiotic prophylaxis and cost among women undergoing cesarean section. Rev Clin Pharmacol Pharmacokinet Int Ed 24: 19-24.

31. Tita AT, Owen J, Stamm AM, Grimes A, Hauth JC, et al. (2008) Impact of extended-spectrum antibiotic prophylaxis on incidence of postcesarean surgical wound infection. Am J Obstet Gynecol 199: 303.

32. Cziraki K, Lucas J, Rogers T, Page L, Zimmerman R, et al. (2008) Communication and relationship skills for rapid response teams at hamilton health sciences. Healthc Q 11(3 Spec No.

33. Gray SH, Hawn MT (2007) Prevention of Surgical Site Infections. Surgical Patient Care Series 2007: 41-51.

34. Bratzler DW, Dellinger EP, Olsen KM, Perl TM, Auwaerter PG, et al. (2013) Clinical Practice Guidelines for Antimicrobial Prophylaxis in Surgery. Am J Health Syst Pharm. 70: 195-283.

35. Willemsen I, van den Broek R, Bijsterveldt T, van Hattum P, Winters M, et al. (2007) A standardized protocol for perioperative antibiotic prophylaxis is associated with improvement of timing and reduction of costs. J Hosp Infect 67: 156-160.

36. Tan JA, Naik VN, Lingard L (2006) Exploring obstacles to proper timing of prophylactic antibiotics for surgical site infections. Qual Saf Health Care 15: 32-38.

37. Alagbe-Briggs OT, Onajin Obembe BO (2013) A survey on selection and administration of perioperative antibiotics by anaesthetists. West Afr J Med 32: 3-7.

32

Ultrasound Guided Supraclavicular Brachial Plexus Block for Arterio-Venous Shunt Surgery in Chronic Renal Failure, Comparative Study between Two Volumes of Bupivacaine

Mona Mohamed Mogahed* and **Mohamed Samir Abd El Ghafar**

Faculty of Medicine, Tanta University, Egypt

***Corresponding author:** Mona Mohamed Mogahed, Faculty of Medicine, Tanta University, Tanta, Egypt, E-mail: monamogahedfr@hotmail.com

Abstract

Background: There are different anesthetic techniques for AVF (Arterio-venous fistula) creation as general anesthesia, regional anesthesia and local anesthetic infiltration. Sympathetic nerve block is produced by regional anesthesia which increases intraoperative venous diameter and vessel flow, both intra-operatively and for several hours post-operatively. Regional anesthesia can maintain adequate blood flow through the fistula post-operatively which can prevent thrombosis and fistula failure and is important in fistula maturation.

Aim: The aim of this study was to evaluate the effect of two different volumes of bupivacaine in chronic renal failure patients with ultrasound-guided supraclavicular brachial plexus block in arterio-venous shunt creation surgery.

Methods: Patients were randomly classified using sealed envelope into two equal groups each of 25 patients; Group I: Patients received plain bupivacaine 0.5% (30 ml), Group II: Patients received plain bupivacaine 0. 5% (20 ml) In all groups, we measured the onset of sensory block, the onset of motor block, success rate , duration of motor and sensory block and complications.

Results: Insignificant difference between both groups according to onset of sensory block, insignificant difference between both groups according to onset of motor block, Significant prolongation in duration of sensory block in group I as compared to group II, significant prolongation in duration of motor block in group I as compared to group II. There was significant increase in the rate of complications in group I as compared to group II and there was no significant difference between the two groups as regard the success rate.

Conclusion: During ultrasound guided supraclavicular block in end stage renal disease (ESRD), administration of 20 ml bupivacaine 0.5% is equal to 30 ml bupivacaine 0.5% as regard the onset of sensory block, motor block and the success rate but with shorter duration as regard the sensory block and motor block and significant decrease in complications.

Keywords: Supraclavicular; A-V shunt ; Bupivacaine

Introduction

It is a difficult process to treat chronic kidney disease patients. Perioperative morbidity and mortality in chronic kidney disease patients can be lowered by understanding how to care for them [1]

Renal replacement therapy (RRT) is necessary for survival in irreversible end stage renal failure patients. Hemodialysis which is the commonest form of RRT and surgical creation of an arteriovenous fistula (AVF) are recommended for those patients [2].

There are different anesthetic techniques for AVF creation as general anesthesia, regional anesthesia and local anesthetic infiltration [3].

Sympathetic nerve block is produced by regional anesthesia which increases intraoperative venous diameter and vessel flow, both intra-operatively and for several hours post-operatively. Regional anesthesia can maintain adequate blood flow through the fistula post-operatively

which can prevent thrombosis and fistula failure and is important in fistula maturation. Also, arterial and venous spasm reduces flow and is more common with local infiltration than regional or general anesthesia [4].

General anesthesia increases intra-operative vasodilatation and hypotension, chronic kidney disease (CKD) patients are known to be at increased risk of peri- and post-operative anesthetic complications. Many of these complications can be avoided if regional anesthesia is employed [5].

Systemic local anesthetic toxicity is still frequent and dose dependent. Therefore, reducing the dose of local anesthetic in regional anesthesia can contribute to the safety of regional anesthesia [6].

Minimum local anesthetic volume required for ultrasound guided supraclavicular block was 23 ml. However, many different dosages are described; an overall volume of 20 to 25 ml of local anesthetic in combination with ultrasound guidance is commonly accepted. Nowadays, many studies aim to prove equal efficacy with a reduction of the necessary volume [7].

The aim of this study was to evaluate the effect of two different volumes of bupivacaine in chronic renal failure patients with ultrasound-guided supraclavicular brachial plexus block in arterio-venous shunt creation surgery as 1ry outcome was onset and duration of sensory and motor block while secondary outcomes were complications and success rate.

Patients and Methods

Study design

This double blind randomized prospective study had been carried out in Anesthesia and Surgical Intensive Care department, Tanta University Hospitals for six months. A written informed consent had been obtained from all patients. Every patient received an explanation to the purpose of the study and had a code number to ensure privacy to participants and confidentiality of data.

Research results were only used for scientific purposes. Procedures had been approved by both the institutional and the regional ethical committees. Any unexpected risks appeared during the course of research had been clarified to the participants and the ethical committee in time.

Sample size

The sample size was calculated using Epi-Info software statistical package created by World Health organization and center for Disease Control and Prevention, Atlanta, Georgia, USA version 2002. The sample size was calculated at N=30.

The criteria used for sample size calculation were as follows:

95% confidence limit, 80% power, The ratio between experimental and control groups is 1:1, Expected outcome in in treatment group is double times better than control groups (40-80% of optimal required).

Study population

Adult patients with chronic renal failure which defined as progressive kidney damage with glomerular filtration rate (GFR)<15 mL/min/1.73 m^2 for 3 months or more irrespective of cause which is the point of needing dialysis with physical status ASA III classification scheduled for elective arterio-venous shunt creation surgery were included in our study. While patients with neurological deficit with upper limb, bleeding disorders (coagulopathy), mental dysfunction, history of drug abuse and chronic analgesic use, history of allergy to local anesthetics were excluded in our study. Patients were randomly classified using sealed envelope into two equal groups each of 25 patients by random selection of envelopes performed in the operating theatre. The envelopes were prepared in advance and contained a computer-generated randomization schedule. The pharmacist (who prepared the medication), the anesthetist (who did the technique), investigator (who did data collection and recording) and patient were blinded about the group assignment. Group I: Patients of this group received plain bupivacaine 0.5% (30 ml), Group II: Patients of this group received plain bupivacaine 0. 5% (20 ml).

Study intervention

Medical & surgical history of the patient were evaluated, clinical examination of the patient was performed, laboratory investigations included complete blood picture, prothrombin time& activity, liver and renal functions and electrolytes.

Routine monitoring of heart rate &rhythm by ECG, arterial blood pressure using non-invasive blood pressure (NIBP) including systolic, diastolic & mean arterial blood pressure, peripheral oxygen saturation (SPO$_2$) using pulse oximeter had been performed.

Equipment used included: Sterile towels and gauze packs, 20 mL syringes with local anesthetic, 25 gauge needle and 2 ml lidocaine 2%, Sterile gloves, gel and marking pen, 20 gauge, 50 mm length needle for infiltration of local anesthetics (visioplex*-vygon-france), Ultrasound machine (sonoscape* SSI-6000) and a 12 MHz linear type probe. The supraclavicular brachial plexus block was performed in supine position.

An intravenous (I.V) line was established with an 18 gauge cannula. While the patient was in supine position the skin was disinfected and a linear probe, high frequency 12 MHz was placed firmly over the supraclavicular fossa , the probe was positioned in the transverse plane immediately superior to the clavicle at approximately its midpoint. The probe was tilted caudally to obtain a cross-sectional view of the subclavian artery. The brachial plexus was seen as a collection of hypoechoic oval structures lateral and superficial to the artery.

Using a 25 gauge needle, 1 to 2 mL of lidocaine was injected into the skin 1 cm lateral to the probe to decrease the discomfort during needle insertion. The needle was advanced along the long axis of the probe in the same plane as the ultrasound beam. The needle shaft and tip can be visualized in real time as the needle was advanced towards the target nerves.

The volume of bupivacaine according to each group was injected under direct vision of ultrasound beams.

In both groups, the followings were measured: Onset of sensory block: checked with a needle every 5 min up to 30 min after injection of local anesthetic in all 5 cutaneous nerve distributions Musculocutaneous nerve: lateral side of the forearm, Radial nerve: dorsum of the hand over the 2nd metacarpophalangeal joint, Ulnar nerve: little finger, Median nerve: medial thenar eminence, and Medial cutaneous nerve: medial side of the forearm) [8]. Onset of motor block : checked every 5 min. up to 30 min. For motor block evaluation, the following nerves were assessed: Radial nerve (elbow extension against resistance), median nerve (flexion of the distal interphalangeal joint of the second finger), ulnar nerve (abduction of the middle and ring fingers), and musculocutaneous nerve (elbow flexion against resistance) [8]. Success rate: success means complete sensory and motor block. Duration of motor and sensory block in hours: checked every 15 min till the end of surgery. And complications: such as Horner's syndrome, chest discomfort, voice changes and pneumothorax.

The patients who had failed blockades that means no sensory block and no motor block received general anesthesia.

Statistical presentation and analysis of the present study was conducted, using the mean ± standard deviation, student´s t test (for quantitative data comparison between studied groups) and chi-square test (for qualitative data comparison between studied groups) by using SPSS software version 16. Statistically significant difference at p.value <0.05 (Figure 1).

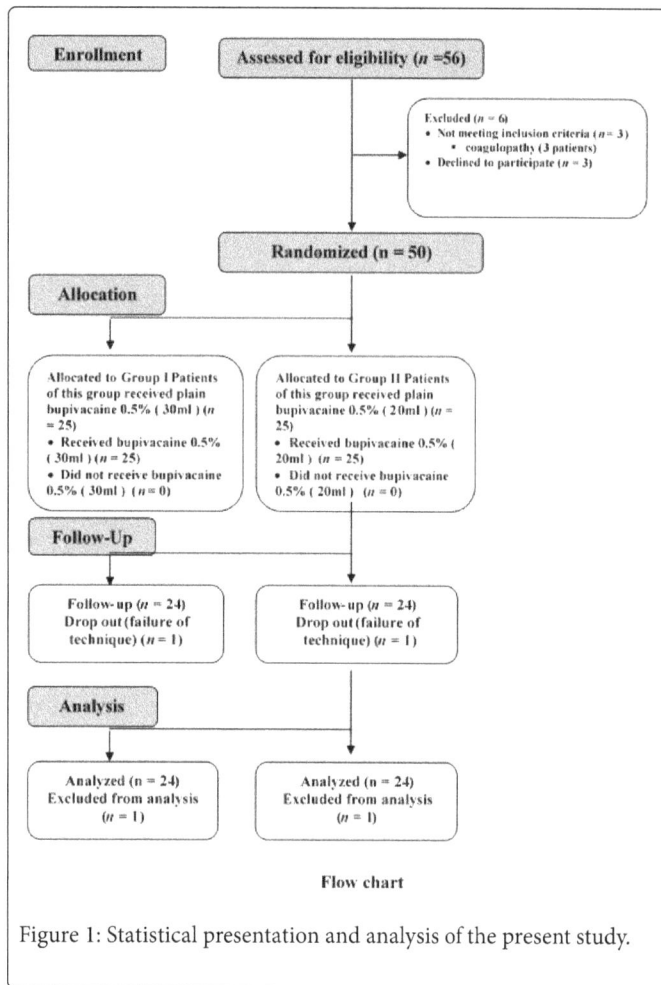

Figure 1: Statistical presentation and analysis of the present study.

Results

The study has been carried out in Tanta University Hospitals on 50 adult patients with chronic renal failure scheduled for elective arterio-venous shunt creation surgery.

Demographic data of patients in both groups shows insignificant difference as regard age, sex and weight (Table 1).

	Age(year)		Wt. (kg)		Sex	
	Group II	Group I	Group II	Group I	Group II	Group I
Mean	50.48	52.08	70.64	70.84	F/M	F/M
SD	5.4	6.3	5.89	6.06	8/17	11/14
t & X2	t=0.964		t=0.118		X2=0.764	
P-value	0.34		0.906		0.382	

Table 1: Demographic data of the studied patients (n=25) in each group.

Onset of sensory and motor block in both groups shows insignificant difference between both groups while duration of sensory and motor block shows significant prolongation in group I as compared to group II (Table 2).

Parameters	Groups	Mean	± SD	T	P-value
Sensory block onset time (mins)	Group I (n=25)	12.3	2.5	0.283	0.778
	Group II (n=25)	12.5	2.6		
Motor block onset time (mins)	Group I (n=25)	22.2	2.1	0.47	0.64
	Group II (n=25)	22.5	2.4		
Duration of sensory block (hours)	Group I (n=25)	33.6	1.19	2.887	0.006*
	Group II (n=25)	2.7	0.75		
Duration of motor block (hours)	Group I (n=25)	2.5	0.7	3.667	0.002*
	Group II (n=25)	1.8	0.73		
*Denotes statistically significant difference at p value < 0.05					

Table 2: The onset and duration of sensory and motor block.

Complications were significantly more in group I compared to group II,

We detected Horner's syndrome in 3 patients complained from red eye t (bloodshot conjunctiva, depending on the site of lesion), ptosis and miosis. These symptoms disappeared within 2 hours and half without any sequelae , voice change (hoarseness) in 2 patients that lasted for minutes & chest discomfort in 2 patients . In group II there was one patient with chest discomfort (Table 3).

	Group I (n=25)		Group II (n=25)	
	N	%	N	%
Horner's syndrome	3	12	0	0
Chest discomfort	2	8	1	4
Pneumothorax	0	0	0	0
Voice changes	2	8	0	0
Total complications	7	28	1	0
X^2	5.357			
P-value	0.021*			

Table 3: Complications in both groups.

The success rate shows no significant difference between the two groups (Table 4).

Success rate	N	%
Group I (n=25)	24	96
Group II (n=25)	24	96

Table 4: Success rate in both groups.

Discussion

One-third of arterio-venous fistulae fail at an early stage. This failure rate is influenced by both the pre-operative arterial and venous diameters and post-operative flow through the AVF. Some anesthetic techniques can directly influence venous diameter as well as intra and post-operative blood flow [4]. General anesthesia, regional anesthesia such as brachial plexus block and local anesthetic (LA) infiltration are all acceptable anesthetic techniques for AVF creation [4]. Many complications can be avoided if regional or local anesthesia is employed. Only regional anesthesia produces an associated sympathetic nerve block which results in an increased intraoperative venous diameter and vessel flow, both intra-operatively and, for several hours, post-operatively. Maintenance of adequate blood flow through the fistula post-operatively can prevent thrombosis and fistula failure and is important in fistula maturation. Furthermore, arterial and venous spasm reduces flow and is more common with local infiltration than regional anesthesia [4].

The most important advantage of ultrasound for peripheral nerve block is the ability to confirm local anesthetic spread around the target nerve [8]. The operator can then manipulate the needle under direct vision to the appropriate depth and place the needle tip immediately adjacent to the target nerve [9]. In addition to imaging the needle and nerve, ultrasound clearly reveals the surrounding hazardous structures, including blood vessels, pleura, and viscera.

In this study the results showed that the success rate in group II with local anesthetic volume 20 ml was 96 %. In agreement with these results Song JG et al. estimated the minimum local anesthetic volume (MEV) for ultrasound-guided supraclavicular block in 95, 90, and 50% of patients were 17, 15, and 9 ml, respectively. However, the location of the needle near the lower trunk of brachial plexus and multiple injections withdrawing the needle should be performed to achieve these results, and very careful injection by a skillful operator is required [10]. Also, a study done by Bigeleisen et al. achieved 100% of success rate with 20 ml of local anesthetic (2.5 mg/ml bupivacaine, 10 mg/ml lidocaine, and 3 µg/ml epinephrine)by ultrasound-guided supraclavicular block that was performed on 55 patients [11]. Furthermore, Duggan et al. estimated minimal effective volume to be successful in 95% of patients (MEV95) and minimal effective volume to be successful in 50% of patients (MEV50) to be 42 ml and 23 ml (1.5% mepivacaine), respectively. According to the study results, it was concluded that they could not reduce the volume of local anesthetic in ultrasound-guided supraclavicular block [12]. Tran et al. showed that the minimum effective volume of lidocaine for ultrasound-guided supraclavicular block to be successful in 90% of patients (MEV90) for double-injection ultrasound-guided supraclavicular nerve block was estimated to be 32 mL lidocaine 1.5% with epinephrine 5 µg/mL. This volume (32 ml) for 90% success rate was lower compared with the conventional technique using 40 ml of local anesthetics [13].

In the current study the results showed that the difference between the two groups regarding to the onset of sensory and motor block was statistically insignificant. In agreement with these results, a study by Raizada et al. showed that there was no significant difference between the onset time of sensory and motor block between the three groups using different volumes and concentrations of mixture of bupivacaine 0.5% and lidocaine 1% [14]. Also, a study was done by Jeon et al. on 102 patients undergoing supraclavicular blocks with different volumes 35 ml, 30 ml, 25 ml, and 20 ml mepivacaine 1%, respectively. The average onset times of Group 35, Group 30, Group 25, and Group 20

were 14.3 ± 6.9 min, 13.6 ± 4.5 min, 16.7 ± 4.6 min, and 16.5 ± 3.7 min, respectively. There were no significant differences [8].

Results showed that the difference between the two groups regarding the duration of sensory and motor block was statistically significant with more prolongation in group I. A study by Raizada et al. showed that there was significant difference between the duration time of sensory and motor block between the three groups using different volumes and concentrations of mixture of bupivacaine 0.5% and lidocaine 1% with more prolongation in large volume group [14]. In a study done by Leonardo et al., they found that the blockades with low doses of local anesthetic 0.5% bupivacaine with 1:200,000 epinephrines were sufficient to perform the procedures with less than 2 h duration [15]. Furthermore, A study by Harper et al., supported the idea that low volumes of anesthetic Lidocaine 1.5% with epinephrine 1:200 000 can achieve the required sensory anesthesia for surgery, while minimizing the duration of the block. We speculate that increasing this volume would produce blocks of quicker onset and longer duration. This could have implications for day surgery, allowing more scope for regional anesthesia [16]. Moreover, Fredrickson et al., showed that low doses of local anesthetic decreased the blockade duration, defined as the time between the onset of blockade installation and the return of motor and sensory functions. Increasing the volume of ropivacaine 0.375% from 10 to 40 mL was estimated to increase median block duration. Increasing the concentration of 20 mL ropivacaine from 0.375% to 0.75% was estimated to increase block duration [17]. In agreement with our results, a study was done by Schoenmakers et al., the patients undergoing axillary blocks with two groups of different volumes showed prolonged duration with larger volume with significant differences between the two groups [18].

The results of this study showed that there were seven patients who complained of chest discomfort , Horner's syndrome, voice changes in group I with 30 ml local anesthetic whereas only one patient who complained of chest discomfort in group II with 20 ml local anesthetic. There was significant difference between the two groups regarding the total complications.

As acidosis decreases the central nervous system threshold to the toxic effects of local anesthetics, the total volume of anesthetic should be decreased by approximately 25 percent in the acidotic patients [19].

As regard to, Arcand et al. mentioned that no pneumothorax has been reported in any study of supraclavicular or infraclavicular block using ultrasound guidance [20]. Furthermore, Cornish et al. checked and evaluated complications, particularly dyspnea by hemidiaphragmatic paresis and observed the possibility of decreased incidence of hemidiaphragmatic paresis in supraclavicular block with a lower local anesthetic volume. Only one patient who received 21 ml of local anesthetic complained of chest discomfort and showed hemi-diaphragmatic paresis on the post-operative chest X-ray. No hemidiaphragmatic paresis was observed in the patients who received a local anesthetic volume<21 ml. Previous studies have reported a 35-60% incidence of hemi-diaphragmatic paresis after supraclavicular block using typical volumes of local anesthetics [21].

Conclusion

During ultrasound guided supraclavicular block in end stage renal disease (ESRD) patients, administration of 20 ml bupivacaine 0.5% is equal to 30 ml bupivacaine 0.5% as regard the onset of sensory block, motor block and the success rate but with shorter duration as regard the sensory block and motor block and significant decrease in complications.

References

1. O'Hare AM, Choi AI, Bertenthal D, Bacchetti P, Garg AX, et al. (2007) Age affects outcomes in chronic kidney disease. J Am Soc Nephrol 18: 2758-2765.

2. Macfarlane AJ1, Kearns RJ, Aitken E, Kinsella J, Clancy MJ (2013) Does regional compared to local anaesthesia influence outcome after arteriovenous fistula creation? Trials 14: 263-265.

3. Hoggard J, Saad T, Schon D, Vesely TM, Royer T, et al. (2008) Guidelines for venous access in patients with chronic kidney disease. A Position Statement from the American Society of Diagnostic and Interventional Nephrology, Clinical Practice Committee and the Association for Vascular Access. Semin Dial 21: 186-191.

4. Shemesh D, Olsha O, Orkin D, Raveh D, Goldin I, et al. (2006) Sympathectomy-like effects of brachial plexus block in arteriovenous access surgery. Ultrasound Med Biol 32: 817-822.

5. Konner K, Nonnast-Daniel B, Ritz E (2003) The arteriovenous fistula. J Am Soc Nephrol 14: 1669-1680.

6. Wedel DJ, Horlokcer TT (2010) Anesthesia (7th ed). Churchill Livingstone, Philadelphia, USA, pp. 1640.

7. Duggan E, El Beheiry H, Perlas A, Lupu M, Nuica A, et al. (2009) Minimum effective volume of local anesthetic for ultrasound-guided supraclavicular brachial plexus block. Reg Anesth Pain Med 34: 215-218.

8. Jeon DG, Kim SK, Kang BJ, Kwon MA, Song JG, et al. (2013) Comparison of ultrasound-guided supraclavicular block according to the various volumes of local anesthetic. Korean J Anesthesiol 64: 494-499.

9. Retzl G, Kapral S, Greher M (2001) Ultrasonographic findings of the axillary part of the brachial plexus. Anesth Analg 92: 1271-1275.

10. Song JG, Jeon DG, Kang BJ (2013) Minimum effective volume of mepivacaine for ultrasound-guided supraclavicular block. Korean J Anesthesiol 65: 37-41.

11. Bigeleisen PE, Moayeri N, Groen GJ (2009) Extraneural versus intraneural stimulation thresholds during ultrasound-guided supraclavicular block. Anesthesiology 110: 1235-1243.

12. Duggan E, El Beheiry H, Perlas A (2011) Minimum effective volume of local anesthetic for ultrasound-guided supraclavicular brachial plexus block. Reg Anesth Pain Med 34: 215-218.

13. Tran de QH, Dugani S, Correa JA (2011) Minimum effective volume of lidocaine for ultrasound-guided supraclavicular block. Reg Anesth Pain Med 36: 466-469.

14. Raizada N, Chandralekha, Jain PC (2002) Does compounding and increase in concentration of local anaesthetic agents increase the success rate of brachial plexus block? Indian J Anaesth 46: 193-196.

15. Ferraro LH, Takeda A, dos Reis Falcão LF, Rezende AH, Sadatsune EJ, et al. (2009) Determination of the minimum effective volume of 0.5% bupivacaine for ultrasound-guided axillary brachial plexus block. Braz J Anesthesiol 64: 49-53.

16. Harper GK, Stafford MA, Hill DA (2010) Minimum volume of local anaesthetic required to surround each of the constituent nerves of the axillary brachial plexus, using ultrasound guidance: a pilot study. Br J Anaesth 104: 633-636.

17. Fredrickson MJ, Abeysekera A, White R (2012) Randomized study of the effect of local anesthetic volume and concentration on the duration of peripheral nerve blockade. Reg Anesth Pain Med 37: 495-501.

18. Schoenmakers KP, Wegener JT, Stienstra R (2012) Effect of Local Anesthetic Volume (15 vs 40 mL) on the Duration of Ultrasound-Guided Single Shot Axillary Brachial Plexus Block: a prospective randomized, observer-blinded trial. Reg Anesth Pain Med 37: 242-247.

19. Tsuchiya H, Mizogami M, Ueno T (2012) Cardiotoxic local anesthetics increasingly interact with biomimetic membranes under ischemia-like acidic conditions. Biol Pharm Bul 35: 988-992

20. Arcand G, Williams SR, Chouinard P, Boudreault D, Harris P, et al. (2005) Ultrasound-guided infraclavicular versus supraclavicular block. Anesth Analg 101: 886-890.

21. Cornish PB, Leaper C (2006) The sheath of the brachial plexus: fact or fiction? Anesthesiology 105: 563-565.

33

Variation of Anesthetic Sedation Requirements in Children Undergoing Auditory Brainstem Response (ABR) Test: A Retrospective Cross-Sectional Study

Hamed Elgendy[1*], **Doaa Ahmed**[4,10], **Soha Elmorsy**[7,8], **Ali Aboloyoun**[3,9], **Ahmad Banjar**[5,6], **Talha Youssef**[5,6] **and Azza Al- Attar**[2,11]

[1]*Department of Anesthesia, Assiut University Hospitals, Egypt*

[2]*Audio-Vestibular Medicine Division, Department of Ear, Nose and Throat-Al-Azhar University Hospitals, Girls Section, Cairo, Egypt*

[3]*Phonetic Division, Department of Ear, Nose and Throat, King Abdullah Medical City, KAMC-HC, Makkah, Saudi Arabia*

[4]*Department of Anesthesia, South Egypt Cancer Institute, Egypt*

[5]*Intern, Umm Al Qura University, Saudi Arabia*

[6]*King Abdullah Medical City, Saudi Arabia*

[7]*Department of Medical Pharmacology Faculty of Medicine, Cairo University, Egypt*

[8]*Research Consultant, King Abdullah Medical City Research Center, Makkah, Saudi Arabia*

[9]*Phonetic Division, Department of Ear, Nose and Throat, Assiut University Hospitals, Egypt*

[10]*Anesthesia Department, King Abdullah Medical City, Makkah, Saudi Arabia*

[11]*AudioVestibular Medicine Division, Department of Ear, Nose and Throat, King Abdullah Medical City, KAMC-HC, Makkah, Saudi Arabia*

*Corresponding Author: Dr Hamed M Elgendy, MD, PhD, Department of Anesthesia, Assiut University Hospitals, Egypt and Anesthesia Department, King Abdullah Medical City, Saudi Arabia, E-mail: helgendy70@gmail.com

Abstract

Background: Varying sedation requirements may impact anesthetic management and patient outcome. Children with brain disorders may have different requirements than unaffected children. The auditory brainstem response (ABR) test is used to estimate hearing sensitivity and as a diagnostic tool to evaluate autism.

Objective: To explore the association between anesthetic requirements of children subjected to ABR test and the degree of abnormality discovered by the test.

Methods: Operative anesthetic data including propofol and midazolam dosages were collected retrospectively for children undergoing ABR tests. Propofol doses were log transformed and entered as dependent variable in linear regression models with weight, height, body mass index, intelligence quotient, CARS score and the extent of lesion by ABR (none, unilateral or bilateral) as covariates and gender as a factor. Independent variables with significant associations were used in multiple regression models.

Results: In 227 total study cases, no lesion was identified in 62 cases, a unilateral lesion was identified in 80 cases, and bilateral lesions were identified in 85 cases. Autism was diagnosed in 31% of children. Simple regression showed significant association of weight, extent of lesion and midazolam dose with the log propofol dose. In multiple regression, the three variables retained their significant association with coefficients and 95% CI of (-0.013) and (-0.024)-(-0.003), 0.111 and 0.034-0.183, and (-0.197) and (-0.271)-(-0.124) respectively. Recovery time was similar among the lesion groups indicating a real need for larger doses.

Conclusion: Children with autistic lesions may require larger doses of propofol for sedation. ABR testing may provide key clinical information about the anesthetic requirements in autistic patients. More studies are required to assess the safety of anesthesia in children requiring larger doses of medication for sedation.

Keywords: Propofol; Midazolam; Pediatric; Sedation; Auditory brainstem response

Introduction

Auditory brainstem response (ABR) refers to electrical activity of the auditory system that occurs in response to appropriate acoustic stimuli. It is an accurate, reliable, and a non -invasive test, which is conducted to estimate auditory sensitivity and integrity of auditory brain stem pathway. ABR consists of a series of seven waves, occurring within 10 min after stimulus. This is a diagnostic test performed outside the operating room and requires sedation to keep a child still during the procedure [1].

Despite early signs, children with autism spectrum disorders often do not seek medical advice until after the second year of age when language delays are observed. Fifty to seventy percent of autistic children have historically been classified as intellectually disabled by nonverbal intelligent quotient (IQ) testing [2].

Moreover, the Childhood Autism Rating Scale (CARS) consisting of 15 questions scored by the parent is commonly used for diagnosis of autism. The CARS can reliably differentiate among children with autism as well as those with mental retardation [3].

Propofol (2,6-diisoproyl-phenol) is commonly used during various procedures for sedation of children with intellectual dysfunction which limits cooperation [4,5].

Currently, there exists a lack of literature describing autistic children and their anesthetic needs, further studies are needed [6].

A previous report suggested that relatively high levels of propofol are required to manage patients with intellectual disabilities [7]. Working in a tertiary center we too have noticed, while managing autistic children undergoing ABR testing, that sedation requirement varies appreciably among these children.

Hence, our aim is to examine the presence of a possible association between the anesthetic requirements of children undergoing this test and the degree of abnormality discovered by the test. The primary objective is to compare the anesthetic requirements among the ABR test result groups, and secondarily to compare the anesthetic requirements between groups of children according to their definitive clinical diagnosis.

Patients and Methods

This retrospective analysis was approved by the Institutional Review Board of our institution and included patients referred for ABR testing based on a preliminary diagnosis of autism. Children sedated with propofol from January 2011 through December 2013 were identified and their records were reviewed. Cases were excluded if they were found to be above 18 years old or if information about their anesthetics or their ABR test were missing.

The following data were extracted from the anesthesia sheets and electronic files: patient's age, gender, weight, height, American Society of Anesthesia (ASA) grading; Intelligence Quotient (IQ) test result; CARS score; past medical history, comorbid diagnoses and medications taken preoperatively. Additional extracted data included types and doses of medications administered intra-operatively with reference to the number and magnitude of propofol doses, (total propofol doses for every kg body weight were calculated), doses of midazolam and perioperative complications.

The following were extracted from the anesthesia record to calculate operative time parameters: "time out", start of the procedure, end of the procedure and fulfilment of the full recovery criteria [8].

Sedation

Procedural sedation at our hospital was performed in accordance with standard guidelines [9]. All patients were nil by mouth for at least 2-8 hours, and had a functional intravenous catheter. Patients were continuously monitored by a combination of one certified anesthetist and anaesthesia technician throughout the procedure. Heart rate, respiratory rate, and oxyhemoglobin saturation were continuously monitored. Noninvasive blood pressure was measured every 5 minutes during the procedure and every 5-15 minutes during recovery. End-tidal CO_2 was monitored via nasal cannula.

Premedication with intravenous midazolam (0.05-0.08 mg/kg) was given to each study patient. Propofol was available in a final concentration of 10 mg/ml and administered intravenously at

increments of 10 mg, flushed with 10 ml of normal saline 0.9%. The increments were continued until the patient was deemed adequately sedated. Incremental dosing followed with flushing was used to avoid overdosing with a continuous infusion. After the procedure, patients were monitored until they returned to their baseline neurological status.

Auditory Brainstem Response (ABR) Test

ABR testing was performed under sedation for all children. Analysis time was 10 seconds. One electrode was placed on each ear lobe and a third on the forehead for grounding. Electrode impedance was less than 5 kOhms and inter-electrode impedance was within 2 kOhms. Click stimuli were presented at 70 dBnHL. The click was averaged across 1000 sweeps and was replicated. Waves I, III, and V were identified and their latencies were measured. Wave I and wave V amplitudes were determined for 70 dBnH click -evoked waveforms.

ABR was detected by placing electrodes on the scalp and separating the response from background electroencephalography measures using averaging and amplification techniques [10].

Although the absolute latencies can be influenced by peripheral hearing loss, the interpeak latencies are generally accepted as measures of central neural conduction time and are influenced by myelination of nerve fibers [11].

Patients were assigned according to the presence of abnormal morphological waveforms into the following groups: Group I, (Normal) who have normal bilateral wave morphology of ABR waves; group II (Unilateral) who had unilateral abnormal ABR wave morphology either in right or left ears; group III (Bilateral) had bilateral abnormal ABR wave morphology in both ears.

For objectivity of patient classification, ABR results, the IQ, and the CARS test results were added to the database only after capturing all data from anesthesia records.

Patients attended Phoniatrics outpatient clinics with parents who observed language delay in their child. Each patient was subjected to a standard protocol of language evaluation. Psychometric evaluation including Stanford-Binet Intelligence Scale for assessment of IQ and CARS test for autism. All patients were referred to audiology unit for hearing evaluation.

Childhood Autism Rating Scale (CARS)

This test consists of 15 questions. A score of 30 to 35 indicates mild autism while a score of 36 and higher indicates moderate to severe autism. Scores are based on direct observation and items are scored from 1-4. A score of 1 indicates age appropriate behavior and a score of 4 indicates severely abnormal behavior. All items contribute equally to the total score that varies from 15 to 60 [12].

Statistical method

Statistical analysis was performed on SPSS version 11.0. Numeric data were presented as mean ± SD, median and interquartile range. Comparison between groups of ABR abnormality (normal, unilateral, and bilateral) was done by the ANOVA or Kruskal Walis test. Alpha values were all set at 0.05 but for multiple comparisons Bonferroni correction was used. Categorical data were presented as percentages and were compared by chi square test. Propofol dosing data were examined for normality of distribution and were converted to the log scale in case of right skewness.

Univariate linear regression models were constructed to test the effect of different variables on log transformed propofol dose. Factors with significant coefficients at a level of 0.05 were incorporated in multiple regression models. The likelihood ratio test was used to explore the relative contribution of different predictors to the multiple regression models.

Results

From January 2011 to December 2013, 227 children were identified to have the ABR test and fulfilled the inclusion criteria; among these 62 had normal ABR while 80 and 85 had unilateral and bilateral abnormalities, respectively. Table 1 shows the demographic and clinical characteristics of the patients. The age ranged from nine months to 13 years with a mean value of 4.3 ± 2.2 and did not differ significantly among the groups.

Parameter (Number)	Total cases (227)	Normal (62)	Unilateral (80)	Bilateral (85)	p value
Age					
(Mean ± SD)	4.3 ± 2.2	4.0 ± 2.2	4.1 ± 1.9	4.7 ± 2.4	
Median	4	3.5	4	4	0.112
Q25- Q75	3.0-6.0	2.8-5.0	3.0-5.0	3.0-6.0	
Gender					
Males No (%)	159 (70.0%)	49 (79.0%)	51 (63.8%)	59 (69.4%)	0.141
Weight in kg					
(Mean ± SD)	16.2 ± 5.4	15.7 ± 5.2	15.0 ± 3.8	17.6 ± 6.4	
Median	15.3	15.1	14.6	16.2	0.006
Q25 - Q75	13.0-18.0	13.0-17.3	12.4-17.0	13.8-16.2	
Height in cm					
(Mean ± SD)	101.5 ± 14.7	100.0 ± 15.0	100.0 ± 12.3	104.2 ± 16.2	
Median	100	99	99.5	104	0.094
Q25 - Q75	91.0 - 111.0	90.4 - 110.0	90.3 - 108.5	94.5 - 115.5	
BMI in kg/m^2					
(Mean ± SD)	15.6 ± 2.9	15.7 ± 3.0	10.0 ± 12.3	10.4 ± 16.2	
Median	15	15.3	9.9	10.4	0.064
Q25-Q75	13.5-16.7	13.5-16.3	9.3-10.9	9.5-11.6	
ASA (NO,%)					
I	177,78%	53,48.3%	61,76.3%	63,74.1%	
II	47,20.7%	9,12.8%	17,21.3%	21,24.7%	0.389
III	3,1.3%	0,0%	2,2.5%	1,1.2%	
IQ total No. of Children	169	39	60*	70	
(Mean ± SD)	67.3 ± 14.6	72.5 ± 13.2	64.7± 14.7	66.5 ± 14.8	
Median	67	73	65	64	0.028
Q25-Q75	57.5-77.0	64.0-85.0	54.3-73.0	58.0-77.0	
IQ class (N)					
NO (%)	169	39	60	70	
Superior	0	0	0	0	0.804
Above average	0	0	0	0	

Average	14 (8.3)	5 (12.8%)	5 (8.3%)	4 5.7%	
Low average	21 (12.4)	6 (15.4%)	5 (8.3%)	10 14.3%	
Slow learner	46 (27.2)	11 (28.2%)	15 (25.0%)	20 28.6%	
Mild MR	74 (43.8)	16 (41.0%)	29 (48.3%)	29 41.4%	
Moderate MR	11 (6.5)	1 (2.6%)	4 (6.7%)	6 8.6%	
Severe MR	3 (1.8)	0 (0.0%)	2 (3.3%)	1 1.4%	
CARS score (Autistic patients)					
NO (%)	52	12	16	24	
(Mean ± SD)	31.8 ± 4.0	31.4 ± 3.6	32.9 ± 4.4	31.2 ± 3.8	0.368
Median	30	30.5	32	30	
Q25-Q75	29.0-32.8	29.0-32.0	30.0-35.3	29.0-31.8	
CARS class (N)					
NO (%)	169	39	60	70	
No autism	117 (69.2%)	27 (69.2%)	44 (73.3%)	46 (65.7%)	
Spectrum autism	18 (10.7%)	4 (10.3%)	3 (5.0%)	11 (15.7%)	0.624
Mild to moderate autism	32 (18.9%)	8 (20.5%)	1 (1.7%)	12 (17.1%)	
Severe autism	2 (1.2%)	0 (0.0%)	12 (20.0%)	1 (1.4%)	
Most variables were presented as mean ± SD; percentage or median ± IQR					
BMI: Body Mass Index, kg/m^2; ASA: American Society of Anesthesiology Classification; IQ: Intelligent Quotient; CARS: Child-hood Autism Rating Scale; IQR: Interquartile Range. CARS score is described for (Autistic patients; n=52).					

Table 1: Demographic and clinical characteristics of study patients stratified by extent of affection assessed by Auditory Brainstem Response (ABR) test.

There was a male predominance in the total population as well as in the individual groups. A little less than half of the patients had positive history of consanguinity; 46.3% in the unilateral and 37.6% in bilateral group (p=0.116).

In addition, less than a half had a positive family history of autism. Most of the children in the three groups were free from congenital mental illness. However, neurological history; anti-convulsant therapy; renal and hepatic diseases were comparable between groups.

A few children had cardiac conditions and many more had respiratory disorders, however associated neurological conditions were most commonly seen, ranging between 11% and 14%. Use of anticonvulsants was recorded in less than 10% in all groups. The group with bilateral ABR abnormality had a significantly higher mean body weight.

ASA score distribution and the CARS score of autism were similar among the study groups. However, the IQ value was significantly higher in the group with unilaterally abnormal ABR readings as compared to the other two groups. The CARS score was not recorded for those with no autism (117 cases); also the score was achievable for comparison only with autistic children (n=52) (Table 1).

A significantly higher proportion of children with unilateral and bilateral ABR abnormality required larger doses of propofol compared to those with bilaterally normal ABR readings; most of children with

abnormal bilateral ABR group required more than two doses (Figure 1A).

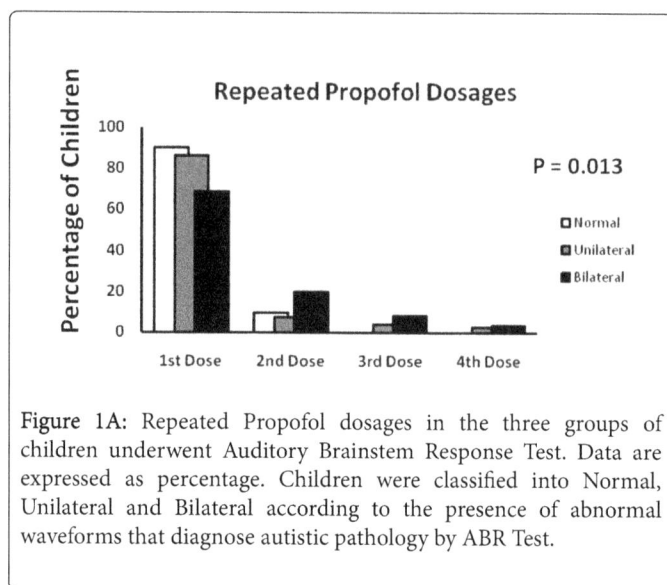

Figure 1A: Repeated Propofol dosages in the three groups of children underwent Auditory Brainstem Response Test. Data are expressed as percentage. Children were classified into Normal, Unilateral and Bilateral according to the presence of abnormal waveforms that diagnose autistic pathology by ABR Test.

None of the procedure time parameters, including the recovery time, differed significantly among groups (Table 2). There was also no significant difference in operative complications among the groups apart from increased percentage of needed additional sedation that was significantly higher in the group with bilateral abnormality (Figure 1B).

Parameter	Total cases	Normal	Unilateral	Bilateral	p value
Midazolam dose in mg/kg					
(Mean ± SD)	0.9 ± 0.7	0.9 ± 0.7	0.9 ± 0.7	0.9 ± 0.7	
Median	1	1	1	1	0.989
Q25 - Q75	0.5-1.0	0.1 -1.0	0.5 -1.0	0.5 -1.0	
Total propofol dose in mg/kg					
(Mean ± SD)	2.3 ± 1.2	2.2 ± 1.2	2.2 ± 1.1	2.5 ± 1.2	
Median	2.1	1.8	2	2.4	0.122
Q25 - Q75	1.5-2.9	1.4-2.9	1.4-2.7	1.7-3.1	
Total Procedure time/ min					
(Mean ± SD)	70.1 ± 41.0	68.0 ± 40.9	69.8 ± 39.6	72.1 ± 42.8	
Median	56	51	56	56	0.833
Q25-Q75	46.0-81.0	45.0-62.3	46.0-81.0	46.0-88.5	
Actual Procedure time / min					
(Mean ± SD)	25.5 ± 9.1	24.2 ± 6.2	26.8 ± 7.4	25.1 ± 11.8	
Median	25	23.5	30	23	0.203
Q25 - Q75	20.0-30.0	20.0-30.0	20.0-30.0	20.0-30.0	
Recovery time/min					
(Mean ± SD)	42.8 ± 39.7	41.7 ± 40.2	41.8 ± 37.0	44.6 ± 42.2	
Median	30	30	30	30	0.866
Q25-Q75	20.0-55.0	20.0-40.0	20.0-53.8	15.5-60.0	
Most variables were presented as mean ± SD; or median ± IQR. Total procedure time=Actual procedure time+Recovery time, Actual procedure time=start of sedation till end of the ABR procedure recording.					

Table 2: Intra-operative parameters of study patients stratified by extent of affection assessed by Auditory Brainstem Response (ABR) test.

Using univariate linear regression with log propofol dose as the dependent variable, only midazolam dose, weight and ABR abnormality were found to show statistically significant association (Table 3). When the three variables were simultaneously incorporated into a multivariate linear model, they all remained significantly associated with the log propofol dose indicating that after adjusting for midazolam dose and for body weight, the extent of ABR abnormality remained an independent predictor for propofol requirement (Table 4).

Likelihood ratio test (Table 5) shows that the midazolam dose seems to be the most important predictor for propofol requirement, however, the extent of the ABR abnormality plays a very important role as well.

Notably, one patient in the bilateral abnormality ABR group experienced vomiting, while cough was reported in one patient in each the normal and unilateral abnormality ABR groups. No patients experienced laryngospasm.

Discussion

Our data revealed that sedation requirements vary for children undergoing ABR in our institution. The extent of autistic pathology in the form of abnormal morphological waves assessed by ABR test was an independent risk factor for increased propofol requirements.

In addition, child's weight and premedication with midazolam were independent risk factors that affected the amount of propofol needed during the ABR procedure.

A few reports described variation in dose requirements of propofol sedation. Asahi et al., in 2009, compared the propofol requirements and its effect during dental treatment in 56 autistic patients.

Their results revealed increased propofol requirements in autistic patients when compared with 56 intellectually impaired patients. But, the study population included both children and adults, and the propofol infusion rates in the intellectually impaired group showed significant decline with age [13].

Other studies too suggested that relatively high levels of propofol are required to manage patients with intellectual disabilities [7,14].

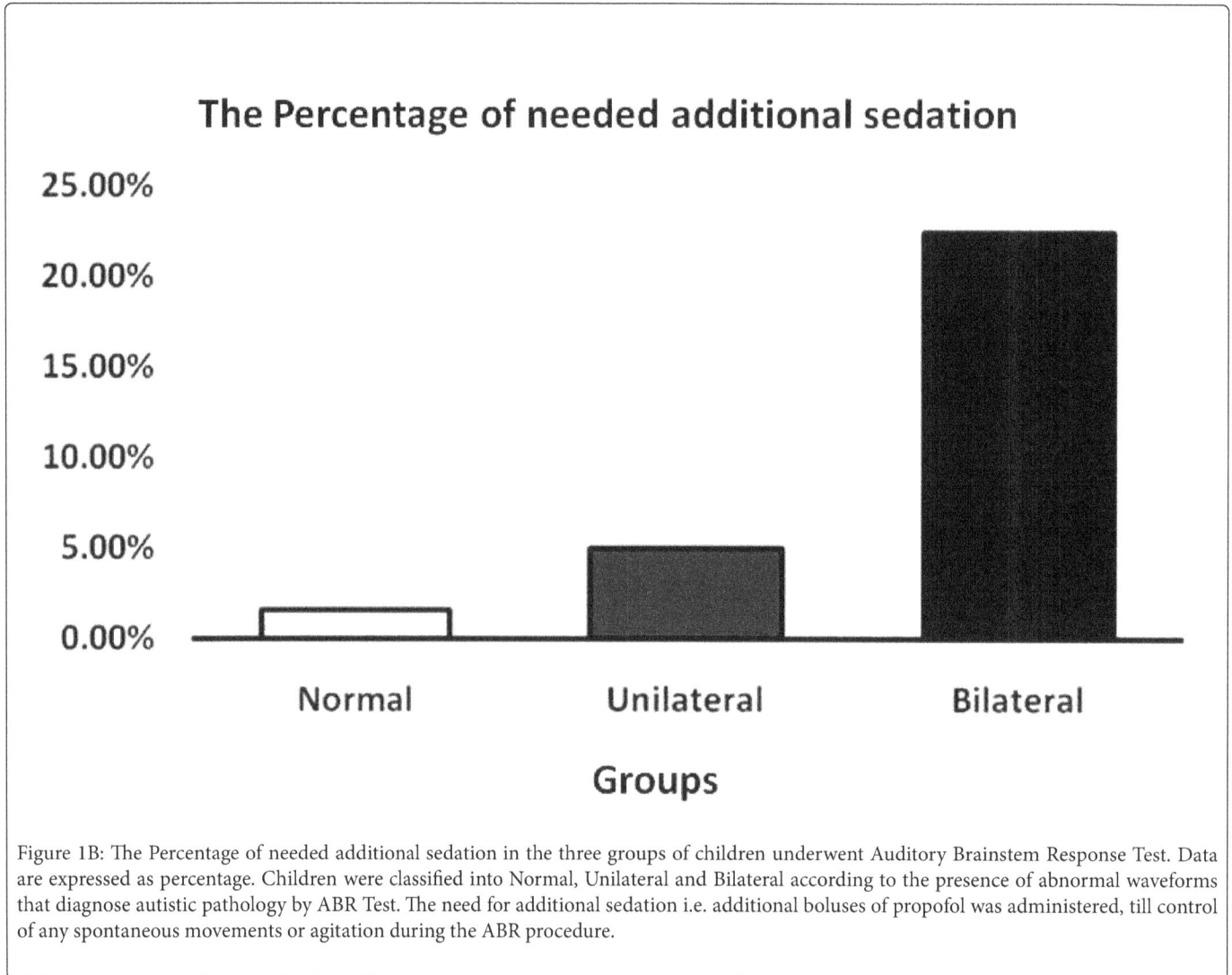

Figure 1B: The Percentage of needed additional sedation in the three groups of children underwent Auditory Brainstem Response Test. Data are expressed as percentage. Children were classified into Normal, Unilateral and Bilateral according to the presence of abnormal waveforms that diagnose autistic pathology by ABR Test. The need for additional sedation i.e. additional boluses of propofol was administered, till control of any spontaneous movements or agitation during the ABR procedure.

Factor entered in regression	Number of observations in the model	Regression coefficient (Beta)	95% CI	p value
Age	227	(-0.006)	(-0.034)-0.022	0.667
Gender	227	0.059	(-0.0734)-0.192	0.379
Weight	227	(-0.012)	(-0.023)-(-0.001)	0.034
Height	227	(-0.003)	(-0.007)-0.001	0.167
BMI	227	(-0.016)	(-.037)-0.005	0.135
IQ absolute value	169	0.001	(-0.004)-0.005	0.822
IQ level	169	(-0.01)	(-0.073)-0.052	0.74
CARS absolute value	169	-0.006	(-0.032)-0.02	0.66
CARS level	169	(-0.074)	(-0.155)-0.008	0.076
Midazolam dose	227	(-0.194)	(-0.27)-(-0.119)	<0.001

| Lesion (normal, unilateral, bilateral) | 227 | 0.084 | 0.009-0.16 | 0.029 |

BMI: Body Mass Index, kg/m^2; IQ: Intelligent Quotient; CARS: Childhood Autism Rating Scale; (95% CI), 95% confidence interval. Children were classified into Normal, Unilateral and Bilateral according to the presence of abnormal waveforms that diagnose autistic pathology.

Table 3: Results of univariate linear regression analysis for the relation of different factors to the log propofol dose.

Factor entered in regression	Adjusted regression coefficient (Beta)	95% CI	p value
Weight	(-0.013)	(-0.024)-0.003	0.015
Lesion (normal, unilateral, bilateral)	0.111	0.034 -0.183	0.002
Midazolam dose	(-0.0197)	(-0.271)-(-0.124)	<0.001

(95% CI): 95% Confidence Interval. Children were classified into Normal, Unilateral and Bilateral according to the presence of abnormal waveforms that diagnose autistic pathology.

Table 4: Results of multiple linear regression analysis for the relation of different factors to the log propofol dose.

Factor removed from the model	Likelihood ratio chi-square	p value for removal
Weight	6.05	0.014
Midazolam dose	26.8	<0.00001
Lesion (normal, unilateral, bilateral)	9.36	0.002

Children were classified into Normal, Unilateral and Bilateral according to the presence of abnormal waveforms that diagnose autistic pathology.

Table 5: Results of likelihood ratio test on the multivariate model for the effect of weight, lesion, and midazolam dose on the log of the propofol dose.

Sedation failure rates of 20-30 % and inadequate sedation of 15-22.5% have been reported depending on the sedation regimen used [15]. Similarly, our study showed that it was needed additional sedation in 20% of autistic children. This percentage was lower in other two groups. This confirms the findings outlined above and the fact that sedation is more difficult in this subset of patients.

Interestingly, Kitt et al. 2015, did not find higher sedative requirements in children with attention-deficit hyperactivity disorder However, it is well established attention-deficit hyperactivity disorder and autism arise from distinct neuronal pathologies [16].

There exist several potential explanations for increased propofol requirements in autistic patients. Autistic children are known to have decreased amplitude of ABR evoked potential. This can be explained on the basis of an increased transmission time due to decrease in the myelination or the synaptic efficiency in the brain stem nuclei [17,18]. A previous study [19] described a maturational defect in myelination within the brain stem in autism. Mastschke et al. demonstrated that myelination takes place in the first year of life and this is necessary for functional maturation [20]. A functional MRI study has revealed that the degree of synchronization was lower for the autistic than for others. This functional under connectivity could be due to microgliosis and

astrogliosis [21] and can result in delayed nerve conduction [22]. It may explain the relatively increased doses of sedatives to achieve the desired level in autistic patients.

Several factors could explain, in particular, the variability in propofol requirements in these children. Propofol is known to act via gamma amino butyric acid (GABA)A receptors [23-26]. The neuro-developmental disorder that accompanies autism involves some structural changes such as delayed cortical development with larger white matter and lack of the mirror neuron system [27]. These abnormalities may involve the GABA inhibitory system. Ma et al. [28], for example, reported that autistic patients have abnormal (GABA) A receptors. Also Yu [29] has stated that there is a change of (GABA) A receptor subunit distribution during brain maturation for autistic children.

The different response of autistic patients to propofol may also correlate with their hypersensitivity to acoustic stimuli and increased serum levels of glutamate [30]. The serum levels of glutamate, an excitatory neurotransmitter, are increased in adult autistic patients [31]. Propofol potentiates the inhibition of glutamate release as described before in experimental studies [32,33] . Thus, an increase in glutamate may be expected to make autistic children in need for bigger propofol doses to achieve the desired pharmacological effect.

In the current study, midazolam was an independent risk factor for propofol dosing. Midazolam is generally used to reduce anxiety in children undergoing ambulatory procedures such as the MRI (Machata et al.). Rainey et al. [6] has used it in autistic children to reduce their delirium. Midazolam is known to possess a synergistic effect with propofol [34-36]. Indeed, Midazolam dose did not show a statistically significant difference between groups of children but there was a significant negative correlation between it and the log propofol dose which is expected since children receiving a bigger dose of any sedative would need a relatively smaller dose of the other. Given the relatively small sample size, we thought it would be safer to include midazolam in the multivariate regression model to adjust for its correlation with propofol.

The positive association between the midazolam dose and the extent of the lesion observed in this study can be explained based on the general increase in sedative requirements and because of the relative resistance to the action of propofol that dictated the increase on midazolam to achieve the desired target.

In the present study, the required propofol dose was found to be significantly associated with the extent of ABR abnormality but not with the autism diagnostic tools including IQ and CARS tests. The increased propofol requirements may be related to structural brain abnormalities which manifests ABR abnormalities. The link to a clinical syndrome may less direct. Follow up studies using larger numbers of patients may reveal other subtle associations.

The association of propofol doses with the extent of ABR abnormality was not accompanied by a significant change in the procedure time parameters. Although children with ABR abnormality received higher propofol doses, they required a similar amount of time to recovery as their peers. This indicates that affected children are in real need of increased propofol dosing.

The current study has its own limitation due to its retrospective nature and limited number of patients. During the period of this study, we have not got target-controlled infusion (TCI) machines at our institution. Future prospective studies should be completed to address the underlying mechanism of increased demand for sedatives in patients with ABR abnormalities. Comparison of different types of sedatives can be also investigated to get suitable combinations that may provide better sedation control in such patients.

The results of our observational study may have an impact on the management of children who are diagnosed with autism. They may frequently undergo anesthesia or sedation for other surgical purposes. ABR testing may provide key clinical information about the anesthetic requirements in autistic patients.

Conclusion

Autistic children may require increased propofol doses. This group of children need careful documentation of their increased requirements for future use in other types of surgeries as this can affect their outcome and safety.

Financial Disclosures

The authors did not receive any grant or financial support for this study.

Authorship

First and Second authors have equally contributed to this work. HE performed the data collection, participated in the study design, statistical analysis and wrote the manuscript. DA participated in the data collection, study design, statistical analysis, and interpretation of data. S. Elmorsy participated in the study design, statistical analysis, and interpretation of data and writing of manuscript. AB participated in the data collection; TY participated in the data collection; Aboloyoun participated in the study design, preparation and critical revision of the manuscript. Al Attar participated in the study design, and in the preparation and critical revision of the manuscript.

A portion of these results was presented at the Australian & New Zealand Society of Anesthesiologists, ASM-ANZCA held in Adelaide, May 2015.

Acknowledgments

Dr Wessam Ahmed, who was the first got observation; Dr Manal Mashaat; Head of Anesthesia department; Dr Bayan Alzahrani; Dr Emran Alsawaf; Dr Tariq Alsubhi; in Umm Al Qura university, for data collection. Dr M. Kareemulla Shariff, MRCP, MD, Dr Abdulhamid Alsaigh for their critical revision of the manuscript. The authors thank Dr. Michael Schnetz, Department of Anesthesiology, University of Pittsburgh Medical Center, for his editorial assistance with the article.

References

1.   [No authors listed] (1992) American Academy of Pediatrics Committee on Drugs: Guidelines for monitoring and management of pediatric patients during and after sedation for diagnostic and therapeutic procedures. Pediatrics 89: 1110-1115.

2.   Asahi Y, Kubota K, Omichi S (2009) Dose requirements for propofol anaesthesia for dental treatment for autistic patients compared with intellectually impaired patients. Anaesth Intensive Care 37: 70-73.

3.   Buggy DJ, Nicol B, Rowbotham DJ, Lambert DG (2000) Effects of intravenous anesthetic agents on glutamate release: a role for GABAA receptor-mediated inhibition. Anesthesiology 92: 1067-1073.

4.   Cressey DM, Claydon P, Bhaskaran NC, Reilly CS (2001) Effect of midazolam pretreatment on induction dose requirements of propofol in combination with fentanyl in younger and older adults. Anaesthesia 56: 108-113.

5.   Dalal PG, Murray D, Cox T, McAllister J, Snider R (2006) Sedation and anesthesia protocols used for magnetic resonance imaging studies in infants: provider and pharmacologic considerations. Anesth Analg 103: 863-868.

6.   Daskalopoulos R, Korcok J, Farhangkhgoee P, Karmazyn M, Gelb AW, et al. (2001) Propofol protection of sodium-hydrogen exchange activity sustains glutamate uptake during oxidative stress. Anesth Analg 93: 1199-1204.

7.   Eaves RC, Milner B (1993) The criterion-related validity of the Childhood Autism Rating Scale and the Autism Behavior Checklist. J Abnorm Child Psychol 21: 481-491.

8.   Eggermont JJ, Don M (1986) Mechanisms of central conduction time prolongation in brain-stem auditory evoked potentials. Arch Neurol 43: 116-120.

9.   Fein D, Skoff B, Mirsky AF (1981) Clinical correlates of brainstem dysfunction in autistic children. J Autism Dev Disord 11: 303-315.

10. Fodale V, Pratico C, Santamaria LB (2004) Coadministration of propofol and midazolam decreases bispectral index value as a result of synergic muscle relaxant action on the motor system. Anesthesiology 101: 799.

11. Gillberg C, Rosenhall U, Johansson E (1983) Auditory brainstem responses in childhood psychosis. J Autism Dev Disord 13: 181-195.

12. Gomot M, Giard MH, Adrien JL, Barthelemy C, Bruneau N (2002) Hypersensitivity to acoustic change in children with autism: electrophysiological evidence of left frontal cortex dysfunctioning. Psychophysiology 39: 577-584.

13. Hadjikhani N, Joseph RM, Snyder J, Tager-Flusberg H (2006) Anatomical differences in the mirror neuron system and social cognition network in autism. Cereb Cortex 16: 1276-1282.

14. Herbert MR (2005) Large brains in autism: the challenge of pervasive abnormality. Neuroscientist 11: 417-440.

15. Hosey MT, Makin A, Jones RM, Gilchrist F, Carruthers M (2004) Propofol intravenous conscious sedation for anxious children in a specialist paediatric dentistry unit. Int J Paediatr Dent 14: 2-8.

16. Just MA, Cherkassky VL, Keller TA, Kana RK, Minshew NJ (2007) Functional and anatomical cortical underconnectivity in autism: evidence from an FMRI study of an executive function task and corpus callosum morphometry. Cereb Cortex 17: 951-961.

17. Kitt E, Friderici J, Kleppel R, Canarie M (2015) Procedural sedation for MRI in children with ADHD. Paediatr Anaesth 25: 1026-1032.

18. Klin A, Pauls D, Schultz R, Volkmar F (2005) Three diagnostic approaches to Asperger syndrome: implications for research. J Autism Dev Disord 35: 221-234.

19. Leitch JA, Anderson K, Gambhir S, Millar K, Robb ND, et al. (2004) A partially blinded randomised controlled trial of patient-maintained propofol sedation and operator controlled midazolam sedation in third molar extractions. Anaesthesia 59: 853-860.

20. Leung A, Kao CP (1999) Evaluation and management of the child with speech delay. Am Fam Physician 59: 3121-3128.

21. Ma DQ, Whitehead PL, Menold MM, Martin ER, Ashley-Koch AE, et al. (2005) Identification of significant association and gene-gene interaction of GABA receptor subunit genes in autism. Am J Hum Genet 77: 377-388.

22. Matschke RG, Stenzel C, Plath P, Zilles K (1994) Maturational aspects of the human auditory pathway: anatomical and electrophysiological findings. ORL J Otorhinolaryngol Relat Spec 56: 68-72.

23. McClelland RJ, Eyre DG, Watson D, Calvert GJ, Sherrard E (1992) Central conduction time in childhood autism. Br J Psychiatry 160: 659-663.

24. Miyawaki T, Kohjitani A, Maeda S, Egusa M, Mori T, et al. (2004) Intravenous sedation for dental patients with intellectual disability. J Intellect Disabil Res 48: 764-768.

25. Norrix LW, Trepanier S, Atlas M, Kim D (2012) The auditory brainstem response: latencies obtained in children while under general anesthesia. J Am Acad Audiol 23: 57-63.

26. Paspatis GA, Charoniti I, Manolaraki M, Vardas E, Papanikolaou N, et al. (2006) Synergistic sedation with oral midazolam as a premedication and intravenous propofol versus intravenous propofol alone in upper gastrointestinal endoscopies in children: a prospective, randomized study. J Pediatr Gastroenterol Nutr 43: 195-199.

27. Rainey L, van der Walt JH (1998) The anaesthetic management of autistic children. Anaesth Intensive Care 26: 682-686.

28. Ramsay MA, Savege TM, Simpson BR, Goodwin R (1974) Controlled sedation with alphaxalone-alphadolone. Br Med J 2: 656-659.

29. Schopler E, Reichler RJ, DeVellis RF, Daly K (1980) Toward objective classification of childhood autism: Childhood Autism Rating Scale (CARS). J Autism Dev Disord 10: 91-103.

30. Sebel LE, Richardson JE, Singh SP, Bell SV, Jenkins A (2006) Additive effects of sevoflurane and propofol on gamma-aminobutyric acid receptor function. Anesthesiology 104: 1176-1183.

31. Shinohe A, Hashimoto K, Nakamura K, Tsujii M, Iwata Y, et al. (2006) Increased serum levels of glutamate in adult patients with autism. Prog Neuropsychopharmacol Biol Psychiatry 30: 1472-1477.

32. Sitar SM, Hanifi-Moghaddam P, Gelb A, Cechetto DF, Siushansian R, et al. (1999) Propofol prevents peroxide-induced inhibition of glutamate transport in cultured astrocytes. Anesthesiology 90: 1446-1453.

33. Stephens AJ, Sapsford DJ, Curzon ME (1993) Intravenous sedation for handicapped dental patients: a clinical trial of midazolam and propofol. Br Dent J 175: 20-25.

34. Wakasugi M, Hirota K, Roth SH, Ito Y (1999) The effects of general anesthetics on excitatory and inhibitory synaptic transmission in area CA1 of the rat hippocampus in vitro. Anesth Analg 88: 676-680.

35. Westphalen RI, Hemmings HC (2003) Selective depression by general anesthetics of glutamate versus GABA release from isolated cortical nerve terminals. J Pharmacol Exp Ther 304: 1188-1196.

36. Yu ZY, Wang W, Fritschy JM, Witte OW, Redecker C (2006) Changes in neocortical and hippocampal GABAA receptor subunit distribution during brain maturation and aging, Brain Res 1099: 73-81.

34

Induction with Propofol Decreases Emergence Agitation in Pediatric Patients

Onur Koyuncu[1*], **Mustafa Ozgur**[2], **Cagla Akkurt**[3], **Selim Turhanoglu**[3], **Bulent Akcora**[4], **Mehmet Emin Celikkaya**[4] and **Alparslan Turan**[5]

[1]*Department of Anesthesiology and Department of Outcomes Research, Mustafa Kemal University Tayfur Ata Sokmen Medicine Faculty, Hatay, Turkey*

[2]*Department of Anesthesiology, Antakya Devlet Hastanesi, Hatay, Turkey*

[3]*Department of Anesthesiology, Mustafa Kemal University Tayfur Ata Sokmen Medicine Faculty, Hatay, Turkey*

[4]*Department of Pediatric Surgery, Mustafa Kemal University Tayfur Ata Sokmen Medicine Faculty, Hatay, Turkey*

[5]*Department of Outcomes Research, Cleveland Clinic, Cleveland, USA*

[*]**Corresponding author:** Onur Koyuncu, Department of Anesthesiology, Mustafa Kemal University, Tayfur Ata Sokmen Medicine Faculty, Serinyol, Hatay, Turkey, E-mail: onurko@yahoo.com

Abstract

Background and objectives: Emergence agitation (EA) is a common complication seen after inhalational anesthesia especially with sevoflurane, with an incidence of 20-80%. The hypothesis of the study was that induction with propofol reduces the incidence and severity of emergence agitation when compared with sevoflurane in children undergoing inguinal hernia surgery.

Methods: 116 Children undergoing inguinal hernia were randomly assigned to two groups: Sevoflurane group received sevoflurane increasing concentrations up to 8% and propofol group received 3 mg kg propofol in induction. Postoperative agitation treatment and analgesia was standardized, and postoperative assessments included Cole Agitation Scale and narcotic consumption for agitation, Wong-Baker Faces Pain Rating Scale for pain, first spontaneous eye opening time, first verbal command follow time, post-anesthesia care unit (PACU) staying time, first analgesic requirement time and parents satisfaction.

Results: The incidence of EA at arrival in PACU and the cumulative incidences at the end of the postoperative two hours were significantly lower in the propofol group. EA scores were lower in propofol group in all measurement times during postoperative 30 minutes. Fentanyl consumption at arrival in PACU and the sum of the two hours were significantly lower in propofol group. Pain scores were lower in propofol group in the postoperative 24 hours. First analgesic requirement time and parents satisfaction were higher in propofol group.

Conclusion: Propofol in accurate dose is effective in reducing the incidence and intense of EA in children undergoing inguinal hernia and maybe preferred in children with high risk of EA.

Keywords: General anesthesia; Sevoflurane; Propofol; Emergence agitation; Children

Background

Currently more than 400000 pediatric patients are admitted for surgery only in United States annually [1]. Recoveries from these surgeries are sometimes complicated with adverse events. Emergence agitation (EA) is one of the most common and terrifying complication seen after inhalational anesthesia, with an estimated incidence of 20–80% [2,3].

Emergence agitation is described as non-purposeful restlessness and agitation, thrashing, crying or moaning, involuntary physical activities, disorientation, and incoherence after extubation [4]. Patients can even harm themselves by disrupting surgical site, and dislocate indwelling catheters [5]. Mechanisms behind EA are still not clear. Suggested mechanisms involve variable rate of recovery of certain brain areas like late emergence of cognitive function when compared with other areas (such as locomotion and audition) causes the confusion state [6], and various animal and human studies demonstrated that sevoflurane exerts transient paradoxical excitatory effects by exciting neurons in the locus coeruleus [7]. Rapid emergence from anesthesia has also been suspected as a risk factor [8].

Various pharmacological agents have been used to reduce the incidence of EA, including propofol, midazolam, α2 adrenoceptor agonists and opioids [9]. Propofol is a short-acting hypnotic agent used in children for induction and maintenance of general anesthesia [10]. Propofol has been used in different studies to decrease EA. Continuous infusion of propofol [11] and the administration of propofol at the end of procedure have been associated with decrease in the incidence of EA [12,13]. However, it has well known inconveniences and not preferred. Even lethal complications have been reported with a dose as low as 4.5 mg.kg.h[-1] after 3 days of administration [14,15].

There are few studies at the literature comparing the effect of propofol and sevoflurane in children and EA [16-19]. But they are limited with sample size and administration time and dose of propofol with no clear conclusion.

Thus, we tested the primary hypothesis that induction with propofol will decrease the incidence and intensity (severity) of emergence agitation when compared with sevoflurane. Secondary hypothesis, we tested that postoperative pain after propofol induction will be lower than sevoflurane.

Methods

This prospective interventional study was conducted at Mustafa Kemal University Hospital, Turkey. The protocol was approved by the Hospital Ethics Committee (number 267, June 2012), and written informed consent was obtained from the parents of all enrolled children. The study used a double-blind methodology with random allocation to the two groups by a computer-generated list. The protocol was registered, Clinical Trials number NCT02110745.

We enrolled 116 American Society of Anesthesiologists Physical Status I-II children scheduled for elective inguinal hernia under general anesthesia over the course of two years. Patients were excluded in the presence of a genetic syndrome, allergy to propofol, neurologic disorder, and use of psychiatric medications and had undergone a series of recent general anesthesia.

Protocol

All patients were inpatients and followed standard fasting guidelines (no solids after midnight and unlimited clear liquids up to 2 hours before premedication). EMLA Cream (Lidocaine HCl, prilocaine, Astra Zeneca, Istanbul, Turkey) was applied to the hands of all the children one hour prior the induction of anesthesia. All the patients were also premeditated with midazolam hydrochloride 0.6 mg/kg orally one hour prior to the surgery. Intravenous cannula was inserted before arrival to the operating room. Heart rate (HR), mean arterial pressure (MAP), and peripheral oxygen saturation (SpO_2) were monitored in operating room. Patients were randomized into two groups using a computer-generated random number table; Group P (Propofol) and Group S (Sevoflurane). 0.25 mg/kg intravenous lidocaine was given to all patients in the induction of anesthesia. Anesthesia was induced with a bolus injection of 3 mg/kg propofol and maintained oxygen (FiO_2 0.50), nitrous oxide (FiO_2 0.50), 1-3% sevoflurane in group P. In group S, anesthesia was induced with oxygen (FiO_2 0.50), nitrous oxide (FiO_2 0.50), and sevoflurane (increasing concentrations up to 8%) via face mask and maintained with 1-3%. To facilitate intubation, 0.5 mg/kg rocuronium and 1 mcg/kg fentanyl were given to all patients. The concentration of sevoflurane was adjusted to maintain the heart rate and blood pressure within 20% of the pre-induction values. All the children received 12 ml/kg 5% dextrose in 0.45% normal saline solution during surgery. Same surgeon performed all the inguinal hernia procedures. No local anesthesia was used during the surgical procedure. At the skin closure, 15 mg/kg acetaminophen was given intravenously to all patients. At the end of the surgery, neuromuscular blockade was reversed with intravenous neostigmine 0.03 mg/kg and atropine 0.01 mg/kg. Anesthesia was discontinued, the stomach was suctioned, and the tracheal tube was removed when airway reflexes returned. The patients were transferred to the post anesthesia care unit (PACU). If agitation exceeded a score of 3 on the Agitation Cole Score [20] (Table1), 1 mcg/kg fentanyl was given intravenously. This score was used to calculate the incidence of agitation, where agitation scores of 1, 2 and 3 were regarded to represent absence of agitation, and scores of 4 and 5 were regarded to indicate presence of agitation. If pain exceeded score of 3 on the Wong-Baker FACES Pain Rating Scale [21], intravenous 15 mg/kg acetaminophen was given and first analgesic requirement time (discontinuation of the sevoflurane anesthesia to postoperative first analgesic need) was recorded. First transition from PACU to surgical

ward was considered safe when patient had achieved a Modified Aldrete Score [22] 9 for at least 10 min, and SpO_2 95% with oxygen 2 l/min or 92% without oxygen, signified recovery of physical, mental, and physiological function to near preanesthetic levels. Postoperative nausea and vomiting (PONV) was treated with ondansetron 0.15 mg/kg intravenously. Patients were discharged only when they had no bleeding, no nausea and vomiting, were able to drink liquids, and had pain scores ≤ 2. Patients stayed at least 24 h in the hospital per surgical routine even in the absence of aforementioned parameters.

Score	Behavior
1	Sleeping
2	Awake, calm
3	Irritable, crying
4	Inconsolable crying
5	Severe restlessness, disorientation

Table 1: Cole scoring system for emergence agitation.

Measurements

Demographic and morphometric characteristics were recorded. An anesthesiologist blinded to group allocation evaluated patients for postoperative agitation using Cole agitation scale at arrival in PACU, 10 min, 20 min, 30 min, 40 min, 50 min, 1 h and 2 h.

All the patients were assessed for pain intensity using the Wong-Baker Faces Pain Rating Scale at arrival in PACU, 10 min, 20 min, 30 min, 40 min, 50 min, 1 h, 2 h, 4 h, 6 h, 12 h and 24 h.

Heart rate, mean arterial blood pressure, oxygen saturation, respiratory rate and side effects were recorded at arrival in PACU, 10 min, 20 min, 30 min, 40 min, 50 min, 1 h, 2 h, 4 h, 6 h, 12 h and 24 h. Side effects including bronchospasm, laryngospasm (characterized by an inability to ventilate the patient's lungs and requiring either administration of continuous positive pressure or a neuromuscular blocking agent to restore ventilation), persistent coughing (duration longer than 15 s), desaturation ($SpO_2<95\%$), re-intubation, postoperative bleeding, and reoperation were recorded. Surgery time and duration of anesthesia (time from the induction to the discontinuation of sevoflurane anesthesia) were recorded. First analgesic requirement time was recorded. First eye opening, following first verbal command follow were recorded in operating room. Total PACU stay time, ambulation time (the time between PACU to first stand up) and first oral intake time were also recorded.

Furthermore, 10-point analogue scales were used to measure parents' satisfaction with their child's overall anesthetic and surgical care (0=not at all satisfied, 10=extremely satisfied).

Data Analysis

The sample size was designed to evaluate the difference in the incidence of EA during recovery. The sample size was determined assuming that the probability of propofol agitation was 30% and sevoflurane agitation was 55%. We wanted to find a significant difference ($P<0.05$) ($α=0.05$, one tailed) with a power of 80% to detect a difference of 25%. Forty-seven patients per group would have been sufficient, but we expected some exclusions from the protocol (which did not happen) and increased this number to 58 (which allowed finding the same significant difference with a power of 80%). For estimation of sample size, a preliminary study was performed [23]. Normal distribution of continuous variables was tested with Kolmogorov-Smirnoff test. Chi-square test was used for comparisons between categorical variables. Mann-Whitney U test and Students' T were used for comparison of groups for continuous variables. Statistical Package for the Social Sciences (SPSS) version 15.0 (SPSS Inc., Chicago, IL, USA) used. P<0.05 was considered significant.

Results

One hundred and sixteen parents consented patients who fulfilled the entry criteria were enrolled; all patients completed the entire study and were included the final analysis. There were no differences between groups in age, body weight, height, ASA physical status, durations of surgery and anesthesia (Table 2).

	Group S (n=58)	Group P (n=58)	P
Age (year)	3 (2-11)	4 (2-10)	0.081
Height (cm)	100 (50-140)	110 (60-163)	0.094
Weight (kg)	17 (10-35)	20 (11-50)	0.089
ASA	53/5	51/7	0.542
Duration of Surgery (min)	20 (10-120)	25 (10-150)	0.196
Duration of Anesthesia (min)	30 (18-145)	30 (15-110)	0.138
Results presented as numbers or median and range.			

Table 2: Baseline characteristics, Duration of surgery, duration of anesthesia.

The incidence of EA was significantly lower in the propofol group when compared with sevoflurane group at arrival in PACU (12 (20%) vs. 22 (37%), P=0.041), however there were no differences in other measurement times. But the cumulative incidences at the end of the postoperative two hours were statistically higher in sevoflurane group (38 (65.5%) vs. 23 (39.7%), p<0.005).

	Group S (n=58)	Group P (n=58)	P
PACU (0.h)	3 (2-5)	3 (1-5)	0.002
Postoperative 10 min	3 (2-5)	2 (2-5)	0.006
Postoperative 20 min	3 (2-5)	2 (2-4)	0.000
Postoperative 30 min	3 (2-4)	3 (2-4)	0.001
Postoperative 40 min	3 (2-4)	3 (2-4)	0.450
Postoperative 50 min	3 (2-4)	3 (2-4)	0.259
Postoperative 1 h	3 (2-4)	3 (2-4)	0.856
Postoperative 2 h	3 (0-3)	3 (2-3)	0.072
Results presented as numbers or median and range.			

Table 3: Postoperative agitation scores.

EA scores were significantly lower in propofol group in all measurements during postoperative 30 minutes (Table 3). Furthermore, fentanyl consumption at arrival in PACU and at the sum of the two hours was statistically lower in propofol group [(0 (0-35) vs. 0 (0-30), P=0.025) (14 (0-60) vs. 0 (0-60), P=0.019)].

Pain scores were significantly lower in the propofol group when compared with sevoflurane at all the measurement times (Table 4).

	Group S (n=58)	Group P (n=58)	P
PACU (0.h)	4 (2-8)	2 (0-8)	0.000
Postoperative 10 min	4 (2-6)	2 (0-6)	0.000
Postoperative 20 min	4 (2-6)	2 (0-6)	0.000
Postoperative 30 min	4 (2-4)	2 (0-6)	0.000
Postoperative 40 min	4 (2-6)	2 (0-6)	0.000
Postoperative 50 min	4 (0-6)	2 (0-6)	0.000
Postoperative 1 h	2 (0-6)	2 (0-6)	0.152
Postoperative 2 h	2 (0-6)	2 (0-4)	0.975
Postoperative 4 h	2 (0-4)	2 (0-4)	0.772
Postoperative 6 h	2 (0-4)	2 (0-4)	0.216
Postoperative 12 h	2 (0-4)	2 (0-4)	0.035
Postoperative 24 h	2 (0-2)	0 (0-2)	0.096
Results presented as numbers or median and range.			

Table 4: Postoperative pain scores.

Table 5 summarizes the speed and the quality of recovery from anesthesia. Sevoflurane provided a faster recovery as evidenced by the time to first spontaneous eye opening, first verbal command follow time and PACU staying time. Ambulation time, first oral intake time was all similar in both groups. Time to first analgesic dose was statistically shorter in sevoflurane group. The overall parents' satisfaction was higher in propofol group. PONV was the most common adverse event; there were no difference between the adverse events in postoperative 24h. Antiemetic consumption in postoperative 24h were also similar in both groups (4 (3%) vs. 3 (2%), p=1.000).

Discussion

The incidence of emergence agitation varies between 20-80% and is more frequently seen in young children and unrelated to gender [24,25]. According to previous studies the incidence of EA after propofol maintenance of anesthesia is between 0-9% [11-26]. The present study showed that the overall frequent incidence is lower in propofol group with a ratio of 39% and approximately 25% difference between two groups. Sun et al concluded that the incidence of EA was significantly higher in sevoflurane group when compared with propofol [27]. Because of different measurement techniques to quantify EA and differing methods of data analysis, the range of ratios accepted for EA is still really wide, makes the comparison of the results of these studies difficult. Time of scoring was another cause, because it is different in studies. Cole et al, [20] explained that the degree of EA is highly dependent on when it is measured.

There are fewer studies assessed both incidence and intense of EA together. This investigation demonstrates that the induction with propofol causes less incidence and intense of EA and postoperative pain when compared with sevoflurane.

	Group S (n=58)	Group P (n=58)	P
First spontaneous eye opening time (min)	5 (1-23)	10 (1-60)	0.008
First verbal command follow time (min)	10 (2-120)	15 (5-60)	0.004
PACU stay time (min)	18 (7-41)	25 (5-60)	0.000
Ambulation time (h)	8 (3-15)	6 (2-12)	0.143
First oral intake time (h)	4 (2-8)	4 (2-9)	0.118
First analgesic dose(ml)	245 (0-575)	292 (0-750)	0.485
First analgesic requirement time (min)	30 (2-180)	55 (5-180)	0.000
Parents satisfaction	8 (5-10)	9 (7-10)	0.000
Results presented as numbers or median and range.			

Table 5: Recovery parameters.

The etiology of EA after general anesthesia with volatile anesthetics is not clear yet. But the probable mechanism between children and EA is about variable rate of neurological recovery in brain and insufficient development of neurons [28]. But the most reasonable explanations for the mechanism of EA were rapid awakening with sevoflurane, desflurane, isoflurane [29,30] and postoperative pain sensation [31,32]. Sevoflurane is the most common well known aggravator anesthetic agent responsible for rapid emergence, with a dissociative state, that is, children awaken with altered cognitive perception [33,34]. The incidence of EA was lower in children after propofol anesthesia than sevoflurane [35]. Therefore, our results and the previous findings question the relationship between induction techniques and EA incidence and intense in children. The analgesic effect of propofol in proper induction doses as 3 mg/kg and fentanyl as 1 mcg/kg given together for all patients may be the probable causes of low incidence of EA in overall, preventing the pain sensation and low EA incidence in current study. It is well known that pain and opioid usage have been shown to change EA incidence [36]. We may only say probably because EA also occurs in pain-free procedures like imaging [37] and pain-free children with caudal analgesia [38]. Dahmani's meta-analysis supported our results that fentanyl is still preventative against EA following sevoflurane anesthesia [39]. In contrast Kararmaz et al [40] reported that fentanyl administration during the induction period does not reduce the incidence of EA. In our study, pain scores are not statistically significant in middle repeated measurement times because of the analgesic effects of fentanyl used as a requirement for EA in early postoperative period.

Postoperative pain scores were lower in postoperative period in propofol group. But it is really impossible to explain the underlying mechanisms simply. Because it may be about the analgesic properties of propofol or hyperalgesic effects of sevoflurane that both of them are recorded in the literature [41,42]. The relation between pain and emergence agitation really needs further investigations.

More emotional children who had difficulties in separation from their parents had higher EA incidence [20-43]. In current study all the patients were premedicated with oral midazolam, which creates inhibitory effects on the central nervous system. Midazolam premedication reduces sevoflurane-associated emergence agitation incidence by 40% [44]. In opposite the other study showed that it has no effect on EA after inhalational anesthesia in postoperative period [45]. But we know very well that midazolam has short duration of action like propofol. So we may explain how to reduce the incidence of EA with the residual effect or combination of the drugs. On the other hand preoperative anxiety is a well-known factor contributing to EA [39]. The effect of midazolam on emergence agitation is still controversial [11]. Maybe it reduces the overall agitation scores but we could not think the opposite, in our opinion mask induction technique is really difficult to accept for children without premedication.

When compared with sevoflurane contrarily propofol usage in children decreases the incidence of EA [28]. The rapid pharmacokinetics of propofol and the low doses (1 mg/kg) given in previous studies would explain why the bolus doses not achieve to prevent EA in induction [39]. Furthermore, 1 mg/kg propofol given after discontinuation of sevoflurane decreased the incidence of EA [10]. Cohen et al reported that induction with propofol 2 mg/kg at the beginning does not decrease EA, probably because of the short duration time of the propofol and low serum level not enough to suppress EA in acute postoperative period. But that is the point that these levels especially may be given after long procedures [35]. If the incidence of EA still reduces after long procedures, probably it may be about residual effect of propofol. Meta-analysis reported that timing in administration is important. Especially continuous administration and a bolus dose at the end of anesthesia were protective because of propofol concentration during emergence [39]. We could not measure the concentration but our study group inguinal hernias are not such long surgical procedures. Propofol, gamma (γ)-aminobutyric acid-A (GABA-A) receptor inhibitor, produces a positive mood or euphoric state postoperatively in adults [46,47].

Tan et al concluded that patients anesthetized with propofol have less postoperative pain compared with sevoflurane in acute postoperative period [48]. Fentanyl is an important opioid routinely used in induction of children. Propofol bolus with fentanyl may prolonged the efficacy of propofol, with the effect of midazolam given in the premedication [2,36]. Likewise there are several studies with lower incidence of EA in propofol group with longer recovery times when compared with sevoflurane [49]. Longer recovery times can be due to residual sedative effect of propofol in the early recover period as well [16]. The recovery times has opposite correlation with agitation scores [50]. First eye opening, first verbal command follow, PACU staying time were shorter in sevoflurane group. It was really important to measure the depth of anesthesia in such conditions because the comparison between propofol and sevoflurane in this regard is really complicated. Rapid awakening in an unfamiliar environment for psychologically underdeveloped children is another major cause of EA [49].

Adverse events may cause EA like hypoxemia, bladder distension, nausea and pain. None of the patients experienced hypoxemia and bladder distension but a few of them had nausea. The most common adverse event in children in postoperative period is nausea and vomiting [51]. Fentanyl and nitrous oxide was used in the same doses in both groups. In current study we gave all patients ondansetron as antiemetic routine. May be it suppressed the reducing effect of propofol about PONV, because there was no statistical difference between two groups. But may be children felt pain however we could not measure, fentanyl given, nitrous oxide cause this adverse effect in a few of them.

Viitanen et al. [52] concluded that the induction of propofol and continued with sevoflurane causes quiter state during acute recovery period. And also it is well known that propofol has sedative and euphoric effects in adults in postoperative periods [46,47] which causes better agitation scores in children during postoperative period. At the same this calmer state may cause the difference between two groups in parents' satisfaction as in current study. Parents' satisfaction was really high in propofol group when compared with sevoflurane.

The current study has several limitations. More than 16 rating scales have been used to measure EA [53]. The major lack of the study like the most of the others done before, we used simple graded measurement [49,28]. It was important that only one blinded observer graded all scores. We also used hemodynamical variables to indicate comparable depths of anesthesia intraoperatively, although these variables are not reliable for monitoring the depth of anesthesia. The patients under 2 years of age were all excluded, because of difficulties in evaluation of emergence agitation state in them. The doses of propofol and sevoflurane are accurate for induction but they are not equipotent in fact. Lidocaine HCl is the most used medication for pain relieve before propofol injection. This medication may achieve preemptive analgesia and reduction of airway reflexes in pediatric patients. So it may cause less EA, from the other aspects it prevents the increase of EA incidence related with propofol pain [54,55].

We concluded that induction with propofol in accurate dose may be effective in reducing the incidence and intense of EA in children undergoing inguinal hernia surgery between 2-12 years old. Propofol may be preferred as an agent in induction for all children undergoing operations with general anesthesia. Future studies should focus on associations of pain and EA.

References

1. Tzong KY, Han S, Roh A, Ing C (2012) Epidemiology of pediatric surgical admissions in US children: data from the HCUP kids inpatient database. J Neurosurg Anesthesiol 24: 391-395.

2. Pieters BJ, Penn E, Nicklaus P, Bruegger D, Mehta B, et al. (2010) Emergence delirium and postoperative pain in children undergoing adenotonsillectomy: a comparison of propofol vs sevoflurane anesthesia. Paediatr Anaesth 20: 944-950.

3. Cravero J, Surgenor S, Whalen K (2000) Emergence agitation in paediatric patients after sevoflurane anaesthesia and no surgery: a comparison with halothane. Paediatr Anaesth 10: 419-424.

4. Sikich N, Lerman J (2004) Development and psychometric evaluation of the pediatric anesthesia emergence delirium scale. Anesthesiology 100: 1138-1145.

5. Veyckemans F (2001) Excitation phenomena during sevoflurane anaesthesia in children. Curr Opin Anaesthesiol 14: 339-343.

6. Kuratani N, Oi Y (2008) Greater incidence of emergence agitation in children after sevoflurane anesthesia as compared with halothane: a meta-analysis of randomized controlled trials. Anesthesiology 109: 225-232.

7. Yasui Y, Masaki E, Kato F (2007) Sevoflurane directly excites locus coeruleus neurons of rats. Anesthesiology 107: 992-1002.

8. Dahmani S, Delivet H, Hilly J (2014) Emergence delirium in children: an update. Curr Opin Anaesthesiol 27: 309-315.

9. Cho EJ, Yoon SZ, Cho JE, Lee HW (2014) Comparison of the effects of 0.03 and 0.05 mg/kg midazolam with placebo on prevention of emergence agitation in children having strabismus surgery. Anesthesiology 120: 1354-1361.

10. De Grood PM, Coenen LG, van Egmond J, Booij LH, Crul JF (1987) Propofol emulsion for induction and maintenance of anaesthesia. A combined technique of general and regional anaesthesia. Acta Anaesthesiol Scand 31: 219-223.

11. Uezono S, Goto T, Terui K, Ichinose F, Ishguro Y, et al. (2000) Emergence agitation after sevoflurane versus propofol in pediatric patients. Anesth Analg 91: 563-566.

12. Abu-Shahwan I (2008) Effect of propofol on emergence behavior in children after sevoflurane general anesthesia. Paediatr Anaesth 18: 55-59.

13. Aouad MT, Yazbeck-Karam VG, Nasr VG, El-Khatib MF, Kanazi GE, et al. (2007) A single dose of propofol at the end of surgery for the prevention of emergence agitation in children undergoing strabismus surgery during sevoflurane anesthesia. Anesthesiology 107: 733-8.

14. Mani V, Morton NS (2010) Overview of total intravenous anesthesia in children. Paediatr Anaesth 20: 211-222.

15. Bray RJ (1998) Propofol infusion syndrome in children. Paediatr Anaesth 8: 491-499.

16. Nakayama S, Furukawa H, Yanai H (2007) Propofol reduces the incidence of emergence agitation in preschool-aged children as well as in school-aged children: a comparison with sevoflurane. J Anesth 21: 19-23.

17. Pieters BJ, Penn E, Nicklaus P, Bruegger D, Mehta B, et al. (2010) Emergence delirium and postoperative pain in children undergoing adenotonsillectomy: a comparison of propofol vs sevoflurane anesthesia. Paediatr Anaesth 20: 944-950.

18. Hofer CK, Zollinger A, Buchi S, Klaghofer R, Serafino D, et al. (2003) Patient well-being after general anaesthesia: a prospective, randomized, controlled multi-centre trial comparing intravenous and inhalational anaesthesia. Br J Anaesth 91:631-7.

19. Hendolin H, Kansanen M, Koski E, Nuutinen J (1994) Propofol-nitrous oxide versus thiopentone-isoflurane-nitrous oxide anaesthesia for uvulopalatopharyngoplasty in patients with sleep apnea. Acta Anaesthesiol Scand 38: 694-698.

20. Cole JW, Murray DJ, McAllister JD, Hirshberg GE (2002) Emergence behaviour in children: defining the incidence of excitement and agitation following anaesthesia. Paediatr Anaesth 12: 442-447.

21. Bailey B, Bergeron S, Gravel J, Daoust R (2007) Comparison of four pain scales in children with acute abdominal pain in a pediatric emergency department. Ann Emerg Med 50: 379-383, 383.

22. American Society of Anesthesiologists Task Force on Postanesthetic Care (2002) Practice guidelines for postanesthetic care: a report by the American Society of Anesthesiologists Task Force on Postanesthetic Care. Anesthesiology 96: 742-752.

23. Kim YH, Yoon SZ, Lim HJ, Yoon SM (2011) Prophylactic use of midazolam or propofol at the end of surgery may reduce the incidence of emergence agitation after sevoflurane anaesthesia. Anaesth Intensive Care 39: 904-908.

24. Jöhr M (2002) Postanaesthesia excitation. Paediatr Anaesth 12: 293-295.

25. Voepel-Lewis T, Malviya S, Tait AR (2003) A prospective cohort study of emergence agitation in the pediatric postanesthesia care unit. Anesth Analg 96: 1625-1630, table of contents.

26. Picard V, Dumont L, Pellegrini M (2000) Quality of recovery in children: sevoflurane versus propofol. Acta Anaesthesiol Scand 44: 307-310.

27. Sun JH, Han N, Wu XY (2008) Systematic evaluation of Sevoflurane in pediatric anesthesia maintenance. Chinese J Evidence-Based Med 11: 988-996

28. Aouad MT, Nasr VG (2005) Emergence agitation in children: an update. Curr Opin Anaesthesiol 18: 614-619.

29. Lerman J, Davis PJ, Welborn LG, Orr RJ, Rabb M, et al. (1996) Induction, recovery, and safety characteristics of sevoflurane in children undergoing ambulatory surgery: a comparison with halothane. Anesthesiology 84:1332-40.

30. Welborn LG, Hannallah RS, Norden JM, Ruttimann UE, Callan CM (1996) Comparison of emergence and recovery characteristics of sevoflurane, desflurane, and halothane in pediatric ambulatory patients. Anesth Analg 83: 917-20.

31. Davis PJ, Greenberg JA, Gendelman M, Fertal K (1999) Recovery characteristics of sevoflurane and halothane in preschool-aged children undergoing bilateral myringotomy and pressure equalization tube insertion. Anesth Analg 88: 34-38.

32. Galinkin JL, Fazi LM, Cuy RM, Chiavacci RM, Kurth CD, et al. (2000) Use of intranasal fentanyl in children undergoing myringotomy and tube placement during halothane and sevoflurane anesthesia. Anesthesiology 93: 1375-83.

33. Silva LM, Braz LG, Módolo NS (2008) Emergence agitation in pediatric anesthesia: current features. J Pediatr (Rio J) 84: 107-113.

34. Yamashita M (2003) Postanaesthetic excitation and agitation. Paediatr Anaesth 13: 641.

35. Cohen IT, Finkel JC, Hannallah RS, Hummer KA, Patel KM (2003) Rapid emergence does not explain agitation following sevoflurane anaesthesia in infants and children: a comparison with propofol. Paediatr Anaesth 13: 63-67.

36. Cohen IT, Finkel JC, Hannallah RS, Hummer KA, Patel KM (2002) The effect of fentanyl on the emergence characteristics after desflurane or sevoflurane anesthesia in children. Anesth Analg 94: 1178-1181, table of contents.

37. Cravero JP, Beach M, Thyr B, Whalen K (2003) The effect of a small dose fentanyl on emergence characteristics of pediatric patients after sevoflurane anesthesia without surgery. Anesth Analg 97: 364-7.

38. Weldon BC, Bell M, Craddock T (2004) The effect of caudal analgesia on emergence agitation in children after sevoflurane versus halothane anesthesia. Anesth Analg 98: 321-326, table of contents.

39. Dahmani S, Stany I, Brasher C, Lejeune C, Bruneau B, et al. (2010) Pharmacological prevention of sevoflurane- and desflurane-related emergence agitation in children: a meta-analysis of published studies. Br J Anaesth 104: 216-223.

40. Kararmaz A, Kaya S, Turhanoglu S, Ozyilmaz MA (2004) Oral ketamine premedication can prevent emergence agitation in children after desflurane anaesthesia. Paediatr Anaesth 14: 477-482.

41. Briggs LP, Dundee JW, Bahar M, Clarke RS (1982) Comparison of the effect of diisopropyl phenol (ICI 35, 868) and thiopentone on response to somatic pain. Br J Anaesth 54: 307-311.

42. Zhang Y, Eger EI 2nd, Dutton RC, Sonner JM (2000) Inhaled anesthetics have hyperalgesic effects at 0.1 minimum alveolar anesthetic concentration. Anesth Analg 91: 462-466.

43. Kain ZN, Caldwell-Andrews AA, Maranets I, McClain B, Gaal D, et al. (2004) Preoperative anxiety and emergence delirium and postoperative maladaptive behaviors. Anesth Analg 99: 1648-1654, table of contents.

44. Lapin SL, Auden SM, Goldsmith LJ, Reynolds AM (1999) Effects of sevoflurane anaesthesia on recovery in children: a comparison with halothane. Paediatr Anaesth 9: 299-304.

45. Breschan C, Platzer M, Jost R, Stettner H, Likar R (2007) Midazolam does not reduce emergence delirium after sevoflurane anesthesia in children. Paediatr Anaesth 17: 347-352.

46. Mortero RF, Clark LD, Tolan MM, Metz RJ, Tsueda K, et al. (2001) The effects of small-dose ketamine on propofol sedation: respiration, postoperative mood, perception, cognition, and pain. Anesth Analg 92: 1465-1469.

47. Tang J, Chen L, White PF, Watcha MF, Wender RH, et al. (1999) Recovery profile, costs, and patient satisfaction with propofol and sevoflurane for fast-track office-based anesthesia. Anesthesiology 91: 253-261.

48. Tan T, Bhinder R, Carey M, Briggs L (2010) Day-surgery patients anesthetized with propofol have less postoperative pain than those anesthetized with sevoflurane. Anesth Analg 111: 83-85.

49. Aono J, Ueda W, Mamiya K, Takimoto E, Manabe M (1997) Greater incidence of delirium during recovery from sevoflurane anesthesia in preschool boys. Anesthesiology 87: 1298-1300.

50. Liang P, Zhou C, Ni J, Luo Z, Liu B (2014) Single-dose sufentanil or fentanyl reduces agitation after sevoflurane anesthesia in children undergoing ophthalmology surgery. Pak J Med Sci 30: 1059-1063.

51. Rose JB, Watcha MF (1999) Postoperative nausea and vomiting in paediatric patients. Br J Anaesth 83: 104-117.

52. Viitanen H, Tarkkila P, Mennander S, Viitanen M, Annila P (1999) Sevoflurane-maintained anesthesia induced with propofol or sevoflurane in small children: induction and recovery characteristics. Can J Anaesth 46: 21-28.

53. Banchs RJ, Lerman J (2014) Preoperative anxiety management, emergence delirium, and postoperative behavior. Anesthesiol Clin 32: 1-23.

54. Elgebaly AS (2013) Sub-Tenon's lidocaine injection improves emer¬gence agitation after general anaesthesia in paediatric ocular surgery. SAJAA 19: 114-9.

55. Seo IS, Seong CR, Jung G, Park SJ, Kim SY, et al. (2011) The effect of sub-Tenon lidocaine injection on emergence agitation after general anaesthesia in paediatric strabismus surgery. Eur J Anaesthesiol 28: 334-339.

35

Hypoglycemia in Laparoscopic Colectomy with Remifentanil Use and Preoperative Intravenous Glucose Infusion: A Prospective, Randomized, Single-Blind, Controlled Trial

Rie Kanamori, Rika Aihara, Nobutada Morioka[*] and Makoto Ozaki

Department of Anesthesiology, Tokyo Women's Medical University, Japan

[*]**Corresponding author:** Nobutada Morioka, Department of Anesthesiology, Tokyo Women's Medical University, 8-1, Kawada-cho, Shinjuku-ku, Tokyo 162-8666, Japan, E-mail: nobutadamorioka@gmail.com

Abstract

Background: The profound effect of a minimally-invasive procedure under general anesthesia with remifentanil contributes to suppression of hyperglycemic responses, which was formerly observed as a stress response. However, intraoperative occurrence of hypoglycemia is considered more of a concern. In addition, depending on preoperative nutritional status, critical hypoglycemia may occur during surgery. There are few reports on perioperative glucose metabolism in patients not receiving glucose infusion under anesthesia with remifentanil. The preoperative fasting period is longer in Japan and preoperative carbohydrate infusion or other pretreatment is not actively performed; thus, the preoperative nutritional status is close to that of starvation. Furthermore, the regulation of glucose metabolism under intraoperative management with potent opioids, such as remifentanil, as well as the fluctuations in metabolism due to perioperative glucose infusion, is important from the viewpoint of nutritional management.

Objective: This study aimed to examine the impact of preoperative intravenous glucose infusion on glucose, lipid, and protein metabolism before and after surgery under general anesthesia with remifentanil.

Methods: Forty patients who were scheduled for elective laparoscopic colectomy were randomly assigned to 2 groups: a glucose group that received 1500 mL of a maintenance solution with 10% glucose (glucose 150 g) and a non-glucose group that received the same amount of an extracellular solution without glucose. Glucose metabolism during and after surgery (blood glucose levels, insulin, C-peptide), lipid metabolism (ketone body fractions, free fatty acids), and protein metabolism (urinary 3-methyhistidine) were also evaluated.

Results: No changes were found in background in either group. Blood glucose levels during surgery remained significantly lower (P=0.003) in the control group than in the glucose group. One patient had a blood glucose level below 40 mg/dL, and 6 patients had blood glucose levels below 60 mg/dL. Lipid catabolism increased before the induction of anesthesia.

Conclusion: The incidence of hypoglycemia and the rate of lipid catabolism would increase before the induction of anesthesia and during surgery in elective laparoscopic colectomy using remifentanil without glucose infusion.

Keywords: Remifentanil; Carbohydrate metabolism; Laparoscopic surgery

Background

Stress induced by surgical procedures causes increased catabolism, which in turn triggers a cascade of enhanced glycogen breakdown, gluconeogenesis, and catabolism of lipids and proteins that eventually leads to increased insulin resistance and postoperative hyperglycemia [1,2]. Persistent postoperative hyperglycemia is a risk factor for infection and various other complications [3].

The Enhanced Recovery After Surgery (ERAS) program, which has been developed mostly in northern-European countries, recommends a preoperative intake of 12.5% carbohydrate-rich drinks (800 mL the night before surgery and another 400 mL up to 2 hours before surgery) to improve postoperative insulin resistance (150 g) [4,5]. However,

studies claiming that preoperative carbohydrate administration reduces postoperative insulin resistance are based on case evaluations of a small number of patients [6-8]. Other studies have shown that postoperative insulin resistance is not affected even with a preoperative carbohydrate load [9,10-12]. The effects of preoperative carbohydrate administration on metabolism during surgery are also unclear. In addition, few studies exist regarding the effects of preoperative intravenous carbohydrate administration in Japanese patients. Recent controversial issues are discussed, such as insulin resistance resulting from various factors, such as surgical invasion, and the associated hyperglycemia. Laparoscopic surgery, which is a minimally invasive procedure, is presently widely performed to reduce surgical invasion. The use of short-acting opioids, such as remifentanil, enables maintenance of adequate blood opioid concentrations during surgery, contributing to further reduction in surgical invasion. In this situation, a new need for glucose infusion presented itself. Unlike the world standard for preoperative treatment, mechanical preoperative treatment and extended fasting continue to be strictly performed in Japan. Additionally, fluctuations in intraoperative blood glucose levels at present differ from those in the past due to anesthetic management geared toward minimizing surgical invasion; however, no studies regarding this had been conducted. Therefore, in our study we administered 150 g of intravenous glucose to patients undergoing elective laparoscopic colectomy during the period between the night before surgery and the start of surgery. We then examined fluctuations in intraoperative blood glucose levels and specifically the impact on glucose metabolism, in addition to lipid and protein metabolism.

Methods

Trial design

This randomized, non-blinded, controlled trial was approved by the Institutional Review Board of Tokyo Women's Medical University and conducted in compliance with the Helsinki Declaration. The patients were fully informed both orally and in writing, and written informed consent was obtained.

Participants

Inclusion criteria: Patients were included if they were 20 years or older; scheduled for elective, morning laparoscopic colectomy in the Department of Gastroenterological Surgery at Tokyo Women's Medical University; and classified as American Society of Anesthesiologists physical status I or II.

Exclusion criteria: Patients were excluded if they had diabetes mellitus or glucose intolerance, severe heart dysfunction, severe renal dysfunction, or severe hepatic dysfunction. Patients were also excluded if they were regarded as inappropriate for the study by the study investigators. The registration period was 2 consecutive years.

Intervention

After informed consent was obtained, each patient's eligibility was assessed. The patients were then randomly assigned to 2 groups: a glucose group and a control group. The patients were radomized by computed numberized assignment for each groups. In the glucose group, the patients were not allowed to eat or drink beginning at 9:00 PM the night before surgery. At that time, they received 1500 mL (glucose 150 g) of a 10% glucose maintenance solution (Physio 35, Otsuka Pharmaceutical Factory, Inc., Tokushima, Japan), which was continued until before induction of anesthesia. Patients in the control group were also not allowed to eat or drink beginning starting at 9:00 PM the night before surgery. They received 1500 mL of an acetate Ringer's solution without glucose (Solyugen F, Nipro Corporation, Osaka, Japan) until the induction of anesthesia.

Outcomes and measurements

The primary endpoints were pre and intraoperative blood glucose levels. Glucose metabolism, lipid metabolism, protein metabolism, and surgical stress were also measured. Glucose metabolism was determined by measuring blood glucose levels, insulin, and C-peptide in blood samples taken before the start of the infusion the night before surgery, before induction of anesthesia the day of surgery, 2 hours after induction of anesthesia, at the end of surgery, and in the early morning the day after surgery. Lipid metabolism was determined by measuring

ketone body fractions and free fatty acids before induction of anesthesia the day of surgery, 2 hours after induction of anesthesia, and at the end of surgery. Protein metabolism was determined by measuring urinary 3-methylhistidine [13-17] from the urine that accumulated between induction of anesthesia and the end of surgery. In addition, surgical stress was determined by measuring catecholamines (epinephrine, norepinephrine, and dopamine) and cortisol in blood samples taken before the induction of anesthesia the day of surgery, 2 hours after the induction of anesthesia, and at the end of surgery.

Treatment

During and after surgery, patients were treated as follows. Before the induction of anesthesia, a thoracic epidural catheter was placed. Anesthesia was induced with 1 mg/kg of propofol, 0.5 µg/kg/min of remifentanil, and 0.6 mg/kg of rocuronium; anesthesia was maintained with 0.25 to 0.5 µg/kg/min and 1.5% of sevoflurane with 0.25 to 0.5 µg/kg/min of remifentanil. During surgery, a Ringer's solution without glucose was administered at a rate of 8 to 15 mL/kg/hr. Blood glucose levels during surgery were measured every hour with the simplified method. Insulin was administered if a patient's blood glucose levels were 200 mg/dL or higher, and glucose was administered if blood glucose levels were 40 mg/dL or lower. At the end of surgery, patients were given a bolus of 5 to 8 mL of 0.25% popscaine, and continuous administration was begun at a rate of 4 mL/hr. Patient-controlled analgesia (PCA) was used for pain control. An epidural PCA device was inserted, and the patients were transferred to their rooms. For 24 hours after surgery, 2500 mL of Ringer's solution without glucose was administered. During the study period, intravenous solutions containing carbohydrates, hetastarch, or amino acids were not administered. Patients who received insulin because of high blood glucose levels (≥ 200 mg/dL), patients who received glucose because of low blood glucose levels (≤ 40 mg/dL), patients who received blood transfusions, and patients who were found not to meet the inclusion criteria were withdrawn from the study immediately after they were disqualified.

Statistical analyses

Data were analyzed for all patients who were not withdrawn from the study. A paired t test was used for paired continuous data, and a student's t test was used for unpaired continuous data. A chi-squared test was used for categorical data. All analyses were performed with two-tailed tests. Significance was considered at $P < 0.05$. The mean ± standard deviation was used to express the variability of data. JMP® (SAS Institute Japan, Ltd., Tokyo, Japan) was used for statistical analyses.

Results

Between April 2010 and March 2012, 40 patients were enrolled in the study; 20 patients each were assigned to the glucose and control groups. Two patients were withdrawn and excluded from the data analysis: one patient whose glucose tolerance met the exclusion criteria and one patient who received glucose because of blood glucose levels ≤ 40 mg/dL. However, analysis also included intraoperative measurements of blood glucose at each measurement point up to the administration of salvage therapy. No differences were found in the patient or surgical characteristics of the groups (Table 1).

	Glucose group n=19	Control group n=19	P value
Men/Women	13/6	11/8	0.35[b]
Age, mean ± SD, yrs	64 ± 12	61 ± 13	0.50[a]
Height, mean ± SD, cm	162 ± 8	168 ± 8	0.48[a]
Body weight, mean ± SD, kg	58 ± 11	59 ± 10	0.80[a]
ASA Classification, I/II	8/11	6/13	0.32[b]
Colon/Rectum	12/7	11/8	0.64[b]
Anesthesia time, mean ± SD, min	252 ± 45	242 ± 35	0.42[a]
Surgical time, mean ± SD, min	178 ± 43	170 ± 35	0.53[a]
Amount of solution infused during surgery, mean ± SD, mL	2179 ± 430	2104 ± 523	0.63[a]
Amount of bleeding during surgery, mean ± SD, mL	20 ± 22	26 ± 42	0.57[a]
Urinary output during surgery, mean ± SD, mL	559 ± 396	548 ± 546	0.95[a]

Table 1: Characteristics of the patients and surgical procedures.

Data for glucose metabolism, lipid metabolism, protein metabolism, and surgical stress were analyzed. Blood glucose as the primary endpoints and insulin levels remained significantly higher in the glucose group than in the control group from the induction of anesthesia to the day after surgery ($P<0.05$ for both parameters, Figure 1). Insulin levels remained significantly higher in the glucose group than in the control group from the induction of anesthesia to end of surgery ($P<0.00001$) (Figure 1). Ketone body fractions remained higher in the control group than in the glucose group from the induction of anesthesia to end of surgery ($P<0,0001$ Table 2). Free fatty acid levels were significantly higher in the control group than in the glucose group at induction of anesthesia ($P=0.00028$, Table 3). Urinary 3-methylhistidine levels were not statistically significant (0.19 ± 0.19 micromol/day, glucose group; 0.25 ± 0.30 micromol/day), control group, $P=0.51$).

	Reference range	Group	At induction of anesthesia	2 hrs after induction of anesthesia	At the end of surgery
Total ketone bodies μmol/L	Below 130	Glucose group	231 ± 306[a]	825 ± 503[ab]	882 ± 587[ab]
		Control group	2033 ± 1482	1979 ± 1206[b]	2728 ± 1784[b]
Acetoacetic acid μmol/L	Below 55	Glucose group	72 ± 84[a]	214 ± 112[ab]	242 ± 168[ab]
		Control group	495 ± 308	544 ± 236[b]	611 ± 294[b]
3-hydroxy butyric acid μmol/L	Below 85	Glucose group	163 ± 222[a]	610 ± 394[ab]	640 ± 434[ab]
		Control group	1661 ± 1160	1729 ± 1172[b]	2107 ± 1513[b]
Free fatty acids mEq/L	140-850	Glucose group	516 ± 332[a]	830 ± 214[b]	702 ± 198[b]
		Control group	1199 ± 634	670 ± 233[b]	754 ± 210[b]

Data are expressed as mean ± SD; a$P < 0.05$ (comparison of means between the groups using the Student's t test); b$P < 0.05$ (comparison of means between the groups using the Student's t test).

Table 2: Time course of parameters used to determine lipid metabolism.

Levels of the stress hormone cortisol were significantly lower ($P=0.038$) in the glucose group than in the control group 2 hours after induction of anesthesia. Dopamine levels were significantly higher ($P=0.053$) in the glucose group than in the control group the day after surgery. However, the values were both within the reference ranges (Table 3).

Discussion

The impact of preoperative glucose infusion on intraoperative blood glucose levels was examined in patients undergoing elective laparoscopic colectomy under general anesthesia using remifentanil. Neither group had increased blood glucose levels the day after surgery. Therefore, we do not believe postoperative glucose level to be increased after elective laparoscopic colectomy nor does administering preoperative intravenous glucose (150 g) affect postoperative carbohydrate metabolism.

	Group	At induction of anesthesia	2 hrs after induction of anesthesia	At the end of surgery	Day after surgery
Adrenaline pg/mL	Glucose group	44 ± 34	14 ± 9	54 ± 83	26 ± 13
	Control group	53 ± 57	28 ± 39	69 ± 115	62 ± 103
Noradrenaline pg/mL	Glucose group	236 ± 147	199 ± 85	159 ± 98	236 ± 156
	Control group	220 ± 150	168 ± 67	130 ± 66	200 ± 112
Dopamine pg/mL	Glucose group	11 ± 6	16 ± 6	19 ± 31	24 ± 24[a]
	Control group	10 ± 8	15 ± 7	7 ± 7	7 ± 5
Cortisol µg/dL	Glucose group	13 ± 5	5 ± 2a	6 ± 6	15 ± 6
	Control group	14 ± 6	7 ± 3	5 ± 2	13 ± 6

Data are expressed as mean ± SD; aP < 0.05 (comparison of means between the groups [Student's t test])

Table 3: Time course of stress hormone levels.

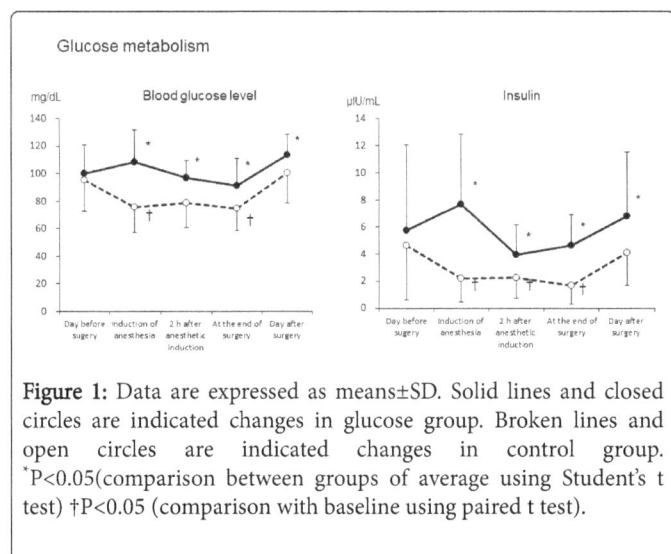

Figure 1: Data are expressed as means±SD. Solid lines and closed circles are indicated changes in glucose group. Broken lines and open circles are indicated changes in control group. *P<0.05(comparison between groups of average using Student's t test) †P<0.05 (comparison with baseline using paired t test).

Studies of patients undergoing cholecystectomy, hip arthroplasty, and colorectal surgery have shown that preoperative carbohydrate load reduced postoperative insulin resistance [6-8]. However, in other studies of patients undergoing cardiovascular surgery preoperative glucose administration did not reduce postoperative insulin resistance [9,10] suggesting that the effects differ with varying degrees of surgical stress. Laparoscopic colectomy, the procedure used in our study, causes less surgical stress than does open surgery. In addition, our patients had been given an enough amount of opioids during surgery because

of the use of remifentanil, and postoperative pain was properly managed with epidural anesthesia, which suppressed the secretion of catecholamines and cortisol [18-20]. All of these factors were thought to have contributed to the fact that postoperative insulin resistance did not increase in our patients.

No changes were seen in blood glucose levels in the glucose group throughout the study period. However, the blood glucose level in the control group was 95.5 ± 22.8 mg/dL the day before surgery and decreased significantly to 75.8 ± 18.6 mg/dL (P=0.005). During surgery, one patient who had a blood glucose level below 40 mg/dL received glucose; 6 patients had blood glucose levels below 60 mg/dL. These episodes of hypoglycemia did not cause clinical symptoms and would have been overlooked had the blood glucose levels not been measured. None of the patients had diabetes mellitus or glucose tolerance before surgery. In Japan, patients who undergo colon surgery are required to fast and mechanical preparation, so their nutritional state is compromised, and they can easily develop hypoglycemia unless glucose is administered before surgery.

Ketone body fractions and free fatty acid levels (parameters for lipid metabolism) were significantly higher before the induction of anesthesia in the control group (P<0.001 for both parameters) and much higher than the upper limit of the reference range, which indicates that lipid is being metabolized due to a lack of glucose. Ketone body fractions increased significantly in both groups until end of surgery because glucose was not administered during surgery. To suppress catabolism, not only preoperative but also intraoperative glucose administration should be considered [21-24].

No difference was found in the levels of urinary 3-methylhistidine, a parameter for protein metabolism, and the values in both groups were within the reference range. Measurements were based on urine samples accumulated between the induction of anesthesia and end of surgery. If protein catabolism started toward the end of the surgical procedure, urinary 3-methylhistidine may have been diluted in a larger amount of accumulated urine, resulting in lower values than the actual values. Also, the time lag for 3-methylhistidine to be excreted in the urine needs to be considered. In evaluating protein catabolism during surgery by using urinary 3-methylhistidine, we believe that more precise results could have been obtained if fresh urine samples obtained at predetermined sampling points, including postoperatively, had been analyzed. In addition, the procedures we studied were relatively short, lasting approximately 3 hours. The time course of blood glucose levels and the degree of lipid breakdown in our patients indicated that protein catabolism might have occurred if the surgical procedures had been longer. While pre- and intraoperative infusion of glucose/carbohydrate has been strongly advocated to prevent postoperative insulin resistance, etc., this study revealed the importance of preoperative infusion of glucose/carbohydrate for prevention of hypoglycemia. In addition, due to advances in minimally invasive techniques typified by the intraoperative use of remifentanil, there has been no further occurrence of intraoperative hyperglycemia as formerly observed. On the contrary, if a patient remains in a starvation-like state from the preoperative period, intraoperative occurrence of hypoglycemia, etc., is more likely to become an issue. Intraoperative measurement of blood glucose levels is necessary and the simple pre- and/or intraoperative infusion of glucose may be a simple and important protocol in the prevention of critical hypoglycemia.

Conclusions

In elective laparoscopic colectomy, preoperative glucose infusion does not induce intra- or postoperative hyperglycemia. However, gastrointestinal pretreatment results in the diminished nutritional status of patients. Unless glucose infusion is performed in the period between the night before surgery and the start of surgery, blood glucose levels will begin to decrease prior to surgery and lipid catabolism will be enhanced. Furthermore, if glucose is not infused during surgery, lipid catabolism may be further enhanced, thereby inducing critical hypoglycemia. In laparoscopic colectomy requiring gastrointestinal pretreatment, perioperative glucose infusion should be considered for the purposes of preventing hypoglycemia and suppressing catabolism.

Acknowledgement

Dr. Kanamori and Dr. Morioka, who are independent of the commercial funder, had full access to all the data and takes responsibility for the integrity of the data and analyses.

References

1. Russo N (2012) Perioperative glycemic control. Anesthesiol Clin 30: 445-466.

2. Thorell A, Efendic S, Gutniak M, Häggmark T, Ljungqvist O (1994) Insulin resistance after abdominal surgery. Br J Surg 81: 59-63.

3. Zerr KJ, Furnary AP, Grunkemeier GL, Bookin S, Kanhere V, et al. (1997) Glucose control lowers the risk of would infection in diabetics after open heart operations. Ann Thorac Surg 63: 356-361.

4. Nygren J, Soop M, Thorell A, Efendic S, Nair KS, et al. (1998) Preoperative oral carbohydrate administration reduces postoperative insulin resistance. Clin Nutr 17: 65-71.

5. Fearon KC, Ljungqvist O, Von Meyenfeldt M, Revhaug A, Dejong CH, et al. (2005) Enhanced recovery after surgery: a consensus review of clinical care for patients undergoing colonic resection. Clin Nutr 24: 466-477.

6. Gustafsson UO, Scott MJ, Schwenk W, Demartines N, Roulin D, et al. (2000) Enhanced Recovery After Surgery Society. Guidelines for perioperative care in elective colonic surgery: Enhanced Recovery after Surgery (ERAS*) Society recommendations. Clin Nutr 31:783-800.

7. Ljungqvist O, Thorell A, Gutniak M, Häggmark T, Efendic S (1994) Glucose infusion instead of preoperative fasting reduces postoperative insulin resistance. J Am Coll Surg 178: 329-336.

8. Nygren J, Soop M, Thorell A, Efendic S, Nair KS, et al. (1998) Preoperative oral carbohydrate administration reduces postoperative insulin resistance. Clin Nutr 17: 65-71.

9. Nygren J, Thorell A, Ljungqvist O (2001) Preoperative oral carbohydrate nutrition: an update. Curr Opin Clin Nutr Metab Care 4: 255-259.

10. Breuer JP, von Dossow V, von Heymann C, Griesbach M, von Schickfus M, et al. (2006) Preoperative oral carbohydrate administration to ASA III-IV patients undergoing elective cardiac surgery. Anesth Analg 103:1099-1108.

11. Järvelä K, Maaranen P, Sisto T (2008) Pre-operative oral carbohydrate treatment before coronary artery bypass surgery. Acta Anaesthesiol Scand 52: 793-797.

12. Matthews DR, Hosker JP, Rudenski AS, Naylor BA, Treacher DF, et al. (1985) Homeostasis model assessment: insulin resistance and beta-cell function from fasting plasma glucose and insulin concentrations in man. Diabetologia 28:412-419.

13. Haffner SM, Kennedy E, Gonzalez C, Stern MP, Miettinen H (1996) A prospective analysis of the HOMA model. The Mexico City Diabetes Study. Diabetes Care 19: 1138-1141.

14. Williamson DH, Farrell R, Kerr A, Smith R (1977) Muscle-protein catabolism after injury in man, as measured by urinary excretion of 3-methylhistidine. Clin Sci Mol Med 52: 527-533.

15. Threlfall CJ, Stoner HB, Galasko CS (1981) Patterns in the excretion of muscle markers after trauma and orthopedic surgery. J Trauma 21: 140-147.

16. Munro HN, Young VR (1978) Urinary excretion of N gamma-methylihistidine (3-methylhistidine): a tool to study metabolic responses in relation to nutrient and hormonal status in health and disease of man. Am J Clin Nutr 31:1608-1614.

17. Elia M, Carter A, Bacon S, Winearls CG, Smith R (1981) Clinical usefulness of urinary 3-methylhistidine excretion in indicating muscle protein breakdown. Br Med J (Clin Res Ed) 282: 351-354.

18. Young VR, Munro HN (1978) Ntau-methylhistidine (3-methylhistidine) and muscle protein turnover: an overview. Fed Proc 37: 2291-2300.

19. Katz A, Nambi SS, Mather K, Baron AD, Follmann DA, et al. (2000) Quantitative insulin sensitivity check index: a simple, accurate method for assessing insulin sensitivity in humans. J Clin Endocrinol Metab 85: 2402-2410.

20. Thorell A, Nygren J, Ljungqvist O (1999) Insulin resistance: a marker of surgical stress. Curr Opin Clin Nutr Metab Care 2: 69-78.

21. Myre K, Raeder J, Rostrup M, Buanes T, Stokland O (2003) Catecholamine release during laparoscopic fundoplication with high and low doses of remifentanil. Acta Anaesthesiol Scand 47: 267-273.

22. Schricker T, Lattermann R, Carli F (2005) Intraoperative protein sparing with glucose. J Appl Physiol (1985) 99: 898-901.

23. Mikura M, Yamaoka I, Doi M, Kawano Y, Nakayama M, et al. (2009) Glucose infusion suppresses surgery-induced muscle protein breakdown by inhibiting ubiquitin-proteasome pathway in rats. Anesthesiology 110: 81-88.

24. Yamasaki K, Inagaki Y, Mochida S, Funaki K, Takahashi S, et al. (2010) Effect of intraoperative acetated Ringer's solution with 1% glucose on glucose and protein metabolism. J Anesth 24: 426-431.

36

How should Beginners Learn Ultrasound In-Plane Needle Techniques? A Randomized Comparison between Directed-and Self-Learning

Daniel Chora de la Garza, Pornpan Chalermkitpanit, Prangmalee Leurcharusmee, Vanlapa Arnuntasupakul, De QH Tran and Roderick J Finlayson[*]

Department of Anesthesia, Alan Edwards Pain Management Unit, McGill University Health Center, Montreal, Quebec, Canada

[*]**Corresponding author:** Roderick J Finlayson, Montreal General Hospital, Department of Anesthesia, 1650 Ave Cedar, D10-144, Montreal, Quebec, Canada, E-mail: roderick.finlayson@mac.com

Abstract

Background: With ultrasound (US) guidance, the in-plane (IP) technique allows operators to track the needle in real time during its advancement towards the target nerve. While mastery of the IP technique is instrumental to the success (and safety) of peripheral nerve blocks, the optimal learning strategy for beginners has not been elucidated. In this randomized trial, using phantom gel models, we compared control-, self- and directed-learning for the acquisition of IP needle skills. We hypothesized that, compared to the 2 other groups, directed-learning would require a shorter performance time and fewer needle passes to complete the post-test.

Methods: Thirty novice operators (experience level<30 US-guided procedures in the 6 months prior to the study) were randomized to 1of 3 groups. In the control group, subjects underwent pre- and post-testing with no training in between. In the self-learning group, subjects underwent 1 hour of independent learning (needling of a practice phantom model) between the pre- and post-tests. In the directed-learning group, 1 hour of learning through coaching and feedback was provided between the pre- and post-tests. Pre-tests and post-tests, which were identical, consisted of needling sonographic targets of varying sizes and depths, which were embedded in a test phantom model. The primary outcomes encompassed performance time and number of needle passes; secondary outcomes included the presence or frequency of 8 quality-compromising behaviors. All study variables were assessed by a blinded observer.

Results: Compared to the pre-tests, post-test performance times improved similarly in all 3 groups. However only subjects randomized to directed-learning showed a reduction in the number of needle passes as well as improvement in several quality-compromising behaviors.

Conclusion: A directed-learning session, integrating coaching and feedback, is pedagogically more productive than self-learning for beginners aiming to acquire US IP technique. Further trials are required to determine the IP technique learning curve for novice operators.

Keywords: Ultrasound; Learning; In-plane technique; Deliberate practice; Randomized trial; Skills

Introduction

Ultrasonography (US) has revolutionized the practice of Regional Anesthesia by enabling operators to visualize the nerve and block needle [1]. More specifically, the in-plane (IP) technique allows anesthesiologists to continuously track the needle in real time during its advancement towards the target nerve. While mastery of the IP technique is instrumental to the success (and safety) of peripheral nerve blocks, the optimal learning strategy for beginners has not been elucidated. To date, two important learning models have been identified: the discovery model (self-learning), whereby the learner discovers and amalgamates information by himself [2], and the deliberate practice model (directed-learning), whereby an instructor provides feedback and coaching to the learner [3]. Because of its simplicity, self-learning is most commonly used [4]; however, directed learning may be pedagogically more productive [5].

Although deliberate practice models have been described for Regional Anesthesia [6,7], a direct comparison between directed and self-learning has not been carried out. Thus, in this randomized trial, using phantom models, we compared self- and directed learning for the acquisition of IP needle skills in novice operators. We also included a third (control) group to account for the learning effect associated with repeated testing (pre-test and post-test). We hypothesized that, compared to its control and self-learning counterparts, the directed-learning group would require a shorter performance time and fewer needle passes to complete the post-test.

Methods

After obtaining ethics committee approval (McGill University Health Center, Montreal, Canada), as well as written and informed consent, 30 novice operators were enrolled in the study protocol. A novice operator was defined as a Fellow, resident or medical student who had performed <30 US-guided procedures in the 6 months prior to recruitment. Exclusion criteria included prior training on an US phantom model. Using sealed envelopes and a computer-generated sequence of random numbers, participants were randomly allocated to a control (CT), self-learning (SL) or directed-learning (DL) group. The Zonare Z.one Ultra sp US machine, L14-5w linear array probe (Zonare Medical Systems, Mountain View, CA), 90 mm, 22-gauge block needles

(Terumo Corporation, Tokyo, Japan) and test phantom models were identical in all 3 groups.

Test and practice phantom models were constructed by inserting wooden pegs of various diameters and lengths into a wooden base. The test models consisted of 3 sets of wooden pegs grouped by diameter (6 mm, 4 mm and 2 mm) and positioned in order of decreasing length (Figure 1A). The latter was calculated to ensure that the top of the pegs were at 2, 4 and 6 cm below the gel surface. An additional 6 mm of depth was added to compensate for compression of the gel medium by the US probe. To facilitate identification of the 2 mm-set, 6 mm marker pegs were placed at both ends of the wooden base. These pegs were not considered US targets. In the practice phantom model (SL and DL groups), the pegs were positioned differently and grouped by length (target depth). Furthermore an additional 12 mm diameter target was added. Thus the practice model displayed 3 sets (2, 4 and 6 cm in depth) and 4 targets of different diameters per set (Figure 1B).

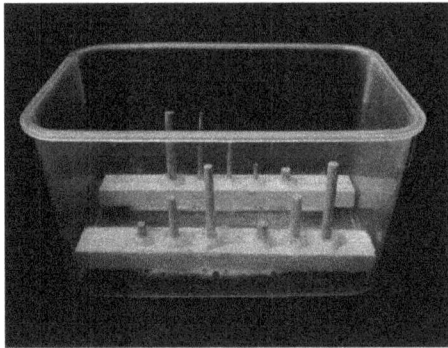

Figure 1A: Test phantom model before the addition of gel medium.

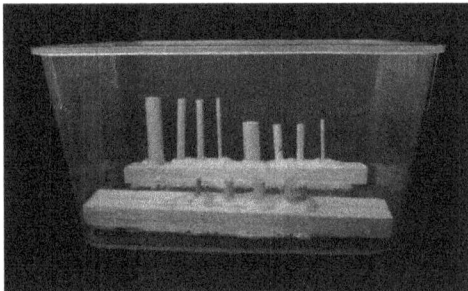

Figure 1B: Practice phantom model before the addition of gel medium.

After the pegs had been secured to the wooden base, the latter was bonded to the bottom of a 2.6 liter plastic container using polyurethane glue. Each container was then filled with a water mixture containing 182 grams of agar gelatin powder, 150 mL of orange colored Metamucil (Procter and Gamble, Toronto, Canada) and 15 mL of chlorhexidine solution. Metamucil served as a US speckling agent and also served to opacify the gel. Chlorhexidine was added as a preservative. Care was taken to remove all undissolved material and air bubbles prior to cooling the mixture. In the resulting phantom model, the top of the wooden pegs appeared as distinct linear targets (Figure 2). Prior to use, the surface of the model was covered with a thin layer of water to optimize imaging and minimize needle tracks.

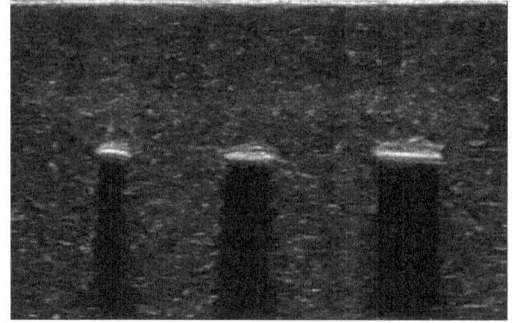

Figure 2: Long axis sonographic view of the practice gel phantom model. The 2 mm-, 4 mm- and 6 mm-targets from the first set (depth=2 cm) can be visualized. The 12 mm-target from the same set is located outside the visual field.

Participants in all 3 groups underwent an identical pre- and post-test. The latter was administered 1 hour after the pre-test (CT group), or 1 hour after the learning session (SL and DL groups). Before the pre-test, all subjects were asked to read the study protocol. All questions were answered to ensure that they understood the test procedure as well as the outcomes that would be measured. Furthermore an IP needle placement was demonstrated and an empty copy of the test model (Figure 1A) was made available throughout the test period to facilitate understanding of the target layout. Participants were asked to complete each of the targets in sequence (from the 6 mm- to the 2 mm-set), moving to the next group only when the needle had been successfully placed in direct contact with the top of each of the 3 wooden pegs (Figure 3). An assessor, who was blinded to group allocation, was present during the pre/posttest periods but only interacted with the participants to confirm the successful completion of each set.

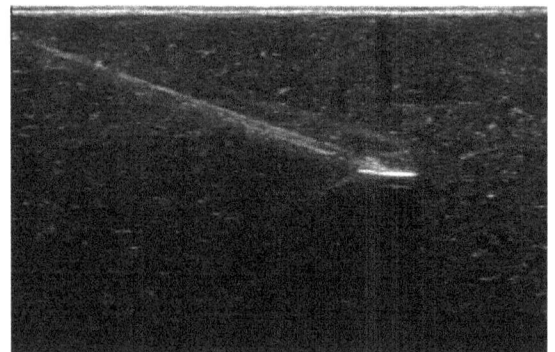

Figure 3: Short axis sonographic view of the test phantom model, demonstrating an in-plane needle placement on the 6 mm-target (depth= 2 cm).

After the pre-test, subjects allocated to the CT group were simply asked to wait 1 hour without further practice/teaching intervention. In contrast, subjects randomized to the SL group were left alone in a room for 1 hour, given a practice phantom model and asked to perform 3 in-plane needle placements on each of the 12 targets. Subjects allocated to the DL group performed a similar number of needle placements during an identical period of time using the same practice phantom model. However, they were provided with coaching and feedback by an instructor (experienced operator who had performed over 250 US-guided nerve blocks). The latter addressed basic issues; such as alignment of the needle and visual axis [8] and ability to troubleshoot an off-course needle. Furthermore he also provided feedback on quality-compromising behaviors (Table 1).

Name	Description	Outcome type
QCB1	Advancement of needle while not visualized	Count
QCB2	Malposition of target on screen	Count
QCB3	Poor probe handling or ineffective probe movement	Yes/No
QCB4	Awkward needle holding	Yes/No
QCB5	Watching hands or needle instead of target	Yes/No
QCB6	Fatigue	Yes/No
QCB7	Failure to correlate sidedness of screen and probe	Count
QCB8	Inappropriate needle insertion site	Count

Table 1: Quality-compromising behaviors (QCBs) (Adapted from Sites et al. [10]).

After completion of the allocated learning intervention, subjects underwent a post-test, which was identical to the pre-test. During both tests, the performance time and number of passes constituted the primary outcomes. Performance time was measured from the moment the probe was first placed on the phantom model, until the last set of targets was successfully completed. A pilot study involving 10 experienced operators (staff anesthesiologists and regional anesthesia Fellows who have performed >200 US-guided procedures in the last 6 months), found a mean performance time of 345 ± 95.8 seconds for completion of the test phantom model. Based on this information, we decided that 16 minutes (960 seconds), i.e., a value 50% greater than 3 standard deviations beyond the average expert performance time, would be the maximum allowable time for beginners to complete the test. Study participants who were unable to complete all 3 target sets within 16 minutes were deemed to have failed and their performance time was fixed at 960 second for the purpose of analysis. The number of passes was determined by looking at the US screen as well as the participant's hand movements. One needle pass was defined as an advancement that was preceded by a withdrawal of more than 1 cm [9]. Secondary outcomes included quality-compromising behaviors, which we adapted from a previous study by Sites et al. [10]. They were recorded as a binary outcome (yes/no), or as a count (number of instances) (Table 1). To ensure consistency, the same blinded observer recorded all primary and secondary outcomes.

Statistical analysis

We hypothesized that the DL group would require a shorter performance time and fewer needle passes to complete the post-test. Based on the performance time (345 ± 95.8 seconds) displayed by expert operators in the pilot study, 10 subjects per group were required to detect a 40%-difference (effect size 0.68) in performance time using the One-Way ANOVA test with an alpha type error of 0.05 and a power of 80%. Statistical analysis was performed using SPSS version 20 statistical software (IBM Armonk, NY). The One-Way ANOVA,

Kruskal-Walis and chi-square tests were used to compare data across groups and all P values were adjusted for multiple comparisons. Pre- and post-test data were analyzed using the paired t-test, Wicoxon's signed ranks or Mc Nemar's tests. All P values presented are 2-sided and those inferior to 0.05 were considered significant.

Results

Thirty novice operators were recruited over a period of 2 months. There were no intergroup differences in terms of demographic variables (Table 2). Performance time, number of passes and success rates are presented in Table 3. The performance time and success rates for the pre- and post-tests were similar. However, the number of passes in the post-test was significantly decreased in the DL group compared to the CT and SL groups ($P=0.011$ and $P=0.025$, respectively), as were the number of QCB1 events ($P=0.005$ and $P=0.027$, respectively) and QCB8 events ($P=0.002$ and $P<0.001$, respectively).

	Control	Self-learning	Directed Learning	P value
Sex (Male/Female)	6/4	6/4	4/6	0.727
Age Mean (SD)	29.0	25.3	28.3	0.514
Level of trainee (medical student/resident/fellow)	4/4/2	7/3/0	6/3/1	0.600
Number of in-plane blocks in last 6 months Mean (SD)	4 (8)	1 (2)	2 (6)	0.530

Table 2: Demographic data; SD: Standard Deviation.

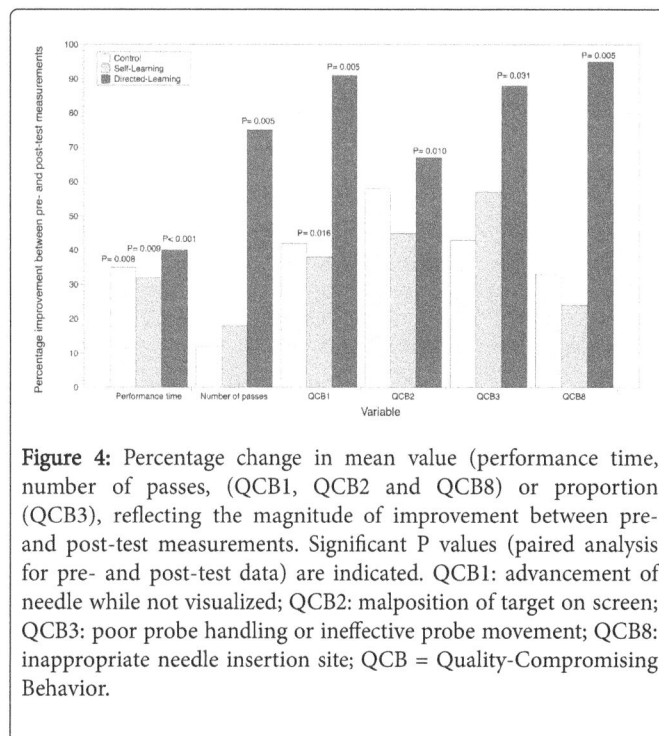

Figure 4: Percentage change in mean value (performance time, number of passes, (QCB1, QCB2 and QCB8) or proportion (QCB3), reflecting the magnitude of improvement between pre- and post-test measurements. Significant P values (paired analysis for pre- and post-test data) are indicated. QCB1: advancement of needle while not visualized; QCB2: malposition of target on screen; QCB3: poor probe handling or ineffective probe movement; QCB8: inappropriate needle insertion site; QCB = Quality-Compromising Behavior.

Results of paired analysis of pre- and post-test variables are presented in Table 4. Compared to the pre-test, the post-test displayed a decreased performance time (all groups), fewer needle passes (DL group) as well as improvement in QCB1 (SL and DL groups) and

QCBs 2, 3 and 8 (DL group). Figure 4 illustrates the proportional improvement between pre- and post-tests for these significant variables.

		Control	Self-learning	Directed Learning	P value
Total performance time Mean (SD)	Pre-test	711.0247.5	713.0193.3	716.3215.5	0.999
	Post-test	463.6219.0	486.6211.1	431.4116.1	0.837
Total number of passes Mean (SD)	Pre-test	58 (32)	61(42)	77(40)	0.501
	Post-test	51(48)	50 (26)	19 (5)	0.006*
Successful performance n/total	Pre-test	7/10	10/10	7/10	0.195
	Post-test	9/10	9/10	10/10	>0.999
*Directed learning vs. self-learning P=0.025, directed learning vs. control P=0.011.					

Table 3: Performance time, number of needle passes and success according to group allocation. SD: Standard Deviation.

Variable		Control	Self-learning	Directed Learning
Total performance time (seconds) Mean (SD)	Pre-test/Post-test	711(247)/463(219)	713(193)/486(211)	716(215)/431(116)
	P value	0.008	0.009	<0.001
Total number of passes Mean (SD)	Pre-test/Post-test	58(32)/51(48)	61(42)/50(26)	77(40)/19(5)
	P value	0.496	0.361	0.005
QCB1 Mean (SD)	Pre-test/Post-test	18.8(17.2)/10.8(11.1)	15.2(12.7)/9.4(8.5)	21.6(20.6)/1.9(1.5)
	P value	0.082	0.016	0.005
QCB2 Mean (SD)	Pre-test/Post-test	2.6(2.5)/1.1(1.5)	2.2(1.8)/1.2(1.9)	3.9(2.7)/1.3(1.4)
	P value	0.156	0.188	0.010
QCB3 Proportion (%)	Pre-test/Post-test	70/40	70/30	80/10
	P value	0.250	0.375	0.031
QCB4 Proportion (%)	Pre-test/Post-test	60/50	50/50	70/10
	P value	>0.999	>0.999	0.063
QCB5 Proportion (%)	Pre-test/Post-test	90/90	50/30	50/30
	P value	>0.999	0.687	>0.999
QCB6 Proportion (%)	Pre-test/Post-test	70/50	30/40	50/10
	P value	0.500	>0.999	0.125
QCB7 Mean (SD)	Pre-test/Post-test	0.9(1.3)/0.3(0.7)	0.6(1.3)/0(0)	0.1(0.3)/0.1(0.3)
	P value	0.313	0.250	>0.999
QCB8 Mean (SD)	Pre-test/Post-test	24.3(28.1)/16.4(26)	18(14.5)/13.6(12.4)	16.7(18.5)/0.9(1.1)
	P value	0.250	0.496	0.005

Table 4: Paired analysis of pre- and post-test variables. SD: Standard Deviation.

Discussion

In this randomized trial, using phantom models, we compared CT, SL and DL for the acquisition of IP needle skills in novice operators.

The performance time and number of passes were selected as primary outcomes because these variables would reflect an improvement in technical ability. Our results show that the performance times similarly decreased in all 3 groups. However the CT and SL groups showed no improvement in the number of passes between the pre- and post-test. In contrast, subjects randomized to DL required markedly fewer passes to complete the post-test than the pre-test. These findings suggest that CT and SL subjects were able to complete the required tasks faster, but not necessarily "better", whereas those in the DL group achieved both. Clinically, a reduction in needle passes may be as important as a decrease in performance time because it could translate into less patient discomfort as well as a decreased risk of needle trauma and vascular puncture. Our findings echo the results of Sites et al [6] who observed rapid improvement of US needling skills when feedback was provided between trials on a phantom model.

Because our protocol compared CT, SL and DL in vitro, the choice of phantom models requires discussion. Several permutations of US phantom models have been previously described [11], essentially they differ both by the embedded targets and the sonographic medium. In our study, the agar gelatin mixture was used because of its low cost and durability. This permitted the fabrication of multiple copies of both test and practice models; in turn, their continuous rotation (after each participant) allowed us to minimize the presence of residual needle tracks, which required 1-2 hours to completely dissipate. Furthermore damaged gel surfaces could be easily repaired by heating the model in a microwave oven. In our protocol, the wooden pegs provided reliable US targets; moreover varying their size and length enabled the creation of multiple configurations in a relatively compact space (plastic container). Extreme caution was taken to ensure that SL and DL subjects would not improve their post-test performance simply by having practiced on the test model itself: that is why the hour-long SL and DL practice session took place on a different (practice) phantom model which displayed different target groupings as well as an additional 12 mm-target.

The QCBs used in our trial were adapted from a previous study by Sites et al. [10]. Quality-compromising behaviors have also been employed in studies investigating the learning curves of skills required for US-guided Regional Anesthesia [7,12]. For the purpose of our trial, we identified 8 behaviors that were applicable to tasks performed on the test phantom models: we used them as outcomes as well as key topics addressed by the instructor during the DL training. Out of these 8 QCBs, QCB1 (needle advancement without visualization) has been identified as the most in common mistake seen in novice operators [10]. In fact, our study reveals that subjects in all 3 groups repeatedly exhibited QCB1 during the pre-test. In the post-test, only DL subjects were able to curtail this behavior.

Our protocol contains some limitations. Firstly, we elected to train and test our study subjects using gel models, which are considered low fidelity. Cadaveric models might have simulated real patients more accurately. However, despite their higher fidelity, the access and storage conditions required by cadavers would severely limit their widespread implementation in common learning settings (classroom, hospital or medical conference). Secondly, we chose to study the IP technique because the ability to visualize the needle constitutes one of the most important technical skills in Regional Anesthesia [1]. Thus our findings may not apply to other US techniques such as the out-of-plane needling technique. Thirdly, we limited SL and DL to an hour-long

session. We cannot rule out the possibility that SL might have compared favorably to DL had a longer period of independent technical discovery (SL) been allowed. However our results do suggest that, when novice operators are faced with a limited learning session (1 hour), DL provides better pedagogical efficiency. Finally, because of the punctual nature of our study intervention, no conclusions can be drawn regarding the learning curve of US IP technique for novice operators.

In conclusion, a directed-learning session, integrating coaching and feedback, is pedagogically more productive than self-learning for beginners aiming to acquire US IP technique. Further trials are required to determine the IP technique learning curve for novice operators.

References

1. Sites BD, Chan VW, Neal JM, Weller R, Grau T, et al. (2009) The American Society of Regional Anesthesia and Pain Medicine and the European Society of Regional Anaesthesia and Pain Therapy Joint Committee recommendations for education and training in ultrasound-guided regional anesthesia. Reg Anesth Pain Med 34: 40-46.

2. Bruner JS (1961) The art of discovery. Harvard Educational Review 31: 21-32.

3. Ericsson KA, Krampe RT, Tesch-Romer C (1993) The role of deliberate practice in the acquisition of expert performance. Psychol Rev 100: 363-406.

4. de Oliveira Filho GR, Helayel PE, da Conceição DB, Garzel IS, Pavei P, et al. (2008) Learning curves and mathematical models for interventional ultrasound basic skills. Anesth Analg 106: 568-573.

5. McGaghie WC, Issenberg SB, Cohen ER, Barsuk JH, Wayne DB (2011) Does simulation-based medical education with deliberate practice yield better results than traditional clinical education? A meta-analytic comparative review of the evidence. Acad Med 86: 706-711.

6. Sites BD, Gallagher JD, Cravero J, Lundberg J, Blike G (2004) The learning curve associated with a simulated ultrasound-guided interventional task by inexperienced anesthesia residents. Reg Anesth Pain Med 29: 544-548.

7. Barrington MJ, Wong DM, Slater B, Ivanusic JJ, Ovens M (2012) Ultrasound-guided regional anesthesia: how much practice do novices require before achieving competency in ultrasound needle visualization using a cadaver model. Reg Anesth Pain Med 37: 334-339.

8. Wilson JM, Germain G, Vaghadia H, Tang R, Sawka A (2014) In-plane ultrasound-guided needle insertion along or across the visual axis hand positions. Br J Anaesth 113: 717-718.

9. Casati A, Danelli G, Baciarello M, Corradi M, Leone S, et al. (2007) A prospective, randomized comparison between ultrasound and nerve stimulation guidance for multiple injection axillary brachial plexus block. Anesthesiology 106: 992-996.

10. Sites BD, Spence BC, Gallagher JD, Wiley CW, Bertrand ML, et al. (2007) Characterizing novice behavior associated with learning ultrasound-guided peripheral regional anesthesia. Reg Anesth Pain Med 32: 107-115.

11. Hocking G, Hebard S, Mitchell CH (2011) A review of the benefits and pitfalls of phantoms in ultrasound-guided regional anesthesia. Reg Anesth Pain Med 36: 162-170.

12. McVicar J, Niazi AU, Murgatroyd H, Chin KJ, Chan VW (2015) Novice performance of ultrasound-guided needling skills: effect of a needle guidance system. Reg Anesth Pain Med 40: 150-153.

37

History and Evolution of Anesthesia Education in United States

Mian Ahmad* and **Rayhan Tariq**

Department of Anesthesiology and Perioperative Medicine, Drexel University College of Medicine, Philadelphia, PA, USA

*Corresponding author: Mian Ahmad MD, Vice-Chair Education, Department of Anesthesiology and Perioperative Medicine, Drexel University College of Medicine, 245 N. 15th Street, MS 310, Philadelphia, PA 19102, USA, E-mail: mian.ahmad@drexelmed.edu

Abstract

Resident education is both, a science and an art. Quality and homogeneity of resident education has a considerable correlation with patient safety. This article appraises how formal training in anesthesiology was started in United States and how it has evolved over the years. A comprehensive literature search was performed to identify journal articles, periodicals and historic documents that detailed the development and progression of academic anesthesiology. Various Anesthesiology Departments were also consulted. In 1927 Dr. Waters established the first ever academic department of Anesthesiology at the University of Wisconsin, Madison. The graduates from that residency programs, the so called "Aqualumni" went on to establish residency programs throughout the country. In 1938 American Board of Anesthesiology was formed, elevating the level of anesthesiology to a distinct specialty. World War II and post war era was a period of rapid growth in anesthesiology in general and academic anesthesiology in particular. In late 1970's and early 80's American College of Graduate Medical Education (ACGME) closely regulated the anesthesiology residency programs by recommending minimum program requirements. Over the years the training model has transformed from a relatively heterogeneous one to a uniform outcome based model with focus on learning and teaching of 6 core competencies. This article explores how the anesthesiology education evolved throughout 20th century to its present form.

Keywords: Academic; Education; Residency; Internship; Anesthesiology history; Training; ABA; ACGME

Introduction

Today residency is considered to be the essential dimension that ensures the transformation of a graduating medical student into an independently practicing physician. The training model was not as clear in early days of medical education. Medicine had utilized the same apprentice based model that other trades were using to train the artisan of the next generation. An interested individual would get attached to a practicing physician, observe him dealing with patients and over time learn the knowledge and skills which enabled him to diagnose and treat conditions that patients presented with. Very slowly this model evolved into a structured and process based training. Anesthesia training however, never really followed that pattern. Initially, surgeons administered anesthetics to their patients and then directed nurses to do the same. Physicians interested in this branch of medicine had to teach themselves and soon felt the need to improve upon the technical and cerebral part of anesthetic administration.

This article is meant to review the differences between these early anesthetists and the physicians certified by American Board of Anesthesiology to be the anesthesiologists practicing this specialty of medicine today. Even more importantly, it is going to examine the content and structure of education as it has evolved overtime.

The Early Years: 1900-1920

Surgery has existed long before anesthesiology, but before anesthesia, surgery was a means of last resort. The notion of undergoing surgery was so painful that many would prefer to allow a disease to run its natural course than going under the knife. The greatest development in history of medicine no doubt is the ability to alleviate pain during surgery and essentially making modern surgical practice possible. Although the first public demonstration of General Anesthesia was in 1846 by a dentist at Massachusetts General Hospital, the growth of anesthesiology as a specialty was slow [1]. For most of the early 20th century Anesthesiology remained a neglected field because of the general perception that very little training was needed to administer anesthetics.

During most of the early part of the 20th century instructions in anesthesia were nonexistent and the specialty was being practiced only by a few self-taught individuals [2]. Among them was James T. Gwathmey who authored the first authoritative text on the subject in 1914. His book "Anesthesia" would remain a valuable educational resource over the next few decades [3]. He was the first president of the American Society of Anesthetists, later renamed American Society of Anesthesiologists (ASA) [4]. He, along with other regional anesthesiology societies emphasized the need to give organized instructions and training in Anesthesia.

In 1924, McMechan started the first journal in the specialty; Anesthesia and Analgesia [5]. Previously American Journal of Surgery used to publish quarterly supplements on anesthesia and analgesia. In 1940 Henry Ruth started Anesthesiology, the official journal of ASA. During these early years there was a gradual movement towards establishment of Anesthesia as distinct medical specialty that should be practiced by physicians. History of Anesthesiology residency training was interlinked with the push for specialty status for Anesthesiology in the late 1920's and 1930's.

A Transition from Nurse Anesthetists to Trained Physician Anesthetist

During the latter part of 19th century and the early part of 20th century anesthesia, usually in the form of ether, was mostly administered by surgical nurse or a medical student/intern. Fortunately the surgical procedures at that time were neither as lengthy nor as complicated so these practices seen as rather safe. However with the evolution of surgical techniques and introduction of new techniques in anesthesia including the use of breathing tube in trachea by Ivan Mcgill and the introduction of Neuraxial Blocks by James Corning, it was becoming apparent that anesthesiology was a specialty of its own and hence needed physicians that were specially trained to optimally deliver anesthesia [6]. Dr. Isabella Herb, chief anesthetist at Rush University was one of the first Individuals with an academic appointment in Anesthesiology. She advocated *"nurses when properly trained make very good anesthetizers but that their lack of medical training prevented them from being able to choose a particular anesthetic technique that would best suit the patient's and surgeon's needs [7]. Also nurses' minimal training in medicine and lack of training in research meant that they were not suited to carrying out research in anesthesia".*

Another contributing factor for this shift was the push from national and local Anesthesiology Societies. Gatch and other early ASA leaders emphasized the need to establish a standardized approach to train interns in Anesthesia [8].

Contributions of Dr. Isabella Herb

There was no formal training for anesthesia as a student or at post-graduate level. What little training was there was mostly through apprenticeship. At that time anesthesia training was essentially a short course of few weeks in which anesthetics agents and equipment was taught entirely in the OR. The physicians were being taught as technicians [9].

Wanting to rectify that while at Rush, Dr. Herb Developed a curriculum for teaching medical students comprised of pharmacology, physiology of Anesthesiology and selection of anesthetics [10]. Dr. Herb believed that this program was to be delivered by a physician who had expertise and training in delivery of anesthetics in that hospital, and not by surgeons [11]. She wrote, *"Unfortunately most anesthetists receive their meager instruction from surgeons during the operations, and it is a notorious fact that the majority of surgeons are poor anesthetists. From the fact that a man operates hundreds of times a year, it does not follow that he is proficient in the art of producing and maintaining anesthesia"* [7].

Although the curriculum was only for medical students and this was not a postgraduate training but it was first of its kind and it set course for further development of education in anesthesia.

Dr. Waters and the First Academic Residency Program in Anesthesiology

In 1927 Dr. Waters established the first ever academic residency program of Anesthesiology in University of Wisconsin, Madison. While Dr. Waters' division of anesthesia at the University of Wisconsin remained a section under the department of surgery until 1952, it truly was the foremost beacon of anesthesia education [12]. The graduates from this residency program who called themselves as the 'Aqualumini'

went on to establish residency programs all over the United States. Dr. Waters focused on education and research along with providing optimum patient care. He inculcated morbidity and mortality analysis and discussion (M&M) and literature review in the residency didactics. He hoped to train physicians in the art and science of anesthesia who would go on to train other physicians in the safe clinical practice of anesthesia [2].

The Aqualumini

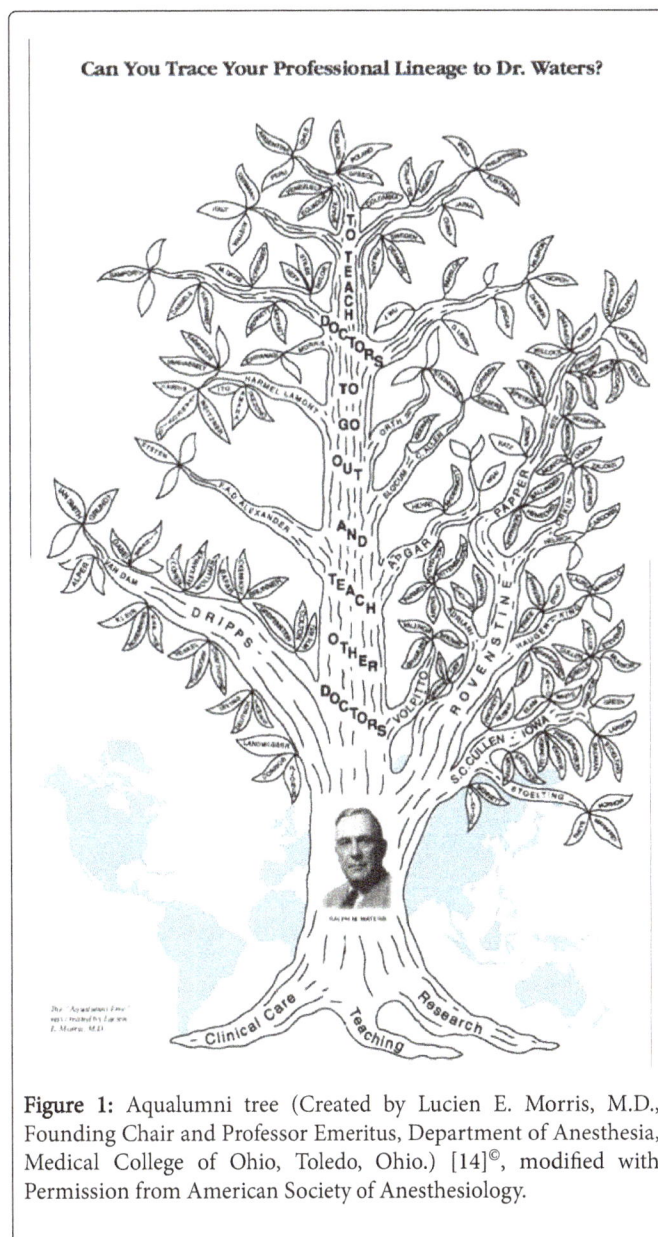

Figure 1: Aqualumni tree (Created by Lucien E. Morris, M.D., Founding Chair and Professor Emeritus, Department of Anesthesia, Medical College of Ohio, Toledo, Ohio.) [14]©, modified with Permission from American Society of Anesthesiology.

Individuals were attracted to anesthesiology from other specialties such as medicine, surgery and pharmacology. Among them is Emery Rovenstine who was Dr. Waters first and most distinguished disciple, he established the anesthesiology residency program at Bellevue/New York University (Figure 1). Among Rosenstein's notable residents were Stuart Cullen, Emanuel Papper, Virginia Apgar, Perry Volpitto, John Adriani, Louis Orkin, Sam Denson, Richard Ament, Gertie Marx, Martin Helrich, Sara Joffe, and Lewis Wright [13]. A genealogical review estimates that more than 80 departmental chairs out of the 120 Medical Schools in US have been of Waters' lineage (Table 1) [14].

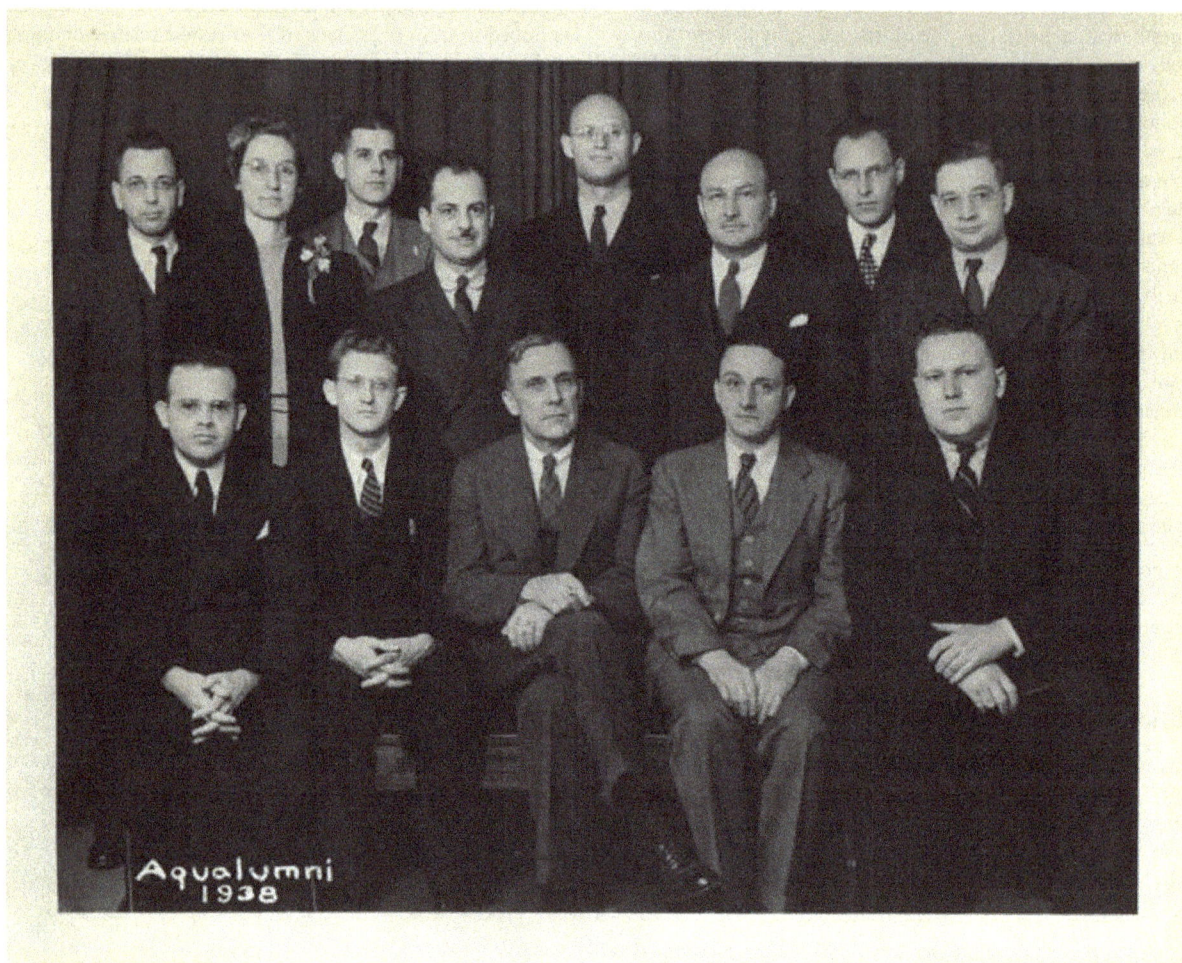

Figure 2: Aqualumini 1938 ©Mount Holyoke College. Archives and Special Collections, Virginia Apgar Papers (MS 0504).

Year Residency Program was Started	Institution/University	The First Chairman of the Department
1927	University of Wisconsin, Madison	Ralph Waters [2]
1929[a]	Hahnemann Medical College (now Drexel University College of Medicine)	Henry Swartley Ruth
1930 [12]	University of Oklahoma	John Alfred Moffitt
1935 [17]		
1935	New York University/Bellevue Hospital	Emery Rovenstine
1938[b]	University of Buffalo	John Evans
1939	Medical College of Georgia	Perry P. Volpitto [16,18]
1941[c]	UCSF	Stuart Cullen [19]
1941	Massachusetts General Hospital	Henry K. Beecher [20,21]
1943	University of Pennsylvania	Robert Dunning Dripps
1947 [22]	Ochsner Clinic Foundation, New Orleans, LA	George Grant
1949[d]	Columbia University	Emanuel Papper [2]

Table 1: Some of the earliest anesthesiology residency programs. [a]From Drexel University website http://drexel.edu/medicine/Academics/Residencies-and-Fellowships/Anesthesiology-Residency/; [b]From University of Buffalo website – Department History -http://www.smbs.buffalo.edu/anest/history.php (retrieved 8/25/2015); [c]From UCSF website – About Us http://anesthesia.ucsf.edu/extranet/about_us/index.php (retrieved 8/25/2015); [d]The Anesthesiology Service was first established as part of the Department of Surgery in 1937 under the direction of Dr. Virginia Apgar.

Dripps Started the Anesthesiology residency program at University of Pennsylvania; Cullen at UCSF; Emeul Papper established the anesthesiology department at Columbia University in 1949. Volpitto [15,16] established the first academic anesthesiology department in the south at medical college of Georgia, which he headed until 1972. The residency training program started slowly with the first resident in 1939 and the second one in 1941. From 1941-45, the majority of the male residents were recruited to a special wartime training program (Tables 1 and 2). John Lundy at Mayo Clinic started teaching anesthesiology as well as carrying out valuable research at that program. It was a chain reaction and soon enough residents graduating from above programs took the responsibility of propagating the knowledge of anesthesiology thorough out the country (Figures 2-4).

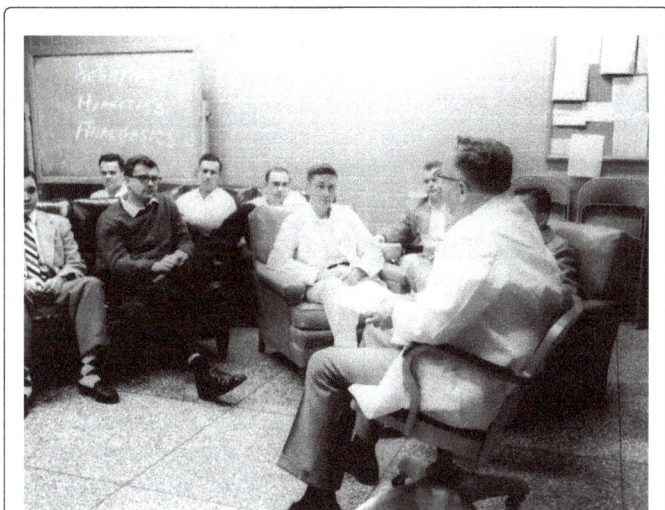

Figure 3: Dr. Volpitto teaching the Anesthesiology Residents©, modified with Permission from Department of Anesthesiology and Perioperative Medicine, Medical College of Georgia, Georgia Regents University.

Year	Number of Residency Programs	Total number of Training Positions
1927	1	Data not available
1943	45	Data not available
1948	214	487
1949	214	650
1964	296	1,858 (of which 1,145 were filled)
1968	148	1,655
2010	132	5,556
2014[a]	133	5,686

Table 2: The growth of residency rrogram with years [23,24]. [a]From FREIDA Specialty training statistics (retrieved 8/28/2015).

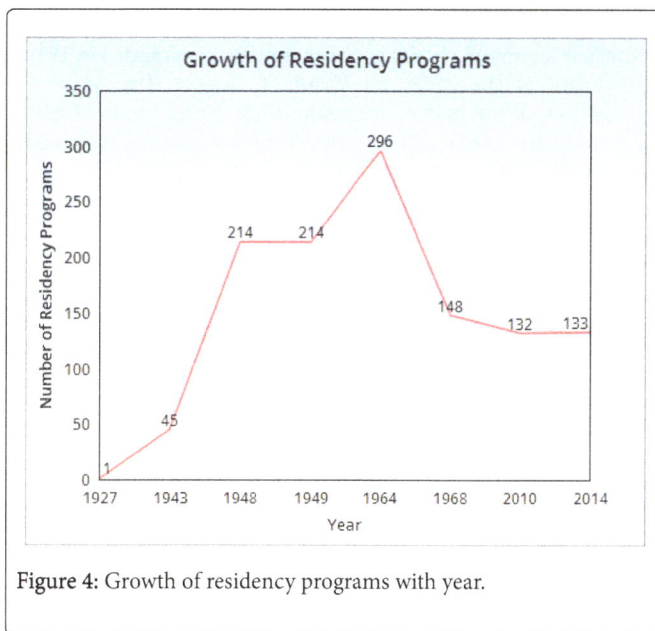

Figure 4: Growth of residency programs with year.

There was an increase in the number of residency programs after World War II which can be explained by the increased interest and increased demand for physician anesthesiologists.

The Influences of John Lundy

John Silas Lundy who is famed for the introduction of IV anesthetics in modern anesthetic practice [25] and the creation of first blood bank in the U.S. was the chair of anesthesia at Mayo Clinic from 1924-1959 [26,27]. Lundy's contribution to anesthesia however is not just the scientific advancement of knowledge but also the promotion of anesthesiology education. In 1925, John Lundy established the first anatomy laboratory at the Mayo Clinic where he taught regional Anesthesia techniques to surgery trainees [28]. He is accredited with creating the Anesthetists' Travel Club in 1929 in order to encourage flow of information between physicians practicing anesthesia. The participants, who were mostly in their thirties, discussed not only the clinical but also the basic research development relevant to anesthesiology. The Club met yearly till the start of World War II [29]. When the American Board of Anesthesiology (ABA) was formed in 1938 eight of the nine directors were members of the Travel Club. In 1941, in a large part due to his lobbying and political connections, the ABMS approved Anesthesia as a distinct specialty [30].

Development of ABA

It took more than a decade of meetings, conferences, and astute politics to convince public and professional organizations that this field merited specialty status. Finally an American Board of Anesthesiology (ABA) was formed as an affiliate of the American Board of Surgery (ABS) in 1937 and approved by American Board of Medical Specialties (ABMS) in 1938. The format of examination was changed to include MCQ within a decade and over time it was transformed to the current format. In 1941 it was approved as an independent primary Board (Table 3).

The First ABA Examination

The first "examining board in anesthesiology" was created in 1937 as a sub-board of the American Board of Surgery. The Board was composed of all the leaders of anesthesiology at that time (Table 5). The Examining Board established criteria for entering the examination process: [33].

1. Medical school graduation.

2. Completion of internship.

3. Two years of training, including 18 months of practical training in anesthesia.

4. Two years in the sole practice of anesthesia.

5. Membership in the AMA or a comparable approved national medical society.

President	Thomas Drysdale Buchanan[a]
Vice-President	Henry Ruth
Secretary-Treasurer	Paul Wood
Other Board Members	John Lundy, Emery Rovenstine, Harry Stewart, Ralph Tovell, Ralph Waters and Philip Wood-bridge.

Table 3: The first ABA committee [31], [a]Thomas Buchanan of the New York Medical Center-Bellevue Hospital was the recipient of ABA certificate number 1.

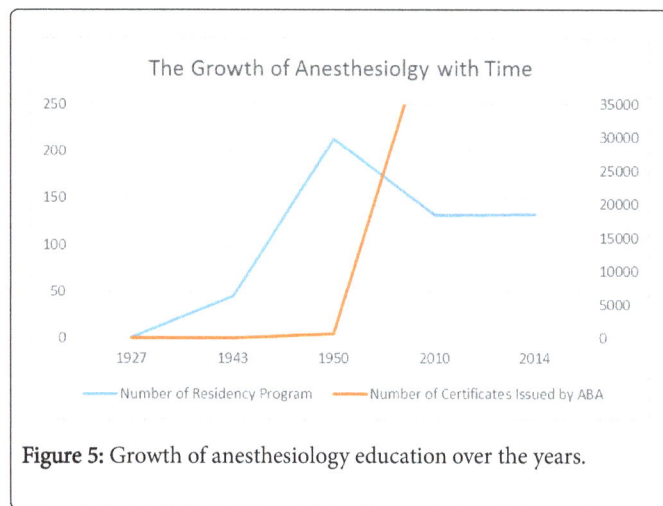

Figure 5: Growth of anesthesiology education over the years.

The process began slowly in the first year, when only 9 physicians were certified. Slowly gaining momentum, 272 anesthesiologists had been accredited by the end of World War II (Figure 5). Initially the Certificate was issued time indefinitely, but starting 2000 the candidates would be certified for a period of 10 years requiring re certification at the end of this period (Table 4).

Year	Number of Cumulative Certificates Issued by ABA
1939	9
1940	105
1950	706
1955	1,324
2015	>50,000

Table 4: Total number of certificates awarded by ABA [24,32].

Founders	Professors and Associate Professors previously elected to Fellowship in the ASA were to be certified without examination.
Group A	Those having practiced for 15 or more years were to appear before the Board and could be certified without examination.
Group B	Those practicing for 7.5 years or more or having administered anesthesia in at least 1500 major procedures could be certified following only an oral examination.
Group C	Those who met the 5 "criteria for entering the examination process" listed above and submitted 150 of their cases for evaluation were allowed to enter the full examination system.

Table 5: Categories for the first candidates for certification [33].

The Contribution of World War II to the Anesthesiology Education

World War II changed the course of American medicine significantly. The residency programs were depleted to meet the need of medical personnel of the U.S armed forces [9]. It was necessary to train more anesthetists (Medical anesthetists was the term used in early part of the 20th century for physicians whose primary responsibility was administration of anesthetics) to meet the war time need. A 12-week course was developed to train military physicians at academic institutions across the country. In addition, U.S Surgeon General mandated all Army officers to take a 2-week course in Surgery and anesthesia, formerly only required of medical officers [31]. Ralph Tovell [34] (Chair of Anesthesiology, Hartford Hospital), was given the task to overlook this Anesthesiology training. Medical Officers, the so-called "90 day wonders" were taught anesthesia in a 12-week course at leading anesthesia departments such as those at Bellevue Hospital, Mayo Clinic, Hahnemann Medical College, and the University of Wisconsin General Hospital [35]. Recommended textbooks included Beecher's Physiology of Anesthesia (1938), Lundy's Clinical Anesthesia (1942), Gillespie's Endotracheal Anesthesia (1941), and Guedel's Inhalation Anesthesia (1937) and Fundamentals of Anesthesia (1942) which was regarded as "Bible for Physician-Anesthetists" at that time [36]. In Great Britain as opposed to the U.S., anesthesia was developed as a physician specialty and was comparatively more developed. This pioneer group of wartime anesthesiologists gained valuable skills and knowledge from their service in European theater of operations. These physician anesthetists proved their competency in the wartime and this led to a greater respect for anesthesia as a profession and it became apparent that this is a field that is more suited for physicians [37]. These veteran anesthesiologists brought back sophisticated Intravenous and regional anesthetics skills. After the war many of these veterans developed an interest in anesthesia and sought more thorough instructions in anesthesia. Many of these "90 day graduates" subsequently joined ASA and/or ABA [38]. Among the trainees was Virgil K. Stoelting, who would go on to become the first chair of anesthesiology at Indiana University. Anesthesiologists nationwide called for a movement to establish independent anesthesiology departments at academic institutions.

This led to creation of Association of University Anesthesiologists (AUA) with aim of promoting free and informal interchange of ideas, development of anesthesia teaching and research. Emeul Papper served as the first president and AUA, whose first meeting took place in Philadelphia, attended by the founding group of eight [39].

Post-World War Years and the Structuring of Graduate Medical Education

In 1955, the ABA required all the applicants to dedicate five years exclusively to the practice of anesthesiology. Also, the applicants were required to submit "case history abstracts of personally conducted anesthesia procedures" to ABA, a predecessor to the online case log system existing today. In addition to the written and oral exam, the ABA also incorporated the "survey exam", in which the applicants were observed in their own practice. The application fee for examination at that time was 125 US$ [32].

The Residency Review Committee (RRC) in Anesthesiology was formed in 1957, with members from both the ABA and American Medical Association. Initially the anesthesiology residency was 2 years but beginning in 1962 the RRC allowed programs to offer a 4-year course, with the extra year spent doing sub-specialty training or doing research. In 1964 ACGME adopted a more standardized approach to the number of years and recommended three-year residency [40]. During the same year doctors of osteopathic medicine were also deemed eligible for ABA certification [40].

In 1966 Citizen's Commission appointed by AMA found serious inadequacies in the current system of graduate medical education (GME) [41]. The commission noted an ineffectiveness of existing institutions of GME and persistence of apprenticeship in training. Citizen's Commission report can be regarded as a significant step forward in development of graduate medical education in general which also naturally effected anesthesiology residency programs. This report led to the formation of the Liaison Committee on Graduate Medical Education (LCGME) in 1972 as a result of collaboration between five concerned authorities namely; AMA, the ABMS, the American Hospital Association, the Association of American Medical Colleges, and the Council on Medical Specialty Societies. The mission of LCGME (later renamed as ACGME in 1981) was to improve healthcare by assessing and advancing the quality of resident physicians 'education through accreditation.

In the late 1970s' and early 1980s' LCGME extensively organized and laid out clear structural framework for anesthesiology residency programs. LCGME emphasized program structure, the amount and quality of formal teaching and promoted a balance between service and education. LCGME achieved this mandate by defining minimum requirements for anesthesiology programs, which became increasingly specific over the coming years. In 1980 the LCGME defined intern year for anesthesiology as the clinical base year which could be spent training in medicine, surgery, neurology, pediatrics or any combination of these with the approval of program director preferably at the same institution as the parent institution [42]. LCGME also recommended the curriculum for post graduate year 2 to 4 (termed as CA1- CA3), suggesting that at least one of the 24 months in CA1-CA2 be dedicated to "recovery room or specialized care unit". Over the recent years ACGME has recommended increased rotation in ICU, as well as mandatory rotation in Pain service. In 1993 [43] ACGME set criteria for the appointment of program director to anesthesiology residency program. ACGME also made recommendations for the qualifications of the faculty, ratio of faculty to number of residents, scholarly activity and resident record maintenance.

1980's was a transformative period for anesthesiology education. In addition to the structural reorganization of anesthesiology by ACGME, ABA also refined its examination process in order to reduce the variability in examination process [33]. During the same time, the Society for Education in Anesthesia (SEA) was formed with an aim of promotion of education in anesthesiology. Over the years, eventually these guidelines and efforts from ACGME, ABA, and anesthesiology societies transformed anesthesiology residency from the rather unstructured model of the past to the well-controlled learning environment of today.

The 80 Hour Work Week Restrictions

Following the death of Libby Zion, purported to be secondary to medical error caused by resident fatigue; Bell Commission recommended an 80 h per week restriction on resident duty hour in 1987. Progress however was slow and the 80 h per week was not officially adopted by ACGME until 2003. As a result of the 80 h work week restriction residents now spend approximately 15,000 h in training compared to 30,000 h before. It is imperative that the sophisticated training techniques should be incorporated into residents training in order to produce well trained anesthesiologist [44]. Interestingly however, Stedman noticed that at Ochsner anesthesiology residency program the work hour restriction caused no loss in total caseload (number of anesthetics administered per resident per year in 2006 was 411 vs. 304 in 1990). He attributed this to the increased OR efficiency and the increased number of cases residents performs in the newly formed regional anesthesia rotation [22].

The ACGME 80 h anesthesia resident work week did cause significant financial implication for Institutions which were used to having inexpensive labor in the form of anesthesia residents. Backeris et al. calculated the cost to replace residents with CRNA was between $236,000 to $581,876, assuming a 50 h resident work week, and $373,400 to $931,001, assuming an 80 h resident work week [45].

The Inoculation of Research in Anesthesia Education

One of the distinctions of an anesthesiologist from their nursing counterparts is the contribution they make to the development of the specialty by continuously trying to improve practice based on evidence. ACGME requires the faculty to create an environment of inquiry and for the programs to provide mechanisms and resources for the residents to conduct research and scholarly activity. There is constant emphasis on participation of the residents in scholarly activity. Residents are expected to learn skills to critically appraise the literature for its validity for future practice. There is however, a concern that there is not enough contribution to research in anesthesiology as compared to some of the peer specialties. Schwinn et al. [46] reported that while anesthesiologist make up 6% of the work force but they only received about 1% of NIH funding. There is a need to train more physician scientists. Incorporating research curriculum into resident education can help them be more academically productive [47-49]. A survey by Ahmad et al. showed that thirty-two percent of programs had a structured resident research education program. While the ACGME places a great deal of emphasis on the importance of research training in a residents' education, it seems that progress is slow in this aspect as well. It would probably require a change in the culture of academic anesthesiology to ensure the mandatory enhancement of resident research education [50]. Sakai et al. [51] observed how the implementation of research didactics including research lectures, research problem based learning discussions, and an elective research rotation translated into greater resident research involvement and publications. Similarly, Freundlich at al. [52] described how a month long research month proved to be a successful educational intervention at University of Michigan anesthesiology residency program. Recently as many as 35/131 (23%) of the approved ACGME residency programs have started offering a dedicated research track [53]. It seems likely that in coming years, anesthesiology departments will continue to devote more time and resources to ensure that anesthesiology residents are well trained in the research methodology; so they can continue to contribute to development of anesthesiology as a profession.

ACGME Core Competencies and Outcome Project

The traditional model of assessment in anesthesiology has been global clinical evaluation and standardized testing. There is a general notion that performance on standardized examinations can be used to predict clinical performance however this claim was not substantiated in any study and there was no direct correlation with actual clinical performance and standardized clinical measures for the same resident [54]. There has been a gradual evolution in anesthesiology education to nontraditional assessment methods that stimulate learning including self-assessment, peer review and simulation based learning.

Over the years the training model transformed from the traditional model to an outcome based model with focuses on learning and teaching of six core competencies [55,56]. These competencies as defined by ACGME are [57]:

1. **Patient Care:** that is compassionate, appropriate, and effective for treating health problems and promoting health;

2. **Medical Knowledge:** about established and evolving biomedical, clinical, and cognate (e.g., epidemiological and social-behavioral) sciences and the application of this knowledge to patient care;

3. **Practice-Based Learning and Improvement:** that involves investigation and evaluation of their own patient care, appraisal, and assimilation of scientific evidence, and improvements in patient care;

4. **Interpersonal and Communication Skills:** that result in effective information exchange and teaming with patients, their families, and other health professionals;

5. **Professionalism:** as manifested through a commitment to carrying out professional responsibilities, adherence to ethical principles, and sensitivity to a diverse patient population;

6. **Systems-Based Practice:** as manifested by actions that demonstrate an awareness of and responsiveness to the larger context and system of health care and the ability to effectively call on system resources to provide care that is of optimal value.

These six core competencies were introduced by ACGME in 1999 and gradually integrated into the residency curriculum in the 2000's. Schwengel et al. [58] described how they introduced Systems-Based Practice (SBP) and Practice-Based Learning and Improvement (PBLI) at John Hopkins Anesthesiology Residency Program. The CA-1 residents participate in a curriculum composed of lectures, interactive sessions and exercises designed to develop conceptual understanding of a wide range of topics, including fundamentals of safety and safe design, how to critically evaluate the literature and how to investigate defects. In the CA 2 and CA 3 years, residents work on an SBP improvement project.

The results of ACGME restructuring gradually became apparent. Variability in the quality of anesthesiology resident education decreased around the country. However, these ACGME minimum program requirements for anesthesiology curtailed the programs from innovation and added administrative burden to the program [59]. The National Interest in patient safety and outcomes measure lead ACGME to come up with The Outcome Project which mandated that residency programs teach six core competencies, create reliable tools to assess learning of the competencies, and use the data for program improvement. In 2014, ACGME implemented Next Accreditation System (NAS) for anesthesiology a program in which accreditation was to be based on educational outcomes in these competencies. It has been suggested that the New Accreditation System will allow better programs to innovate while allowing struggling programs to improve; all while decreasing the amount of administrative work done by the program director [60].

A key element of the NAS is the measurement and reporting of outcomes through the educational milestones. As the ACGME is moving toward continuous accreditation outcomes-based milestones which are specific for anesthesiology, are used for determining resident and fellow performance within the six ACGME Core Competencies [61]. These milestones result from a close collaboration among the ABA, the review committees, medical- specialty organizations, program-director associations, and residents.

The Development of Subspecialty Anesthesia

During 1960's interest increased in research and in sub-specialty anesthesiology training. A small number of anesthesiologists mostly at the larger academic centers would spend time focusing on, and doing research on particular cohort of patients. All these factors lead to advancements in knowledge of physiology and pharmacology with introduction of drugs such as fentanyl and ketamine. Similarly considerable scientific progress was made in critical care and the pediatric anesthesia. In 1959 Peter Safar established first multidisciplinary adult and pediatric ICU in the US at Baltimore City Hospital. In 1967 John Downes and Leonard Bachman established the first pediatric Intensive Care Unit (PICU) in US at Children's Hospital of Philadelphia [62].

Keeping up the development in subspecialty Anesthesiology, ABA mandated subspecialty rotations starting in 1980. In 1985 ABA began to issue certificate in Critical Care. In 1991 Pain Management (renamed Pain Medicine in 2002) was recognized as a subspecialty by ABA. And most recently in 2012 ABA approved an additional time-limited pediatric anesthesiology certificate. Currently the ACGME requires all residents to have a specified minimum recommended amount of subspecialty anesthesia rotations.

Combined Anesthesia Residencies

In 2009 American Board of Pediatrics and ABA announced combined training in pediatrics and anesthesiology. This program requires five, rather than six, years of training and allows physicians to be fully qualified and certified in both specialties [63]. As of 2014, there are 7 combined Anesthesiology/Pediatrics program training about 22 residents (FREIDA Online specialty training [https://freida.ama-assn.org/]). Interest in combined pediatrics-anesthesia training is growing among applicants [64].

The American Board of Internal Medicine (ABIM) and the ABA began a combined training program in Internal medicine and Anesthesiology in January 2012. As of 2016, there are 5 approved programs for combined residency training in Internal medicine and Anesthesiology [65].

Future of Anesthesiology Education-A Blended Educational Model

The advents in information technology in the past decades have also impacted anesthesiology education. Simulation has become an integral part of residency training. Simulation allows residents to experience clinical scenarios that are infrequent in daily practice, but critical to anesthesia practice such as anaphylaxis, airway fire or the use of bronchial blockers and double-lumen endotracheal tubes (ETT) for single lung isolation [66]. As of 2014 ACGME requires at least one simulation training session for residents every year.

With the 80 h work limit, educators are hard pressed to make anesthesiology training as enriching as possible. Educators are trying to find new and innovative ways to introduce technology in anesthesia education. Tanaka et al. [67] showed how the use of an iPad® in a two week anesthesiology rotation at Stanford University objectively increased residents' perception of overall teaching quality of the rotation. Educators are trying to shift to a blended educational model with podcasts, videos, online quizzes and other online educational modalities [68]. This has been somewhat difficult to achieve owing to the intrinsic nature of anesthesiology which requires face to face and hands-on training. There have been varying results on usefulness of different modalities and the effectiveness of these tools depends more on the learning style of the resident. However, it seems likely that with coming time anesthesiology training will evolve to utilize and incorporate more technological advances such as simulation training and e-learning. In conclusion, it is remarkable to see how a specialty that had its humble origins in a self-taught and practiced unstructured training has evolved into this well-planned and regulated educational system producing highly competent physicians that have been trained in all the domains that will help them succeed in providing high quality patient care as well as advance this discipline in the future.

References

1. Rushman GB, Davies NJH, Atkinson RS (1996) A Short History of Anaesthesia: The First 150 Years. Butterworth-Heinemann.

2. Bacon DR, Ament R (1995) Ralph Waters and the beginnings of academic anesthesiology in the United States: the Wisconsin Template. J Clin Anesth 7: 534–543.

3. Gwathmey JT (1914) Anesthesia. Appleton 1st ed.

4. Gwathmey JT (1913) The American Association of Anaesthetists. Ann Surg 58: 865–876.

5. Editorial Foreword (1922) Anesth Analg 1: 1.

6. Eckenhoff J (1966) Anesthesia from colonial times a history of anesthesia at the University of Pennsylvania. Montreal: Lippincott.

7. Herb IC (1911) Administration of General Anesthetics With Special Reference To Ether and Chloroform. JAMA J Am Med Assoc LVI: 1312–1315.

8. WD G (1911) Instructions of medical students and Hospital interns in Anesthesia. Am J Surg 30: 98–99.

9. ROVENSTINE EA, PAPPER EM (1947) Graduate education in anesthesiology. J Am Med Assoc 134: 1279–1283.

10. Strickland RA (1995) Isabella Coler Herb an early leader in anesthesiology. Anesth Analg 80: 600–605.

11. Herb IC (1921) Anesthesia in relation to medical schools and hospitals. Am J Surg 50–51.

12. Rao VS, Schroeder ME, Sim PP, Morris DC, Morris LE (2011) The University of Oklahoma: The First Independent Academic Anesthesia Department? Bull Anesth Hist 29: 40–48.

13. Wang B, Orkin CL, Sutin KM, Blanck, Thomas JJ (2003) The Contribution of Doctor Emory A. Rovenstine to Anesthesiology. Anesthesiology 99: A1271.

14. Morris LE, Ralph M (2001) Waters' Legacy: The Establishment of Academic Anesthesia Centers by the "Aqualumni." American Society of Anesthesiologists Newsletter. 21–24.

15. Steinhaus JE, Perry P, Volpitto (1999) The South's First Academic Anesthesiologist. Bull Anesth Hist 17: 1–8.

16. Bacon DR, Vachon CA (2002) Perry P Volpitto: Bringing the Waters Tradition South. Anesthesiology 96: A1161.

17. Bause GS (2011) The End of the Road for "Huron Road." J Am Soc Anesthesiol 115: 1062.

18. Steinhaus JE (1999) Perry P Volpitto, M.D. The South's First Academic Anesthesiologist. Bull Anesth Hist 17: 1–8.

19. Hamilton WK, Larson CP (1980) Stuart C. Cullen 1909-1979. Anesthesiology 52: 111–112.

20. Gravenstein JS (1998) Henry K. Beecher: The Introduction of Anesthesia into the University. Anesthesiology 88: 245–253.

21. Mizrahi I, Desai SP (2015) Establishment of the Department of Anaesthesia at Harvard Medical School-1969. J Clin Anesth 28: 47–55.

22. Stedman RB (2011) Core program education: tracking the progression toward excellence in an anesthesiology residency program over 60 years. Ochsner J 11: 43–51.

23. Approved Internships and Residencies in the United States 1949. J Am Med Assoc 140: 157–230.

24. Pardo M The Development of Education in Anesthesia in the United States. The Wondrous Story of Anesthesia pp: 483–496.

25. Lundy JS (1936) Intravenous anesthesia. Am J Surg 34: 559–570.

26. Joseph Rupreht, Lieburg MJV, Lee JA, W Erdmann (2012) Anaesthesia: Essays on Its History. pp: 42–44.

27. Nelson CW, Dr John S (1999) Lundy and the 75th anniversary of anesthesiology at Mayo. Mayo Clin Proc 1999. 74: 650.

28. Ellis TA, Narr BJ, Bacon DR (2004) Developing a specialty: J.S. Lundy's three major contributions to anesthesiology. J Clin Anesth 16: 226–229.

29. Lennon R, Lennon RL, Bacon DR (2009) The Anaesthetists' Travel Club: an example of professionalism. J Clin Anesth 21: 137–142.

30. Bacon DR, John S, Lundy, Ralph Waters, Paul Wood (1995) The founding of the American Board of Anesthesiology. Bull Anesth Hist 13: 1–5.

31. Rosenberg H, Axelrod JK (1993) Henry Ruth: pioneer of modern anesthesiology. Anesthesiology 78: 178–183.

32. Directory of Approved Internships and Residencies (1955). J Am Med Assoc 159: 251–377.

33. Eger II EI, Saidman LJ, Westhorpe RN (2014) The Wondrous Story of Anesthesia.

34. Little DM (1967) Ralph Moore Tovell 1901-1967. Anesthesiology 28: 307–308.

35. Parks CL, Schroeder ME (2013) Military anesthesia trainees in WWII at the University of Wisconsin: their training, careers, and contributions. Anesthesiology 118: 1019-1027.

36. Waisel DB (2001) The role of World War II and the European theater of operations in the development of anesthesiology as a physician specialty in the USA. Anesthesiology 94: 907-914.

37. Ruth HS (1945) Postwar Planning in Anesthesiology. J Am Soc Anesthesiol 6: 316-317.

38. Martin DP, Burkle CM, McGlinch BP, Warner ME, Sessler AD, et al. (2006) The Mayo Clinic World War II Short Course and Its Effect on Anesthesiology. J Am Soc Anesthesiol 105: 209-213.

39. Papper EM (1992) The origins of the Association of University Anesthesiologists. Anesth Analg 74: 436-453.

40. Directory of Approved Internships and Residencies 1964- Annual Report On Graduate Medical Education In The United States.

41. The graduate education of physicians⊠: the report of the Citizens Commission on Graduate Medical Education⊠: commissioned by the American Medical Association. Chicago: Council on Medical Education. American Medical Association 1966.

42. 1980/1981 Directory of Residency Training Programs ACCREDITED BY THE LIAISON COMMITTEE ON GRADUATE MEDICAL EDUCATION. Chicago, Illinois Available.

43. 1993-1994 Graduate Medical Education Directory-Accreditation Council for Graduate Medical Education. Chicago, Illinois: American Medical Association.

44. Ramsay M (2007) The new generation of graduating anesthesia residents: what is the impact on a major tertiary referral private practice medical center? Curr Opin Anaesthesiol 20: 568-571.

45. Backeris ME, Forte PJ, Beaman ST, Metro DG (2013) Financial Implications of Different Interpretations of ACGME Anesthesiology Program Requirements for Rotations in the Operating Room. J Grad Med Educ 5: 315-319.

46. Schwinn DA, Balser JR (2006) Anesthesiology physician scientists in academic medicine: a wake-up call. Anesthesiology 104: 170-178.

47. Moharari RS, Rahimi E, Najafi A, Khashayar P, Khajavi MR (2009) Teaching critical appraisal and statistics in anesthesia journal club. QJM 102: 139-141.

48. Mills LS, Steiner AZ, Rodman AM, Donnell CL, Steiner MJ (2011) Trainee participation in an annual research day is associated with future publications. Teach Learn Med 23: 62-67.

49. Vinci RJ, Bauchner H, Finkelstein J, Newby PK, Muret-Wagstaff S, et al. (2009) Research during pediatric residency training: outcome of a senior resident block rotation. Pediatrics 124: 1126-1134.

50. Ahmad S, Oliveira GS De, McCarthy RJ (2013) Status of anesthesiology resident research education in the United States: structured education programs increase resident research productivity. Anesth Analg 116: 205-210.

51. Sakai T, Emerick TD, Metro DG, Patel RM, Hirsch SC, et al. (2014) Facilitation of resident scholarly activity: strategy and outcome analyses using historical resident cohorts and a rank-to-match population. Anesthesiology 120: 111-119.

52. Freundlich RE, Newman JW, Tremper KK, Mhyre JM, Kheterpal S, et al. (2015) The impact of a dedicated research education month for anesthesiology residents. Anesthesiol Res Pract 2015: 623959.

53. Nagle PC (2011) Improving outcomes in anaesthesiology education on research. Best Pract Res Clin Anaesthesiol 25: 511-522.

54. Ferland JJ, Dorval J, Levasseur L (1987) Measuring higher cognitive levels by multiple choice questions: a myth? Med Educ 21: 109-113.

55. Mainiero MB, Lourenco AP (2011) The ACGME core competencies: changing the way we educate and evaluate residents. Med Health R I 94: 164-166.

56. Stephens MB (2010) ACGME core competencies: Who knows what and does it matter? Fam Med 42 :574.

57. Kavic MS (2002) Competency and the six core competencies. JSLS 6: 95-97.

58. Schwengel DA, Winters BD, Berkow LC, Mark L, Heitmiller ES, et al. (2011) A novel approach to implementation of quality and safety programmes in anaesthesiology. Best Pract Res Clin Anaesthesiol 25: 557-567.

59. Oliveira GS De, Almeida MD, Ahmad S, Fitzgerald PC, McCarthy RJ (2011) Anesthesiology residency program director burnout. J Clin Anesth 23: 176-182.

60. Nasca TJ, Philibert I, Brigham T, Flynn TC (2012) The next GME accreditation system-rationale and benefits. N Engl J Med 366: 1051-1056.

61. ACGME Anesthesiology Milestones (2015) The Accreditation Council for Graduate Medical Education and The American Board of Anesthesiology.

62. Mai CL, Coté CJ (2012) A history of pediatric anesthesia: a tale of pioneers and equipment. Paediatr Anaesth 22: 511-520.

63. Pediatrics-Anesthesiology Program (2009) The American Board of Pediatrics.

64. Sanford EL (2013) Pediatrics-anesthesia combined residency training: an applicant's perspective. Anesth Analg 116:1386-1388.

65. Internal Medicine & Anesthesiology. The American Board of Anesthesiology.

66. Lim G, McIvor WR (2015) Simulation-based Anesthesiology Education for Medical Students. Int Anesthesiol Clin 53: 1-22.

67. Tanaka PP, Hawrylyshyn KA, Macario A (2012) Use of tablet (iPad*) as a tool for teaching anesthesiology in an orthopedic rotation. Rev Bras Anestesiol 62: 214-222.

68. Kannan J, Kurup V (2012) Blended learning in anesthesia education: current state and future model. Curr Opin Anaesthesiol 25: 692-698.

Permissions

List of Contributors

Ahmed Hassanein and Josef Zekrly
Department of Anesthesiology, Al-Minia University, Egypt

Hosam Moharram
Department of Ophthalmology, Al-Minia University, Egypt

Khaled Ahmed Yassen, Eman Kamal EL-Deen Awaad, Emad Kamel Refaat, Neveen Mostafa Soliman and Magda Fouad Yehia
Anaesthesia and Intensive Care Unit Department, National Liver Institute-Menoufiya University, Egypt

María Carolina Cabrera Schulmeyer, Jaime De la Maza, Ignacio Fernández, Cristián Ovalle and Carlos Farias
Anesthesiology Department, Universidad de Valparaíso, Hospital Clínico FACH, CINTO Santiago de Chile, Chile

Hoefnagel AL, Lopez M, Mitchell K, Smith DI, Feng C and Nadler JW
University of Rochester Medical Center, Rochester, NY, USA

Alexandra Saraiva, Sónia Duarte, Filipa Lagarto, Helena Figueira, Paulo Lemos and Humberto S Machado, Sílvia Pinho, Marta Carvalho, Maria Soares, Daniela Pinho and Carla Cavaleiro
Departamento de Anestesiologia, Emergência e Cuidados Intensivos, Centro Hospitalar do Porto, Porto, Portugal
Servico de Anesthesiologia, Centro Hospitalar do Porto, Portugal
Instituto de Ciencias Biomedicas Abel Salazar, Universidade do Porto, Portugal

Catarina S Nunes
Universidade Aberta, Departamento de Ciências e Tecnologia, Delegação do Porto, Porto, Portugal

Naglaa Khalil and Hesham M Marouf
Faculty of Medicine, Tanta University, Egypt

Matthew R Kaufman
The Center for Treatment of Paralysis and Reconstructive Nerve Surgery, Jersey Shore University Medical Center, Neptune, New Jersey, USA
The Institute for Advanced Reconstruction, Shrewsbury, New Jersey, USA

Division of Plastic and Reconstructive Surgery, David Geffen UCLA Medical Center, Los Angeles, California, USA

Ryan Fields
Department of Anesthesiology, Jersey Shore University Medical Center, Neptune, New Jersey, USA

John Cece, Catarina P Martins and Kameron Rezzadeh
The Institute for Advanced Reconstruction, Shrewsbury, New Jersey, USA

Andrew I Elkwood
The Center for Treatment of Paralysis and Reconstructive Nerve Surgery, Jersey Shore University Medical Center, Neptune, New Jersey, USA
The Institute for Advanced Reconstruction, Shrewsbury, New Jersey, USA

Reza Jarrahy
Division of Plastic and Reconstructive Surgery, David Geffen UCLA Medical Center, Los Angeles, California, USA

Abdelraouf M S Abdelraouf
Department of Anaesthesia and Critical Care, Assuit University, Egypt

Tiffany Leite Costa
Instituto de Ciencias Biomedicas Abel Salazar, Universidade do Porto, Portugal

Angela Mota, Sonia Duarte, Marta Araujo, Patricia Ramos and Paulo Lemos
Serviço de Anestesiologia, Centro Hospitalar do Porto, Portugal

Aktham Shoukry and Assem Moharram
Department of Intensive Care and Pain Management, Faculty of Medicine, Ain Shams University, Anesthesia, Cairo, Egypt

Osama Shahawy
Department of Pediatric Dentistry, Faculty of Oral and Dental Medicine, Cairo University, Cairo, Egypt

Abla Aly, Heba Morgan and Fayrouz Soliman
Department of Pediatric Dentistry, Faculty of Oral and Dental Medicine, Future University, Cairo, Egypt

Daniel A Hansen, Karl A Poterack, M'hamed Temkit, Mary B Laney CRNA and Terrence L Trentman
Mayo Clinic Arizona, USA

Montaser A Mohammad, Diab Fuad Hetta, Rania M Abd Elemam, Shereen Mamdouh Kamal and Doaa G Ahmed
Department of Anesthesia and Pain Management, South Egypt Cancer Institute, Assuit University, Egypt

Joseph Colao and Daniel Rodriguez-Correa
Department of Anesthesiology, Rutgers New Jersey Medical School, Newark, NJ, USA

Phakapan Buppha, Nuj Tontisirin, Supalak Sakdanuwatwong and Wanida Sodsee
Department of Anesthesiology, Ramathibodi Hospital, Mahidol University, Bangkok, Thailand

Pawin Numthavaj
Department of Otorhinolaryngology, Ramathibodi Hospital, Mahidol University, Bangkok, Thailand

Megumi Kageyama, Shinsuke Hamaguchi and Shigeki Yamaguchi
Department of Anesthesia and Pain Medicine, Dokkyo University School of Medicine, Tochigi, Japan

Dewi Yulianti Bisri, Caroline Wullur and Tatang Bisri
Department of Anesthesiology and Intensive Care, School of Medicine, Universitas Padjadjaran, Hasan Sadikin Hospital-Bandung, Indonesia

Diana Ch Lalenoh
Department of Anesthesiology and Intensive Care, School of Medicine, Prof. R.D. Kandou Hospital-Manado, Universitas Sam Ratulangi, Indonesia

Wosenyeleh Sahile Admassu, Amare Gebregzi Hailekiros and Zewditu Denu Abdissa
Department of Anesthesiology and Critical Care, Addis Abeba University & University of Gondar, Ethiopia

Annekathrin Hausmann and Rupert Schupfner
Surgery II, Klinikum Bayreuth, Germany

Kelley Dixon, Austin Broussard, Mellisa Roskosky and Michael Shuler
Athens Orthopedic Clinic, Athens, Georgia, USA

Mona Mohamed Mogahed, Jehan Mohamed Ezzat Hamed, Jehan Mohammad Ezzat Hamed, Mohamed Shafik Elkhawagy, Atteia Gad Anwar, Mohamed Samir Abd El Ghafar and Wessam Nassar Abo-elazm
Faculty of Medicine, Tanta University, Tanta, Egypt

Sabry Mohamed Amin and Rabab Mohamed Mohamed
Departments of Anesthesiology and Surgical Intensive Care, Faculty of Medicine, Tanta University, Egypt

Aynur Şahin, Serkan Doğru, Fatih Altıparmak and Mustaffa Süren
Department of Anesthesiology and Reanimation, Tokat, Turkey

İsmail Okan
Department of General Surgery, Gaziosmanpaşa University, Tokat, Turkey

Rahaf DA, Hisham Shakhashero and Mohamad Basier Al-Monaqel
Damascus University, Syrian Arab Republic

Hunduma Jisha
Department of Anesthesiology, Jimma University, Ethiopia

Hamed Elgendy
Department of Anesthesia, Assiut University Hospitals, Egypt

Doaa Ahmed
Department of Anesthesia, South Egypt Cancer Institute, Egypt
Anesthesia Department, King Abdullah Medical City, Makkah, Saudi Arabia

Soha Elmorsy
Department of Medical Pharmacology Faculty of Medicine, Cairo University, Egypt
Research Consultant, King Abdullah Medical City Research Center, Makkah, Saudi Arabia

Ali Aboloyoun
Phonetic Division, Department of Ear, Nose and Throat, King Abdullah Medical City, KAMC-HC, Makkah, Saudi Arabia
Phonetic Division, Department of Ear, Nose and Throat, Assiut University Hospitals, Egypt

Ahmad Banjar and Talha Youssef
Intern, Umm Al Qura University, Saudi Arabia
King Abdullah Medical City, Saudi Arabia

Azza Al- Attar
Audio-Vestibular Medicine Division, Department of Ear, Nose and Throat-Al-Azhar University Hospitals, Girls Section, Cairo, Egypt
AudioVestibular Medicine Division, Department of Ear, Nose and Throat, King Abdullah Medical City, KAMC-HC, Makkah, Saudi Arabia

Onur Koyuncu
Department of Anesthesiology and Department of Outcomes Research, Mustafa
Kemal University Tayfur Ata Sokmen Medicine Faculty, Hatay, Turkey

Mustafa Ozgur
Department of Anesthesiology, Antakya Devlet Hastanesi, Hatay, Turkey

Cagla Akkurt and Selim Turhanoglu
Department of Anesthesiology, Mustafa Kemal University Tayfur Ata Sokmen Medicine Faculty, Hatay, Turkey

Bulent Akcora and Mehmet Emin Celikkaya
Department of Pediatric Surgery, Mustafa Kemal University Tayfur Ata Sokmen Medicine Faculty, Hatay, Turkey

Alparslan Turan
Department of Outcomes Research, Cleveland Clinic, Cleveland, USA

Rie Kanamori, Rika Aihara, Nobutada Morioka and Makoto Ozaki
Department of Anesthesiology, Tokyo Women's Medical University, Japan

Daniel Chora de la Garza, Pornpan Chalermkitpanit, Prangmalee Leurcharusmee, Vanlapa Arnuntasupakul, De QH Tran and Roderick J Finlayson
Department of Anesthesia, Alan Edwards Pain Management Unit, McGill University Health Center, Montreal, Quebec, Canada

Mian Ahmad and Rayhan Tariq
Department of Anesthesiology and Perioperative Medicine, Drexel University College of Medicine, Philadelphia, PA, USA

Index

www.ingramcontent.com/pod-product-compliance
Lightning Source LLC
Chambersburg PA
CBHW080642200326

41458CB00013B/4710